TENTH EDITION

Managing
Stress

Skills for Self-Care,
Personal Resiliency, and
Work-Life Balance in a
Rapidly Changing World

Volume 3

Brian Luke Seaward, PhD
Paramount Wellness Institute
Boulder, Colorado

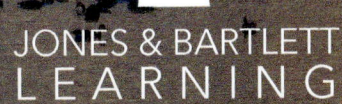

JONES & BARTLETT
LEARNING

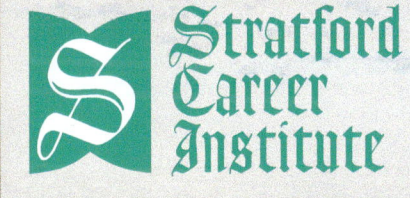

Stratford
Career
Institute

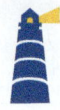

World Headquarters
Jones & Bartlett Learning
25 Mall Road
Burlington, MA 01803
978-443-5000
info@jblearning.com
www.jblearning.com

Jones & Bartlett Learning books and products are available through most bookstores and online booksellers. To contact Jones & Bartlett Learning directly, call 800-832-0034, fax 978-443-8000, or visit our website, www.jblearning.com.

Production Credits
VP, Product Management: Christine Emerton
Director of Product Management: Cathy L. Esperti
Product Manager: Whitney Fekete
Content Strategist: Ashley R. Malone
Content Coordinator: Elena Sorrentino
Project Manager: Kristen Rogers
Project Specialist: Meghan McDonagh
Digital Project Specialist: Rachel DiMaggio
Director of Marketing: Andrea DeFronzo
Content Services Manager: Colleen Lamy
VP, Manufacturing and Inventory Control: Therese Connell
Composition: Exela Technologies
Cover Design: Briana Yates
Senior Media Development Editor: Troy Liston
Rights Specialist: Rebecca Damon
Cover Image (Title Page, Chapter Opener): © Inspiration Unlimited. Used with permission.
Printing and Binding: LSC Communications

Library of Congress Cataloging-in-Publication Data
Names: Seaward, Brian Luke, author.
Title: Managing stress : principles and strategies for health and well-being / Brian Luke Seaward.
Description: 10. | Burlington, MA : Jones & Bartlett Learning, [2021] | Includes bibliographical references and index. | Summary: "Managing Stress with Navigate 2 Advantage Access provides a modern, comprehensive approach to stress management, honoring the balance and harmony of the mind, body, spirit, and emotions. Referred to as the "authority on stress management" by students and professionals, this book equips students with the tools needed to identify and manage stress while teaching them how to strive for health and balance. The holistic approach taken by internationally acclaimed lecturer and author Brian Luke Seaward gently guides the reader to greater levels of mental, emotional, physical, and spiritual well-being by emphasizing the importance of mind-body-spirit unity"– Provided by publisher.
Identifiers: LCCN 2020020982 | ISBN 9781284199994 (paperback)
Subjects: MESH: Stress, Psychological–psychology | Stress, Psychological–prevention & control | Adaptation, Psychological | Mind-Body Therapies–methods | Holistic Health
Classification: LCC RC49 | NLM WM 172.4 | DDC 616.08–dc23
LC record available at https://lccn.loc.gov/2020020982

6048

Printed in the United States of America
27 26 25 24   10 9 8 7 6 5 4 3 2

Brief Contents

Contents

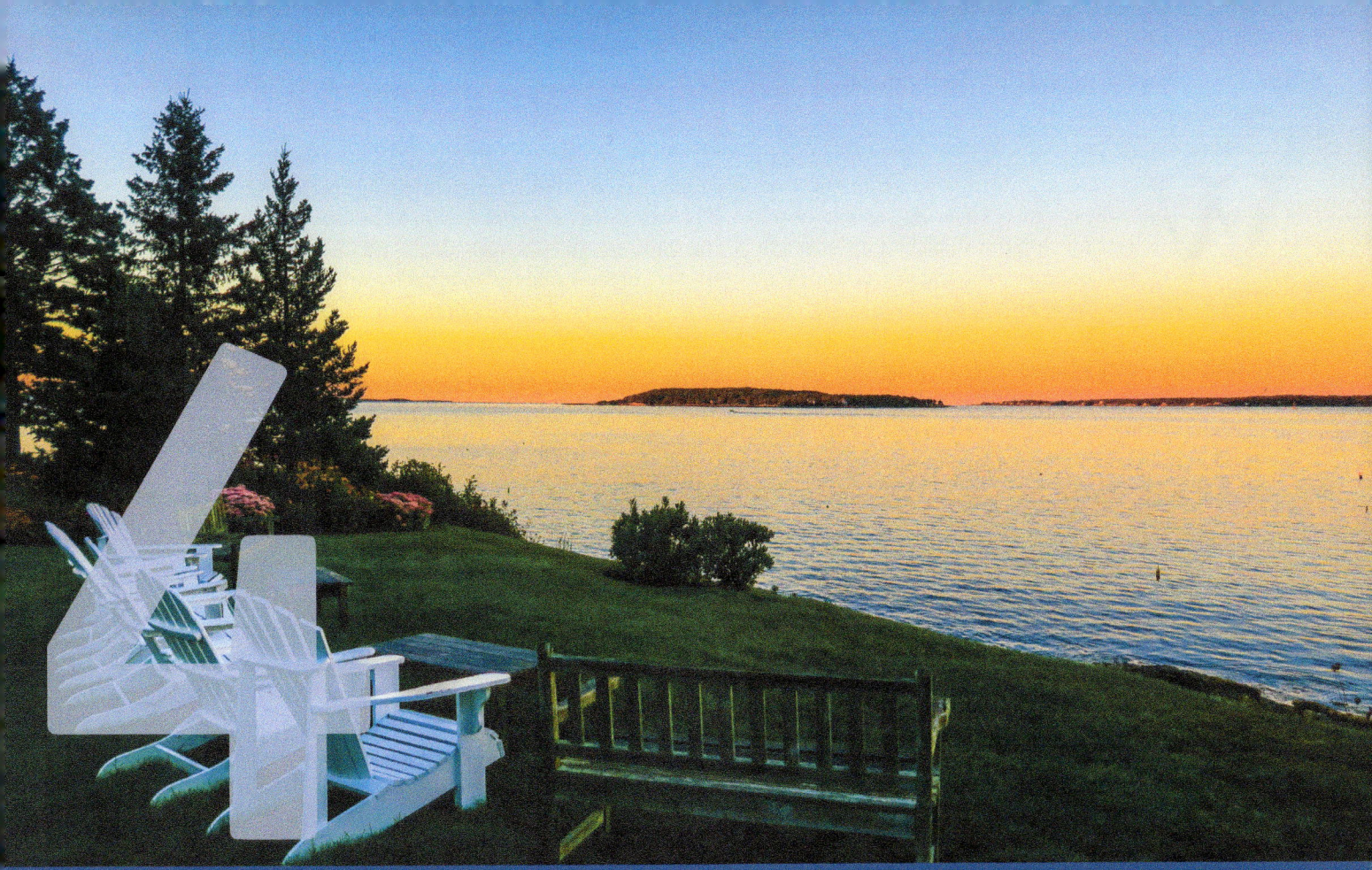

PART FOUR

Relaxation Techniques

That the birds fly overhead, this you cannot stop. That they build a nest in your hair, this you can prevent.

—Ancient Chinese proverb

We process information from the five senses: vision, hearing, smell, taste, and touch. Stimuli picked up through one or more of these senses are then delivered to the cerebral cortex and deciphered, and then processed by the subcortex of the brain. Each piece of information tracked by the senses is labeled with a perception, which is interpreted as either a threat or a nonthreat. If a stimulus is perceived to be a threat, then an alarm is sounded and the body is activated as a means of survival.

To relax the body from a heightened state of physical arousal to homeostasis, action must be taken to alter both the quality and the quantity of stimuli taken in by the five senses. In other words, the five senses must be deactivated or reprogrammed, temporarily, to allow the body to calm down. The purpose of relaxation techniques is to do just that: to deactivate the body's sensory system, decrease stimuli and their associated perceptions, and replace these with nonthreatening sensations that promote the relaxation response. In effect, the primary purpose of relaxation techniques is to *intercept* the stress response, specifically at the neurological and hormonal levels, and return the body to physiological homeostasis.

Of the five senses, two are paramount in the acquisition of sensory information for processing: vision and hearing. By no coincidence, these same two senses are targeted for deactivation during relaxation, through various relaxation techniques such as mental imagery and music therapy, to name two. In addition, because muscle tension is considered the most common symptom of stress, touch is targeted through techniques such as progressive muscular relaxation, massage, and physical exercise.

When the field of stress management unfolded in the early 1970s, the emphasis of attention and instruction was placed solely on relaxation techniques because of the apparently strong association between stress-related symptoms and ensuing diseases. As mentioned in Chapter 1, this is still the common medical approach to the treatment of disease and illness: to first treat the symptoms of the problems. Originally, relaxation techniques were used in both prevention of and intervention for stress-related health problems. What was discovered through this approach, however, was that relaxation techniques alone offered only temporary solutions to long-term problems or chronic stressors. Moreover, if the relaxation techniques were practiced irregularly or discontinued, then stress-related symptoms returned. Thus, by themselves, relaxation techniques are only half the solution. To effectively deal with stress in a preventive or interventive manner, techniques for relaxation must be integrated with positive coping techniques.

Unfortunately, relaxation techniques are not magic. What may provide a calming effect for one person may offer nothing but added frustration for others. The ability to relax (even heal) is largely dependent on the individual. Experts in the field of stress management suggest that you become acquainted with several different techniques and add these to your arsenal of stress defense. As you might expect, some techniques and their intended reactions are less suited to certain situations than others are. For example, you cannot easily plug yourself into a biofeedback machine during a traffic pile-up on the highway, but you can try some mental imagery and diaphragmatic breathing. Ultimately, the choice is up to you and your experience as to how you should employ relaxation techniques. In addition, relaxation techniques, similar to playing the piano or shooting hoops, are skills; skills require regular practice to achieve proficiency. Experts agree that regardless of which technique is chosen (and many may be used in combination), you must practice some form of relaxation every day, usually for 20 minutes. Done effectively, these skills will serve your goal to achieve inner peace.

Because the mind-body connection is so strong, relaxation techniques promote not only physical calming, but also rebound to calm mental processes, creating mental homeostasis. This allows for greater self-awareness. For this reason, several relaxation techniques provide fertile ground for the seeds of several coping strategies. When Jim Fixx wrote the best-seller *The Complete Book of Running* (1977), he thought he would address the physiological relationship between cardiovascular fitness and coronary heart disease. However, with virtually every runner interviewed by Fixx, the first topic mentioned was not the physiological effects of running, but the mental and emotional effects—the runner's high. Renowned runner and 1968 Boston Marathon winner Amby Burfoot, editor of *Running World* magazine and author, is no stranger to the mental well-being aspects of running either (Burfoot 2004). At first, researchers dismissed runner's high as an extraneous effect. Now, a more serious approach has been adopted to understand the mysteries of this profound connection between mind and body. As you will see in Chapter 27, there is a strong crossover between the two, and we have only scratched the surface of the wealth of knowledge to be learned about this unique relationship.

The origins of relaxation techniques span many continents and cultures over many centuries. In Part 4, East meets West as techniques from the Orient dating back thousands of years are paired with contemporary techniques from the New World. Over the past 20 years, some components of the older techniques have begun to merge with the newer techniques, lending them depth and strength. Some methods are best suited as intervention techniques, to be done right on the spot in the face of stress. Others are more appropriate when postponed to later in the day. Yet all the techniques are preventive in nature. So, read through these techniques and try them. See what you think. Chances are, there are some you will take an immediate liking to, whereas others won't do much for you. Once you have tried them all, select one or two that seem very effective and begin to incorporate these into your daily routine. With regular practice, you will be amazed at how your body responds, not only in terms of immediate effects, but also over time. Should there come a time that your favorite relaxation technique seems to lose its ability to bring calmness, then select an alternative technique. There are many to choose from.

Like Part 3, most chapters in this section include a historical introduction to each relaxation technique, as well as a full description of the technique, specific physiological (and psychological) effects induced by the technique, and best steps to take to incorporate the technique into your personal strategy for stress management. Because of the association between stress and chronic pain, a section on this topic is also included in appropriate chapters.

REFERENCES AND RESOURCES

Burfoot, A. 2004. *Runner's World Complete Book of Running: Everything You Need to Run for Fun, Fitness, and Competition*. New York: Rodale Books.

Fixx, J. 1977. *The Complete Book of Running*. New York: Random House.

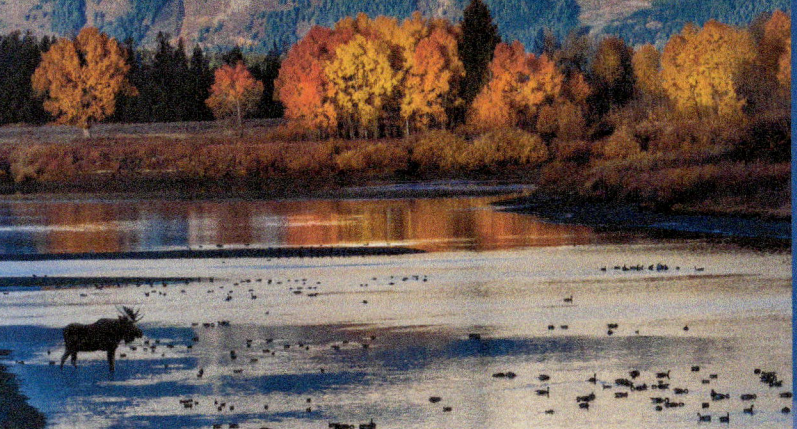

Diaphragmatic Breathing

Let the air breathe for you.

—Emmett Miller, M.D.

Diaphragmatic breathing is unequivocally the easiest method of relaxation to practice. It is easy because breathing is an action that we do normally without thought or hesitation. In its simplest form, **diaphragmatic breathing** is controlled deep breathing. It is symbolic of a deep sigh or a big breath taken when one is about to regroup one's thoughts, gain composure, or direct one's energies for a challenging task. What makes normal breathing different from diaphragmatic breathing is its emphasis on expansion of the chest. Diaphragmatic breathing involves the movement of the lower abdomen. In the practice of yoga, this technique is called **pranayama**, or the restoration of one's energy or life force, the breath behind the breath.

Most Americans breathe emphasizing upper chest and thoracic cavity movement while deemphasizing abdominal movement. This is thought to be a learned behavior influenced by cultural preferences for a large chest and small waist. As children mature, they shift from abdominal to thoracic breathing. When fast asleep, however, without the influence of the conscious mind, all individuals revert back to breathing by distending the stomach, as the diaphragm is allowed to expand and contract without inhibition.

Over the past two decades, the use of diaphragmatic breathing has become well accepted in childbirth (Nakahata 1993). A major tenet of the Lamaze childbirth method is controlled **belly breathing**. In Lamaze classes, expectant mothers (and fathers) are taught to place the emphasis of their breathing on the lower stomach. Then, during the several hours of labor and delivery, this breathing skill is employed to ease pain. And what is taught and practiced for the stressful event of childbirth is now taught and practiced for several other stressful situations as well.

Diaphragmatic breathing: The most basic relaxation technique; breathing from the lower stomach or diaphragm rather than the thoracic area.

Pranayama: A Sanskrit term to describe diaphragmatic breathing that restores one's vital life force of energy.

Belly breathing: The most common form of relaxation by means of placing the emphasis of one's breathing on the lower stomach area (belly or diaphragm) rather than the upper chest (thoracic area), thereby decreasing sympathetic response and inducing a greater sense of relaxation.

■ The Mystery of Breathing

Under normal resting conditions, the average person breathes approximately 14 to 16 times per minute. In a state of arousal, breathing is fast-paced and shallow, with pronounced muscular contractions of the chest cavity (**BOX 18.1**). During heavy exercise, ventilations per minute can increase to as many as 60 as the body tries to meet the increased demand for oxygen (Sherwood 2006). In a relaxed state, the body's metabolism is significantly decreased, allowing for a slower and deeper breathing cycle. Physiologically speaking, when pressure resulting from the expansion of the chest wall and muscular contraction is taken off the thoracic cavity, sympathetic drive decreases. Parasympathetic drive overrides the sympathetic system, and homeostasis results. Itzhak Bentov (1988) offers a second explanation for the pacifying effect of diaphragmatic breathing, which he relates to vibrations emitted from the heart. The force of contractions of the left ventricle and the blood that it ejects sends a vibration through the aorta, which then reverberates throughout the body. A pause in the breathing cycle causes the reverberation to cease. Breathing from the diaphragm, which accents long pauses, decreases this resonance, creating a calming effect. Some Himalayan yogis, in a state of complete relaxation, are reported to take in as few as one or two breaths per minute (Green 2003). As you can imagine, this requires much concentration and practice. Typically, when people learn to modify their breathing from thoracic to diaphragmatic breathing, they can comfortably reduce the number of breaths to between four and six per minute.

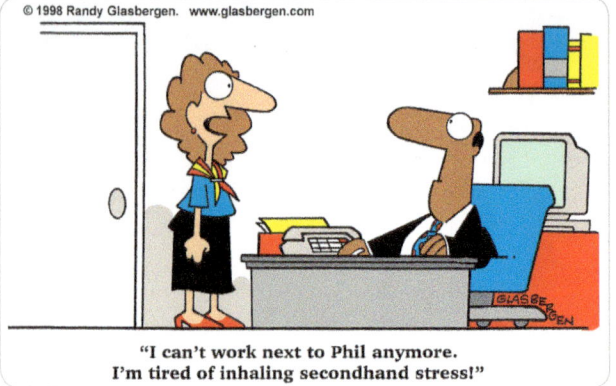

© 1998 Randy Glasbergen. www.glasbergen.com

"I can't work next to Phil anymore. I'm tired of inhaling secondhand stress!"

FIGURE 18.1 Inhale calm peaceful air, exhale stress and tension, just not on someone else.

Diaphragmatic breathing is as old as the ancient exercises of yoga and T'ai chi ch'uan, and it is a fundamental component of these practices. The therapeutic power of breathing is often associated with higher consciousness or spirituality. In fact, the word *spirit* in many cultures is described as "the first breath." Currently, diaphragmatic breathing is itself a form of relaxation, but because of its simplicity and compatibility, it is often incorporated into other techniques, including progressive muscular relaxation, autogenic training, and mental imagery, for a combined relaxation effect (**BOX 18.2**).

BOX 18.1   Are You a Breath Holder?

In times of stress our rate of breathing tends to increase; however, many people who suffer bouts of anxiety tend to hold their breath, forgetting to exhale. This is also called anxiety breathing. Although breath holding may serve pearl divers well in the South Pacific, this behavior puts undue stress on the nervous system, which then secretes more epinephrine, causing an increase in resting heart rate and blood pressure. Stress! Most breath holders are not even aware that they are holding their breath and have to be taught how to breathe normally. What they are taught are the basics of diaphragmatic breathing—slow, comfortable, deep breaths to calm the body (**FIG. 18.1**).

BOX 18.2   Insomnia and Diaphragmatic Breathing

When you stop and think about it, counting sheep is merely a simple form of guided visualization to promote sleep, but it's not always effective. The problem is that most people's minds start wandering off with the sheep. If you are having trouble sleeping, here is a suggestion: Try counting your breath cycles instead. Before you start counting, lie comfortably on your back. Then, take the emphasis of your breathing off your upper chest (this tends to increase the stress response) and place it instead on your lower stomach. Try to make each breath comfortably slow and comfortably deep. Counting backward from 100 also seems to help tire the mind, as the body relaxes. Diaphragmatic breathing is perhaps the simplest way to initiate the relaxation response. If you find your mind wandering, redirect your thoughts back to your breathing, and release each wandering thought with each exhalation.

Many people consider diaphragmatic breathing to be the first recognized mantra; a singular repetitive thought or motion to cleanse the mind. Among those who practice yoga and T'ai chi ch'uan, diaphragmatic breathing is thought to be more effective when inhalation and exhalation occur through the nasal passages because there is a greater ability to regulate air flow that way. Respiratory and sinus problems, however, invite use of both mouth and nose for this style of breathing. In any case, diaphragmatic breathing promotes concentration on one body sensation to the exclusion of all other sensory stimuli: feeling air slowly pass through the nose or mouth, down into the lungs, and then return via the same pathway.

Scientists have observed that over the course of a single day, barring colds or sinus problems, one nostril dominates the breathing cycle for several hours before allowing the other nostril to take over (Searleman et al. 2005). Several studies now suggest that these changes in breathing patterns can actually enhance brain lateralization and their respective modes of thinking (Neimark 1985). The right side of the brain controls and is influenced by the actions of the left side of the body. Scientists suggest that allowing air to enter and exit through your left nostril will access right-brain functions more readily. Thus, when right-brain thinking is preferred, as in the use of imagination, this style of breathing is advocated.

Breathing and Chronic Pain

An expression in China states there are more than 40 different ways to breathe. Whereas most Westerners think there are only two (inhale and exhale), Asians have studied and worked with breathing as a healing modality for thousands of years, primarily combining mental imagery with diaphragmatic breath work. Although few, if any, studies have investigated the relationship between diaphragmatic breathing and the treatment of chronic pain, energy healers who treat patients with a host of diseases use breath work as the core of their energy work (Rosen 2002; Swayzee 1998). Rosen describes a concept called **Bandha**, a series of respiratory contractions to unlock the cause of pain. It is also suggested by healers that clients not merely practice diaphragmatic breathing, but combine imagery with their breath work and visualize inhaling and exhaling "through" that specific area for pain relief.

Steps to Initiate Diaphragmatic Breathing

The following steps can be used to initiate diaphragmatic breathing.

Step 1: Assume a Comfortable Position

The beauty of this technique is its simplicity. It can be done anywhere, at any time. To benefit most, first learn and then practice diaphragmatic breathing in a comfortable position, either sitting or, preferably, lying down on your back with your eyes closed (**FIG. 18.2**). To enhance this position, loosen constrictive clothing around the neck and waist. When first learning this technique, it is suggested that you place your hands over your stomach and feel the rise and fall of your abdomen with each breath. Once the technique is practiced with proficiency, it can be performed just about anywhere, under any circumstances, including while driving in heavy traffic, waiting in line at the post office, giving a public speech, or taking a final exam.

Step 2: Concentration

As with all relaxation techniques that offer respite to the body, diaphragmatic breathing requires focused concentration. Concentration can easily be interrupted by both external noises and internal thoughts. Whenever possible, take steps to minimize external interruptions by finding a nice quiet place to practice this technique. When first learning this and other techniques that require total concentration, you will notice that on occasion your mind begins to wander. This is common. When you notice competing thoughts, allow them to dissipate and refocus your attention on your breathing. One suggestion is to allow these interrupting thoughts to metaphorically escape your body as you exhale.

Bandha: A series of breathing exercises to unlock chronic pain.

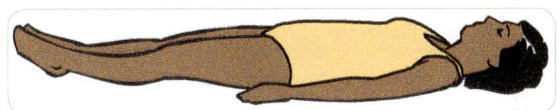

FIGURE 18.2   Lie on a carpeted floor with arms by your sides, back straight, and eyes closed.

Stress with a Human Face

"You know, I really thought all this breathing stuff was a crock," said Tom, a lieutenant in the Navy. "Yup! You could say I have a stressful life right about now." Tom was about to graduate from college, start flight school in Florida, and become a father.

All three events converged about 2 weeks later. Whatever mental toughness Tom had attained in boot camp melted away when the first labor pain arrived. What otherwise seemed like a short drive to the hospital became a comedy of errors as Tom faced traffic of biblical proportions on the Capital Beltway. And it only got worse when the right front tire was punctured by some glass by the side of the road. "I just kept telling Kathy, 'Take a deep breath, keep breathing, it will be all right.' I was breathing right along with her. I'm not sure who it helped more, me or her. You know, you always hear about babies being born in the back seat of a car, but I never thought mine would be one of those."

Normal breathing is for the most part an involuntary, unconscious act. It is regulated by the medulla oblongata of the brain, allowing the conscious mind to focus on other aspects of functional survival. Diaphragmatic breathing, though, necessitates a conscious decision to redirect your attention to this basic physiologic function and turn off the autonomic influence that normally controls it. One approach to deeper awareness is to mentally follow the flow of air as it enters the body and travels to its destination in the lower lobes of the lungs and back out again. Sometimes a mental suggestion can help: "Feel the air come into my nose (or mouth), down into my lungs, and feel my stomach rise and then descend as I exhale the air, feeling it leave my lungs, throat, and nasal cavity." Repeat this with each breath.

Concentration can be augmented further by focusing on the components of each breath. Each ventilation is said to be composed of four distinct phases:

- *Phase 1*: Inspiration, or taking the air into your lungs through the nose or mouth

- *Phase 2*: A very slight pause before exhaling

- *Phase 3*: Exhalation, or releasing the air from your lungs through the passage it entered

- *Phase 4*: Another very slight pause after exhalation before the next inhalation is initiated

These phases can be experienced to a greater extent by exaggerating the breathing cycle, taking a very slow and comfortable deep breath. When trying this technique, try to isolate and recognize the four phases as they occur. Remember not to hold your breath at any time during each phase. Rather, learn to regulate your breathing by controlling the pace of each phase in the breathing cycle. Diaphragmatic breathing is not the same as hyperventilation; this style of breathing is slow, relaxed, and as deep as feels comfortable. It is commonly agreed that the most relaxing phase of diaphragmatic breathing is the third phase, exhalation. At this phase, the chest and abdominal areas relax, sending the relaxing effect throughout the whole body. It requires no effort whatsoever. So, when focusing on your breathing, feel how relaxed your whole body becomes during this phase, especially your chest, shoulders, and abdominal region.

In addition to acknowledging the four phases of each breath, become aware of your capacity to breathe. In the tradition of yoga, there are said to be three regions of the lungs: the upper, middle, and lower lobes. During normal breathing, we typically use only the upper lobes. During the initial stages of relaxed breathing, both the upper and middle lobes are filled with air. But in deep breathing, all three lobes of the lungs are used. As you monitor your breathing, become conscious of filling each layer or region of your lungs.

Step 3: Visualization

Breathing and imagery are dynamic partners in the art of relaxation. Many images can be combined with this breathing technique. The following are two common ones accompanied by suggestions often used in Asian relaxation practices.

Visualization Exercise 1: Breathing Clouds. This technique can be traced back to the origins of yoga in Asia and Zen meditation in Japan. It was introduced as a cleansing process for the mind and body (Shiamora 1992).

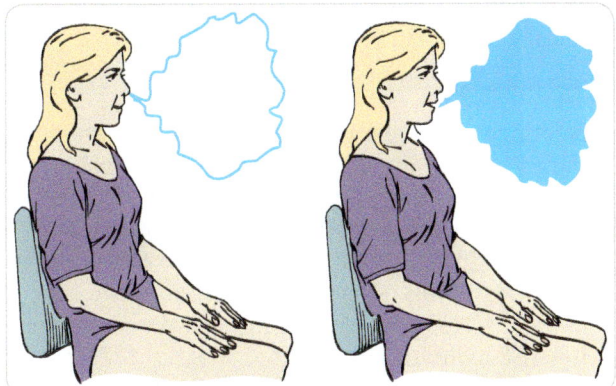

FIGURE 18.3   Breathing clouds exercise.

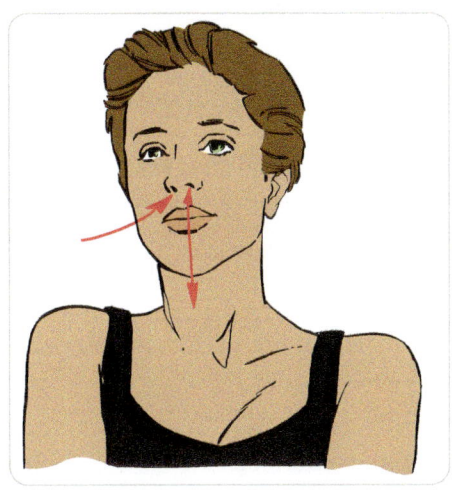

FIGURE 18.4   Alternate nostril breathing exercise.

To begin (**FIG. 18.3**), close your eyes and focus all your attention on your breathing. Visualize the air that you take into your lungs as being clean, fresh air; pure and energized air; clean air with the power to cleanse and heal your body. As you breathe in this clean, fresh air, visualize and feel air enter your nose (or mouth), travel up through the sinus cavities to the top of your head, and down your spinal column to circulate throughout your body. Now, as you exhale, visualize that the air leaving your body is dirty air—dark, cloudy smoke that symbolizes all the stressors, frustrations, and toxins throughout your mind and body. With each breath you take, allow the clean, fresh air to enter, circulate, and rejuvenate your body, and expel the dirty air to help rid your body of its stress and tension. Repeat this breathing cycle for 5 to 10 minutes. As you repeat the breathing clouds exercise, you may notice that, as the body becomes more relaxed through the release of stress and tension, the color of the exhaled air begins to change from gray to an off-white, symbolic of complete relaxation and cleansing.

Visualization Exercise 2: Alternate Nostril Breathing. This technique dates back to the origins of yoga and is also called *nadi shadhanam*. It may seem very difficult if not impossible at first, but with repeated practice it will enhance the relaxation response. To begin, close your eyes and focus all your attention on your breathing. Feel the air enter your mouth or nose and travel down into your lungs. Feel your stomach rise as the air enters, and then slowly descend as you exhale. After becoming relaxed from the sensations of your breathing, take a slow, deep breath. Exhale, allowing the air to leave exclusively through your left nostril (**FIG. 18.4**). When your lungs feel completely empty,

begin your next breath by inhaling air exclusively through your right nostril. Repeat this cycle for the next 15 to 20 breaths by continuing to exhale air through your left nostril and draw air in through your right nostril.

When you feel completely comfortable with this air flow, take a very slow but comfortably deep breath through the right nostril again, but change the direction of the air flow: exhale through the right nostril and inhale through the left. Repeat this cycle for the next 15 to 20 breaths. Throughout the whole process, try to visualize the flow of air as you breathe. You may want to hold a finger to your nose to feel the effectiveness of this visualization. Even if you don't feel a difference, keep trying. Although it may take a while, the nasal passages will begin to open up as a result of these suggestions. Although normally the two nostrils take turns dominating the breathing cycle, you can learn to control this as a relaxation technique.

Visualization Exercise 3: Energy Breathing. Energy breathing is a way to vitalize your body by not only taking in air through your nose or mouth, but, in effect, breathing through your whole body as well. In essence, your body becomes one big lung, taking in air and circulating it throughout. You can do this technique either sitting or lying down. This exercise has three phases. First, get comfortable and allow your shoulders to relax. If you choose to sit, try to keep your legs straight. Now, imagine that there is a circular hole at the top (crown) of your head. As you breathe in, visualize energy in the form of a beam of light entering the top of your head (**FIG. 18.5**). Bring the energy down from the crown of your head to your abdomen as you inhale. As you exhale,

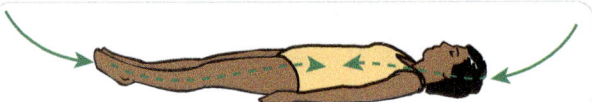

FIGURE 18.5   Energy breathing exercise.

allow the energy to leave through the top of your head. Repeat this 5 to 10 times, coordinating your breathing with the visual flow of energy. As you continue to bring the energy down to your stomach, allow the light to reach all the inner parts of your upper body.

When you feel comfortable with this first phase, you are ready to move on to the second phase. Imagine that there is a circular hole in the center of each foot. Again think of energy as a beam of light. Concentrate only on your lower extremities, and allow the flow of energy to move up from your feet into your abdomen as you inhale with your diaphragm. Repeat this 5 to 10 times, coordinating your breathing with the flow of energy. As you continue to bring the energy up into your stomach area, allow the light to reach all the inner parts of your lower body (**FIG. 18.6**). Today there are many apps to help promote diaphragmatic breathing (**BOX 18.3**).

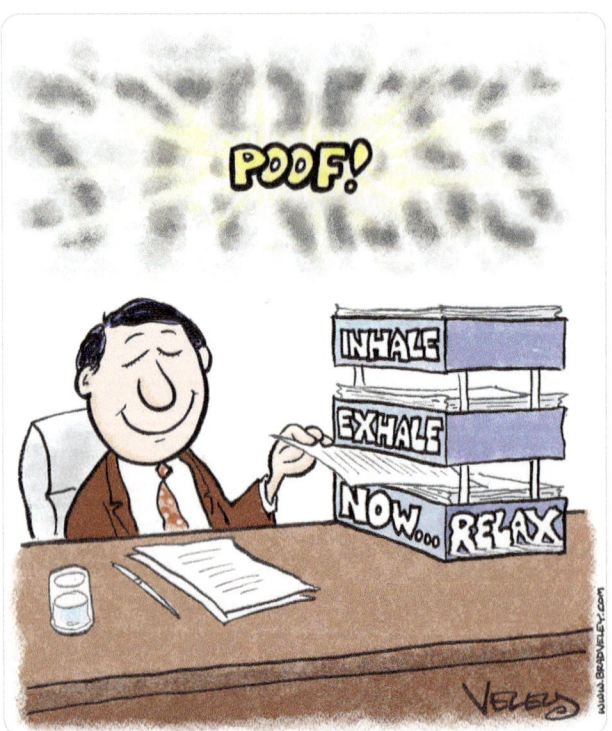

FIGURE 18.6   Take time for belly breathing exercises each day.

© Bradford Veley, Marquette, MI.

BOX 18.3   Breathing Apps

Breathing may seem like one of the most natural things to do, but in our fast-paced, fear-based, stress-prone society this may not be the case. For this reason (and perhaps others), many apps are available to help you breathe easier and lower your stress levels. (The current count is nearly 300 in Apple's App Store.) Headspace; Calm; Insight Timer; Buddhify; Sattva; Stop, Breathe & Think; and 10% Happier all have five-star ratings and were noted as some of the Best Meditation Apps of 2019.

Regardless of which app you choose to use, pay attention to how your body feels as it takes you through a progression of steps. Find an app that works for you. If you become bored with one app after several weeks, consider using another one. Relaxation apps should be considered like training wheels when learning to ride a bike. After several attempts you should be able to relax on your own and not become dependent on a device to achieve peace and quiet.

Once you feel you are coordinating your breathing and the visual flow of energy to your lower extremities, combine the movement of energy from both the top of your head and your feet, and bring it to the center of your body as you inhale with your diaphragm. Then, as you exhale, allow the flow of energy to reverse direction, leaving the way it came. Repeat this 10 to 20 times. Each time you move the energy through your body, feel each body region, each muscle and organ, and each cell become energized. At first it may be difficult to visually coordinate the movement of energy coming from opposite ends of your body, but with practice this will come more easily (**BOX 18.4**).

BOX 18.4   Benefits of Breathing

1. Decreases resting heart rate.
2. Promotes feelings of relaxation.
3. Decreases muscle tension.
4. Improves mental clarity.
5. Increases oxygen capacity in lungs.
6. Helps deal with stress overload.

SUMMARY

- Diaphragmatic breathing is thought to be the easiest method of relaxation. When the emphasis of breathing is centered in the lower abdomen rather than the thoracic cavity, less sympathetic neural activity is generated, causing a greater relaxation effect.

- Diaphragmatic breathing, or belly breathing, is the basic relaxation technique taught in childbirth classes.

- In a normal state of consciousness, the average number of breaths is 12 to 16 per minute. In a relaxed state, this number can be reduced to as few as three to four breaths very comfortably.

- Breathing is thought to be paramount to relaxation in nearly every culture, especially Asian cultures, where breath (*prana* or *chi*) is thought to give the body energy. Diaphragmatic breathing is incorporated into nearly every relaxation technique.

- Diaphragmatic breathing takes little more than a comfortable position, focused concentration, and a little mental imagery.

- Diaphragmatic breathing is known to decrease episodes of chronic pain.

- Diaphragmatic breathing can be done anywhere, under any condition where stress arises. For this reason alone, diaphragmatic breathing is said to be the most accessible (and perhaps effective) technique to initiate the relaxation response.

STUDY GUIDE QUESTIONS

1. What is diaphragmatic breathing?

2. Why is diaphragmatic breathing thought to be an effective relaxation technique?

3. What are the four phases of each breath cycle?

4. What three steps are important to engage in this technique?

REFERENCES AND RESOURCES

Bentov, I. 1988. *Stalking the Wild Pendulum: On the Mechanics of Consciousness*. Rochester, VT: Destiny Books.

Birkel, D. 1991. *Hatha Yoga: Developing the Body, Mind, and Inner Self*. Dubuque, IA: Eddie Bowers.

Borysenko, J. 1987. *Minding the Body, Mending the Mind*. New York: Bantam Books.

Brown, R. P., and P. L. Gerbarg. 2012. *The Healing Power of the Breath*. Boston, MA: Shambhala Publications.

Calihan, L., M. Braga, Y. Matsuo, and E. D. Hernandez. 2002. "Efficacy of Diaphragmatic Breathing in Persons with Chronic Obstructive Pulmonary Disease." *Journal of Cardiopulmonary Rehabilitation* 22: 7–21.

Caponigro, A. 1996. "Healing with the Breath of Life." *Body Mind Spirit* 15(1): 6–11.

Christopher, L. 2016. *Upgrade Your Breath, Upgrade Your Health*. Seattle, WA: Create Space Publishing.

Courtney, R. 2000. "Breathe Easy Eucapnic Breathing: A Powerful Tool for the Somatic Therapist." *Massage & Bodywork* 15(4): 12–16.

Davis, M., M. McKay, and R. Eshelman. 1988. *The Relaxation and Stress-Reduction Workbook* (3rd ed.). Oakland, CA: New Harbinger Press.

Engle, B. T., and R. A. Chism. 1967. "Effects of Increases and Decreases in Breathing Rate on Heart Rate and Finger-Pulse Volume." *Psychophysiology* 4: 83–89.

Farhi, D. 1996. *The Breathing Book: Good Health and Vitality Through Essential Breathwork*. New York: Owl Books.

Fixx, J. 1977. *The Complete Book of Running*. New York: Random House.

Funderburk, J. 1977. *Science Studies Yoga: A Review of Physiological Data*. Honesdale, PA: Himalayan International Institute of Yoga Science and Philosophy.

Green, E. 1992. Personal communication. Stress Physiology of Swami Rama. ISSSEEM Conference, Boulder, CO, June 22.

Hendricks, G. 1995. *Conscious Breathing*. New York: Bantam Books.

Iyengar, B. K. 1981. *Light on Pranayama*. New York: Crossroad.

Iyengar, B. K. 1995. *Light on Pranayama: The Yogic Art of Breathing*. New York: Crossroad/Herder & Herder.

Kabat-Zinn, J. 1990. *Full Catastrophe Living*. New York: Delta Books.

Miller, R. 1989. "Working with Breathing." *Yoga Journal*, September/October, pp. 67–75.

Nakahata, A. K. 1993. "Mastering Lamaze Skills: Discover Breathing and Relaxation Skills to Help You Through Labor and the Years to Follow." *Lamaze Parents Magazine* 12: 36–37.

Neimark, J. 1985. "Brain Rhythms: What the Nose Knows." *American Health*, May.

Peper, E. n.d. "Effortless Diaphragmatic Breathing." https://www.bfe.org/protocol/pro10eng.htm.

Rama, S., R. Ballentine, and A. Hymes. 1998. *The Science of Breath*. Honesdale, PA: Himalayan Institute Press.

Rosen, R. 2002. *The Yoga of Breathing: A Step by Step Guide to Pranayama*. Boston, MA: Shambhala Books.

Searleman, A., D. Hornung, E. Stein, and L. Brzuszkiewicz. 2005. "Nostril Dominance." *Laterality: Asymmetries of Body, Brain, and Cognition* 10(2): 111–112.

Seaward, B. L. 2002. "Breathing Clouds Meditation." *A Change of Heart: Meditations and Visualizations* (audio CD). Boulder, CO: Inspiration Unlimited.

Seaward, B. L. 2004. "Dolphin Breath Meditation." *A Wing and a Prayer: Meditations and Visualizations* (audio CD). Boulder, CO: Inspiration Unlimited.

Shannohoff-Khalsa, D. 1986. "Breathing for the Brain." *American Health* 5: 16–18.

Sherwood, L. 2006. *Fundamentals of Physiology: A Human Perspective*. San Francisco, CA: Thomson Brooks/Cole.

Shiamora, S. 1992. Personal communication. The American University, Washington, DC, January 25.

Spreads, C. 1978. *Breathing: The ABCs*. New York: Harper & Row.

Stern, R. M., and C. Anschel. 1968. "Deep Inspirations as Stimuli for Responses of the Autonomic Nervous System." *Psychophysiology* 5: 132–141.

Straub, W. 2003. "The Effects of Diaphragmatic Breathing and Sleep Training on Sleep, Jet Lag, and Swimming Performance." *The Sports Journal* 6(1).

Stringer, H. 2001. "Breathing Lessons: Yoga Helps Busy Nurses Find Physical Freedom, Maximize Relaxation." *Nurseweek* 6(1): 17–18.

Swami Rama, R. Ballentine, and A. Hymes. 1979. *Science of Breath*. Honesdale, PA: Himalayan International Institute of Yoga Science and Philosophy.

Swayzee, N. 1998. *Breathworks: Strengthening Your Back from the Inside Out*. New York: Avon Books.

Taylor, K. 2003. *Exploring Holotropic Breathwork*. Santa Cruz, CA: Hanford Mead Publishers.

Weil, A. 1999. *Breathing: The Master to Self-Healing*. Boulder, CO: Sounds True.

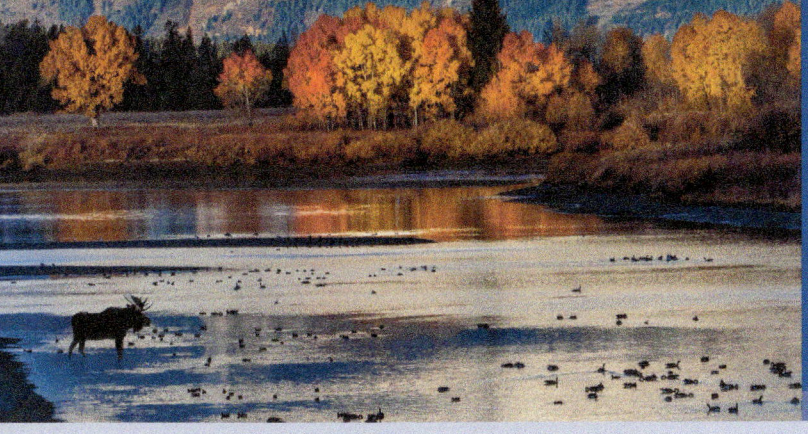

Meditation and Mindfulness

When the pupil is ready, the teacher will come.

—Ancient Chinese proverb

In case no one has officially said this to you yet, "Welcome to the digital-Wi-Fi-YouTube-GPS Information Age." Today more than ever before, the human mind is barraged with bits and bytes every waking hour, practically nonstop. The once humorous cries of "too much information" are not quite so funny anymore as we become deluged in information, with nonstop access to the Internet, smartphones, texts, tablets, and information technology that is being invented as I write this but that will be commonplace by the time you read these words. Although the ability to access information is wonderful, the inundation of information is deafening to the mind. The result is **sensory overload**.

If you were to listen to people talk about the negative aspects of technology (smartphones, email, texts, podcasts, Twitter, Facebook, and such), you surely would hear the word *distraction* used repeatedly. It is hard to focus your mind when there are countless constant distractions begging for your attention every waking moment. Distractions have always been part of the human condition, primarily fear-based thoughts created by the ego. In the twenty-first century, however, the number of distractions has grown exponentially, due

in part to the cyber world. The result is that today people are less focused, less mindful, less patient, and more cynical. Meditation isn't a cure for the world's ills, but the purpose of meditation is to train the mind to minimize distractions, both internal (ego-based thoughts) and external, so that one becomes more focused, more mindful, and more patient and experiences a higher degree of happiness and well-being. Simply stated, meditation is a way to detoxify the mind from sensory bombardment, sensory overload, and the multitude of daily distractions that interfere with clear thinking.

In every age of humanity, the mind has always needed a respite from thoughts, worries, and external stimuli. **Meditation** is the quintessential respite to calm the mind from sensory overload (**FIG. 19.1**). Today, meditation is rapidly gaining recognition in the West as a powerfully effective relaxation technique. What at one time may

> **Sensory overload:** An inundation of information and distractions that overwhelm the mind.
>
> **Meditation:** A practice of focused concentration that leads to increased awareness; a solitary practice of reflection on internal rather than external stimuli.

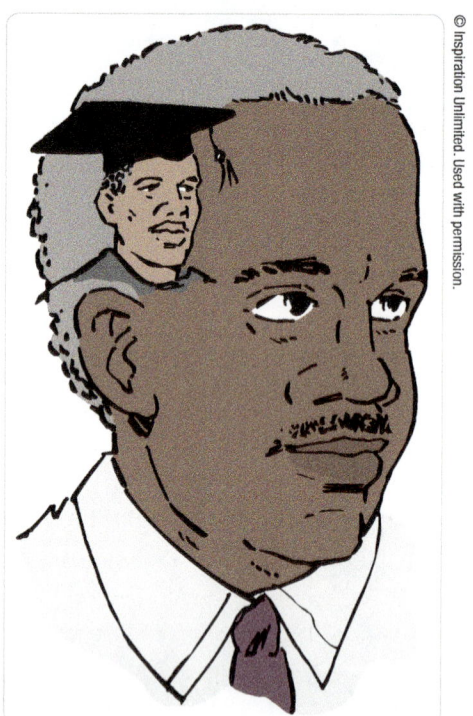

© Inspiration Unlimited. Used with permission.

FIGURE 19.1 We are guided by our inner wisdom only when we take the time to stop and listen.

have been considered a fringe behavior by "new agers" is now considered an American mainstream habit. So declared *Time* magazine in a cover story, with nearly 30 million people citing meditation as a formal practice of relaxation. In that same month, *BusinessWeek* highlighted several CEOs of *Fortune* 500 companies who meditate regularly. The surge in corporate meditation practice correlates with a rise in occupational stress, yet CEOs see meditation as a means to gain not only mental clarity, but also a sharper creative edge in the business world. Those who follow basketball know that former Los Angeles Lakers coach Phil Jackson is a big advocate of meditation as well. Actor Richard Gere, Sting, and former President Jimmy Carter also meditate regularly. Moreover, a random browse through recent social media posts as well as various news headlines offers some insight into the power and practice of meditation: "Canadian Police Taught to Meditate," "Meditation Rather Than Detention for Children," and "Meditation Taught to Wounded Warriors and Military Veterans." With the rise in the number of people practicing yoga, this practice, too, has had an impact.

By all confirmed reports, meditation is not a religion. Rather, it is a solitary practice of reflection on internal rather than external stimuli. Technically speaking,

meditation is an increased concentration and awareness—a process of living in the present moment to produce and enjoy a tranquil state of mind. The practice of meditation is the oldest recognized relaxation technique known. So accepted are several components of meditation that they have become tightly integrated into virtually every relaxation technique known and practiced today.

Shakespeare once said, "The eyes are the windows to your soul." By consciously closing the eyes now and again, the soul is given a chance to pause and cleanse itself. Indeed, all the body's senses are ports of entry bringing in stimuli from outside for the mind to interpret and censor. Human beings are visually oriented animals; we take in more than two-thirds of our sensory information through vision alone. Stimulation from any sensory organ bombards the conscious mind, and under the influence of stress, the mind juggles many thoughts produced both externally and internally as they compete for attention. Quite often, the result of this abundance of sensory stimulation is sensory overload. You have probably experienced this at the end of a long day of classes or work, or perhaps during a visit to an art museum, where after 2 hours every painting looks about the same. Sensory overload is like a blackboard filled to capacity with notes and scribbles that are quite difficult to organize and assimilate into use. When our minds are overloaded with information, concentration is compromised. The term *polyphasia* (also known as multitasking) is used to describe an abundance of simultaneous thoughts cluttering the mind, and there is a strong association between a cluttered mind and a stressful mind.

To use a simile, meditation is like an eraser that cleans the mind's blackboard. In fact, some would say, meditation gets rid of the blackboard as well. Meditation is a tool to unclutter the mind and bring about mental homeostasis (**FIG. 19.2**). In the language of information technology (IT), meditation increases the bandwidth of human consciousness. When the mind is clear of thought, it is more receptive to new information, new perspectives, and new ways of dealing with unresolved problems. In the acclaimed book *The Prophet* (1981), Kahlil Gibran writes, "No man can reveal to you aught but that which lies half asleep in the dawning of your knowledge." In other words, the student is also the teacher. But before lessons can be taught, the proper learning environment must be created. This is the primary purpose of meditation: concentration promoting self-awareness. Thus, as expressed in the ancient Chinese proverb, when the student is ready, the teacher will come.

COSMIC BREADCRUMBS

After several attempts, Jason finally gets the hang of meditation.

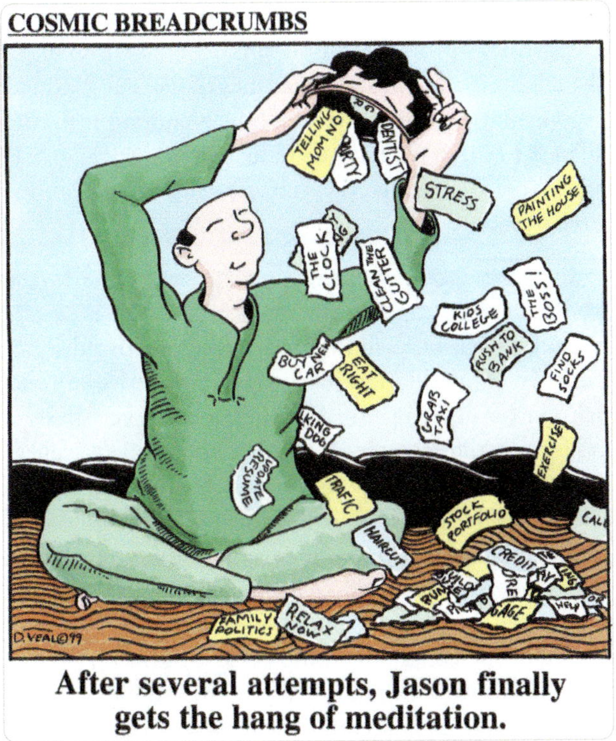

FIGURE 19.2 There are many descriptions of meditation, clearing your mind of ego-based thoughts and feelings is one of the best.

■ Historical Perspective

Although it is likely that the practice existed much earlier, the roots of meditation can be traced back to Asia in the sixth century B.C., when several individuals traveling separate paths to enlightenment took refuge and solace in contemplative and reflective thought. The fruits of this thought became the cornerstones of several philosophies, which gathered many followers eager to learn and share them. These followers, in turn, established rules and guidelines to live by, which evolved into several prominent religious philosophies; namely, Hinduism, Buddhism, Taoism, Confucianism, and the Essenes. Meditation, or self-reflective thought, was integrated into the practices of these religions as a means to cleanse and purify the soul. From this perspective, we can see that although meditation has been adopted by nearly every religion, it is not a religion in itself (Allen 1983).

Self-reflection is considered essential to the maturation process. Every culture and every religious sect has some element of meditation or self-reflective practice, including Judaism, Catholicism, Protestantism, Islam, and the worship of several Native American tribes. There are subtle but significant differences between Eastern and Western cultures in their approach to meditation. Western views promote a search for inner peace through external means, whereas Eastern philosophies direct thoughts inward for harmony and atonement. This dichotomy of approaches has resulted in a high degree of perceived mysticism, and perhaps misunderstanding, in the West. In simple terms, like the mind it affects, meditation appears to have several layers. Initially, meditation has a calming effect on the mind's basic thought processes. Once this layer is peeled away, a deeper series of layers is unveiled to reveal insights of the soul, intuition, or enlightenment (Levey and Levey 1999).

Eastern cultures have accepted the essence of meditation and all its many principles. Western cultures, more skeptical by nature, have only recently begun to appreciate meditation as a means to calm the mind and all its thought processes to achieve inner peace. Meditation became popular in the United States during the 1960s by way of the Beatles, whose music and lifestyles included meditation, thus influencing many people (Woo 2008). Meditation gained additional momentum from the counterculture movements of the 1960s, specifically the human potential movement, which sought to elevate all humanity to a higher level of consciousness. The materialism of the 1980s and 1990s, however, nearly derailed this movement. With the dawning of the twenty-first century, a revival of interest in the advancement of human potential and a quest for spiritual growth and development have emerged. Meditation has again become a major component of this movement, particularly in various self-help workshops, motivational retreats, and corporate seminars. In essence, meditation is now a mainstream practice in America, with more than 30 million people claiming to practice it on a regular basis (Stein 2003). One researcher, José Silva, has taken the concept of meditation one step further, integrating it into a technique to enhance what he calls personal mind control. In the Silva method, meditation is used to access great thinking power and memory function (Silva and Miele 1975). The premise of meditation has also been adapted to a concept called alpha thinking, named for the state of mind physiologically represented by alpha waves, in which specific meditation concepts are integrated with other relaxation techniques, including breathing, biofeedback, and mental imagery, to promote deep relaxation and improved memory.

The medical profession has now adopted meditation as its own behavior-modification technique to combat rising morbidity and mortality from stress-related heart disease. Originally doubtful of claims that meditation promotes physical calmness as well as inner peace, the American Heart Association now advocates it as a preventive health measure in conjunction with proper diet and aerobic exercise to reduce modifiable risk factors for coronary heart disease. In fact, Dr. Dean Ornish (1998) has proven that coronary heart disease is reversible in some cases in people who combine meditation with changes in diet and exercise. The National Institutes of Health advocates meditation for the mental and emotional relief of cancer. Slowly, as Eastern and Western cultures become more closely integrated, the basic concepts of meditation as a relaxation technique will become even more readily accepted for achieving both mental and physical homeostasis.

Although some see meditation as a means only for personal enlightenment, others value it for its greater potential—to raise the collective human consciousness. According to Lyall Watson's Hundredth Monkey theory (Keys 1987) and Rupert Sheldrake's morphogenic field theory (1995), once a critical mass of conscious thought is reached, the direction of human evolution will shift to a higher (stress-free) level. Moreover, it is believed that when a critical mass of people engage in meditation for world peace and ecological harmony, more and more people will eventually resonate with this mind frame to the point of significant positive influence (Hagelin 2007). Can a collective think tank (or non–think tank, as the case may be) of meditators make a difference? Many practitioners of Transcendental Meditation are known to travel collectively to various cities for weeks on end and use meditation as a means to decrease violent crime; the results of their efforts appear promising. As ironic as it sounds, some groups of Pentagon employees meditate

for world peace using a practice known as "human peace shields" for the moral protection of humanity (Winchester 2007). Although they have not claimed responsibility for the demise of Soviet communism, the fall of the Berlin Wall, or the reduction of nuclear armaments, they do feel that their efforts were partially influential in these events.

■ Types of Meditation

From the seeds of Eastern philosophy grew two distinct branches of meditation: exclusive (or restrictive) and inclusive (or opening-up). Although the two vary in style and format, the processes of concentration and awareness are paramount to achieving the benefits they both offer. The end result is the same: a cleansing of the mind that leads to inner peace. Once the conscious mind is calm and without ego chatter and clear of distracting thoughts, new insights bubble up from the unconscious mind to the surface of the conscious mind; these insights often give subtle direction for the next step of our human journey (the aha moment of meditation). Whether one practices a form of exclusive or inclusive meditation, people often refer to these modalities as **insightful meditation** because of the nature of the intuitive thought processes that follow when the mind is disciplined to listen.

Exclusive Meditation

Consider this metaphor: The mind is a sky full of clouds, with several layers superimposed on one another above the earth. Each cloud layer represents a multitude of thoughts that compete for conscious attention. **Exclusive meditation** (also known as concentration meditation) involves the restriction of consciousness to focus on a single thought. This single thought becomes a device to wipe all other thoughts from the conscious slate. A single thought is like a gentle wind that blows the clouds away, leaving a clear blue sky. The power of this single thought is repetition, which continually breaks the surface of attention to the exclusion of all other thoughts. Restrictive meditation advocates a closed awareness to the external senses and all outside stimulation, and directs the focus of one's thoughts inward. In most cases, exclusive meditation is practiced with the eyes closed to prevent visual distractions. Five actions are used to refine one's attention on a single focused thought: mental repetition, visual concentration, repeated sounds, physical repetition, and tactile repetition.

1. *Mental repetition:* Mental repetition means a thought is produced over and over again. Mental

Insightful meditation: An expression given to any type of meditation (inclusive or exclusive) whereby a person, once clearing the mind of interrupting thoughts and ego chit-chat, begins to expand his or her awareness to the intuition, or the deep-seated wisdom of the collective unconscious, thus giving insight into the person's life.

Exclusive meditation: A form of meditation wherein concentration is focused on one object (e.g., *mantra*, *tratak*) to the exclusion of all other thoughts as a means to increase self-awareness and promote relaxation.

repetition is most commonly done by use of a **mantra**, which is a one-syllable word (e.g., *Om*, *one*, *peace*, or *love*), and should be done in conjunction with exhaling. A mantra can also be a short positive phrase (e.g., "I feel good," "I am worthy of love," or "My body is calm and relaxed") to reinforce positive self-esteem. In some cases, prayers are also considered a type of mantra. In cultures where yoga meditation is practiced, it is believed that certain sounds (audible energy) have the power to heal. Thus, chanting in a soft whisper or silently repeating the word *Om* is believed to access the highest level of concentration, that which represents the essence of truth, love, and peace. *Om* and other yoga mantras are based on special sounds that are thought to help release blocked energy that is impeding mental homeostasis. Chanting the word *Om* is thought to produce a vibration that draws the body's rhythm into synchrony with the earth's magnetic field, thus evoking a feeling of oneness with nature. Western philosophy suggests that the vibrations from any one word can have a calming effect. Regardless of philosophical bent, it is commonly accepted that when practiced regularly the repetition of a one-word mantra will clear all other thoughts from the conscious mind.

2. *Visual concentration:* Visual concentration involves visually focusing on or staring at an object or image. In yoga meditation, this is called steady gazing or ***tratak***. Visual concentration is like a visual mantra. The practice of *tratak* involves staring at an object about 3 to 5 feet away, without blinking, until it is etched on the mind's blackboard to the exclusion of all other thoughts. The suggested duration is about 60 seconds. Then, close your eyes and visualize the object. If the mental image fades or vanishes, open your eyes and repeat this again. Common visual mantras include a candle flame, flower, seashell, beautiful scene, or **mandala** (**FIG. 19.3**)—a circular object that is intricately designed, intense in color, and often divided into four quarters.

3. *Repeated sounds:* In some forms of meditation, a sound is repeated continually to help focus the mind's attention. The term for this is ***nadam***. Examples of sounds are a beating drum, chimes, Tibetan bells, or Gregorian chants. Natural sounds such as the rush of a waterfall, ocean

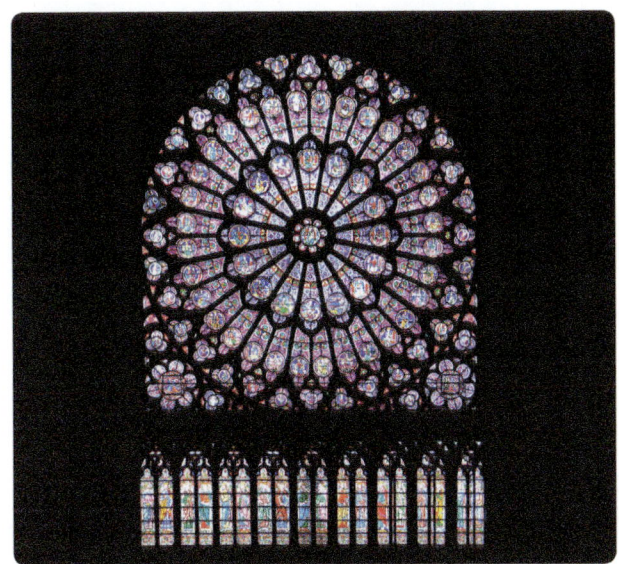

FIGURE 19.3   A mandala is a circular object symbolizing wholeness that can be used as a visual mantra. (This is the famous stained glass window design of Notre Dame Cathedral in Paris, France.)

waves on the shore of a beach, or rolling thunder are also examples of *nadams*. In Western culture, some types of repetitive New Age music may be considered *nadams*.

4. *Physical repetition:* Repetitive motion such as the sensation of breathing or some forms of rhythmic aerobic exercise (e.g., running, swimming, or walking) are believed by many to produce a meditative state (runner's high) either from the sound of breathing or from the rhythmic motions of the feet and arms. Physical repetition is thought to shift the mind to an altered state of consciousness

Mantra: Typically a one-syllable word (e.g., *Om, peace, love*) or a short phrase that acts like a broom to sweep the mind of nonessential (ego-based) thoughts.

Tratak: A visual type of mantra, such as a seashell, a colorfully designed mandala, or any object that is used by the eyes to focus attention and ignore distracting thoughts.

Mandala: A circular-shaped object used as a visual mantra for the purpose of clearing the mind of unnecessary (ego-based) thoughts.

Nadam: An auditory mantra for which a repetitive sound is used to help clear the mind of unnecessary (ego-based) thoughts.

or a relaxed mode of thinking. Some people say that their most creative thoughts come during this type of exercise. In Sufi religious practice, the whirling dervish dance is said to induce a trance-like state through the repetitive circular motion. Pranayama or diaphragmatic breathing is also used extensively as a physical repetitive mantra in virtually every relaxation course. This approach, where there is repetitive motion, is also called **active meditation.**

5. *Tactile repetition:* Holding a small object, such as a tumble stone or seashell, also brings focus to the mind. Hindu yogis use a strand of beads called a *mala* (108 small beads and 1 large *meru* bead), holding it in their right hand and rolling the beads one by one between the thumb and third finger as they meditate. In Western culture, rosary beads offer a similar focus of concentration.

Meditation Position. In all forms of meditation, but particularly in restrictive meditation, correct body position is essential. Perhaps the most recognized posture is the lotus position. In the lotus position, an individual sits with his or her legs crossed and folded, each foot resting on the alternate thigh. A more comfortable position for beginners is the half-lotus position (**FIG. 19.4**), with the legs simply crossed in a comfortable manner. In this passive position, one sits with the back (spinal column) completely aligned from the crown of the head to the tail bone. This alignment minimizes neural firing to the muscles and thus allows for increased (active) concentration on the mental focus. The hands can be placed on the thighs either with the palms down (to center oneself with the earth's energy) or facing up with thumb and index finger joined (to receive energy). Breathing is regulated by placing emphasis on the expansion of the stomach area, rather than the chest, during inhalation. The position should be comfortable enough to maintain for approximately 30 minutes or more without interfering with your ability to concentrate. You may notice some pain in the muscles and joints of your

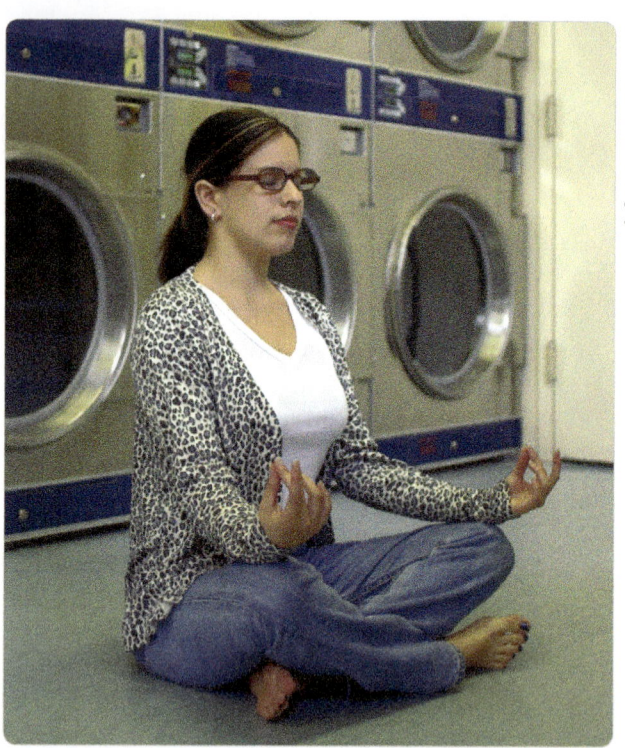

© Thinkstock/Index Stock Imagery.

FIGURE 19.4   A meditation posture based on the lotus position.

hips and knees. If this occurs, stretch your legs to find a more comfortable position. Pain is not conducive to meditation.

There are several types of restrictive meditation. Transcendental Meditation and the relaxation response are two examples (**BOX 19.1**).

Transcendental Meditation. **Transcendental Meditation (TM)** is a classic example of exclusive meditation. TM was developed by the Hindu Maharishi Mahesh Yogi (2001). The story of the development of TM reads like an ancient fable. A young Hindu gentleman named Mahesh Prasad Varma yearned to become a scientist, and in 1942 he received a degree in physics. But the winds of change soon brought him to study with the famed religious leader Swami Brahmanada Saraswati, with whom he spent the next 13 years in divine worship. In this calling, he accepted the challenge to create a simple version of Hindu meditation, one that "anyone" could learn and practice. His life mission became to sow the seeds of world peace through the trained, tranquil soul of each individual. Off he went to the Himalayas, taking refuge in an abandoned cave. After a 2-year retreat, he returned to India with the new technique we

Active meditation: Meditation that uses repetitive motion from physical activity (e.g., walking, swimming) to promote the cleansing of the mind.

Transcendental Meditation (TM): This meditation is the epitome of exclusive meditation in which all thoughts are eliminated save the mantra itself.

> ### BOX 19.1   How to Meditate: The Basics
>
> 1. Find a quiet place.
> 2. Sit comfortably. (A sore butt is a distraction.)
> 3. Remove all distractions (e.g., smartphone).
> 4. Close your eyes.
> 5. Focus all attention on your breathing.
> 6. Take slow, deep, comfortable breaths.
> 7. If your mind wanders, that's OK. Redirect your thoughts back to your breathing. (Consider keeping a pad of paper and pen nearby to jot down important thoughts you don't want to forget.)
> 8. Repeat.
>
> Start small, perhaps just 1 to 2 minutes. Add a minute each time you practice, with a goal of reaching 30 to 40 minutes. Remember, boredom is part of the experience. It is OK to be bored doing this. If you mind races all over the place, congrats. You are in great company. The hardest part is to remove distractions, both external, such as text alerts and noisy roommates, and internal, those produced by your own ego. Meditation (mental training) is many things, but first it is domestication of the ego. Keep practicing. Meditation is a skill. The more you do it, the better you become at it.

know today as TM. This technique, a simplified version of yoga meditation stripped of its spiritual dogma, was introduced into the United States in the late 1960s as a secular practice and gained instant popularity. It was the favorite alternative for those whose recreational drug habits produced nasty side effects, as well as those who were seeking inner peace during the tumultuous and rocky years of the Vietnam War. In the practice of TM, individuals are given a "special mantra" and taught to focus their thoughts on that one word. The mantra, the Maharishi and his teachers instructed, must remain secret to be effective, a statement later proved unfounded (Russell 2001).

Within 10 years' time, more than a million Americans had learned this technique. People reported that it indeed brought inner peace and harmony to their lives when practiced with regularity. TM became the object of scientific curiosity, and inner peace soon became measured by significant decreases in resting

blood pressure as well as the absence of many disease symptoms associated with stress. Intrigued by the possibility that TM could be a new relaxation technique, a team of medical researchers headed by Robert Keith Wallace and Herbert Benson (1972) investigated the effects of TM. To their surprise, they found that it proved quite effective as a mediating factor for chronic stress. In a Harvard laboratory, Wallace asked 36 subjects well trained in TM to practice this technique for three 20- to 30-minute sessions. Before, during, and after meditation sessions, oxygen consumption (VO_2), blood lactate, electrical skin conduction (sweating), and alpha brain waves were measured. Results revealed that TM did, in fact, induce a profound state of physiologic homeostasis. Perplexed at the incongruity between its simplicity and the expensive price tag to learn TM (currently priced at $2,500), Benson Americanized the technique and called it the **relaxation response**.

The Relaxation Response. In his book *The Relaxation Response* (1975), Benson describes four basic steps to follow to promote physiological homeostasis. These same four components can be found in virtually every relaxation technique, from mental imagery to progressive muscular relaxation. They include:

1. *A quiet environment:* A quiet environment can be any room with minimal distractions. It should be a room or area in which you feel completely comfortable. The premise of meditation is to reduce all sensory stimuli, including external stimuli such as ringing phones and doorbells, blaring televisions or radios, and outside street noise. A quiet environment also is interpreted to mean a reduction of internal stimuli, such as tense muscles and physical discomfort.

2. *A mental device:* A mental device is any object or tool used to replace all other thoughts. It is a focal point to direct all attention. A mental device can include repetition of a mantra, concentrated breathing, or a *tratak* or *nadam*. Benson suggests the word *one* for a mantra. He also suggests that if your mind wanders, use the word *no* to discontinue the free association.

> **Relaxation response:** A term coined by Dr. Herbert Benson, who Americanized Transcendental Meditation to make it more accessible to the Western world.

3. *A passive attitude:* A passive attitude is a receptive attitude. A passive attitude is a frame of mind in which you are open to thoughts rather than blocking them out. At first this may sound contradictory to the exclusive nature of restrictive meditation. But without this frame of mind, the walls of the ego censor any effort to relax completely.

4. *A comfortable position:* The earliest meditation advocates stated that to relax the mind, one must first relax the body. So, you must first find a comfortable position. Benson advocates a sitting position with most of the body weight supported. The body should be relaxed with no signs of muscular tension. Positions conducive to sleep should be avoided (**BOX 19.2**).

Inclusive Meditation

The second type of meditation is **inclusive meditation**. It is also referred to as access meditation, insightful meditation, and **mindfulness**. Inclusive meditation appears to be very similar to free association, where the mind wanders aimlessly. In the practice of inclusive meditation, the mind is free to accept all thoughts; no attempt is made to control the mind's content. The conscious mind simply accepts spontaneous thoughts that make themselves available from the unconscious mind. There is one condition to this receptivity, however: All thoughts that enter the conscious mind must do so objectively and without judgment or emotional directive. This process is called **detached observation**. No emotional reaction can be connected with these thoughts. In effect, the mind becomes a movie screen with thoughts projected as images, and the individual observes without judgment

---

Inclusive meditation: A form of meditation where all thoughts are invited into awareness without emotional evaluation, judgment, or analysis. Zen meditation is an example.

Mindfulness: A type of meditation where all senses concentrate on the activity being performed during the present moment, like eating an apple or washing the dishes.

Detached observation: A term derived from inclusive meditation during which the individual observes himor herself meditating, in essence detaching from the ego's desire.

Zen (Zazen) meditation: A form of meditation wherein one learns to detach from one's emotional thoughts by becoming the observer of those thoughts.

BOX 19.2 Insomnia and Meditation

It has been long recognized that meditation is a viable antidote for insomnia. Given that meditation is a vehicle for mental discipline, perhaps it should come as no surprise that people who meditate on a regular basis admit to sleeping soundly. By training the mind to release thoughts and feelings that constantly compete for attention, a deep sense of peace is achieved in an awakened state, a skill that carries over to presleep conditions. In essence, the ability to elicit mental clarity appears similar, if not identical, to the presleep state of consciousness. Research has demonstrated that people who meditate on a regular basis achieve the theta (brain wave) state of consciousness, which is closest to the delta wave pattern observed when sleeping. Sleep/insomnia studies reveal that subjects who lay awake at night or who repeatedly wake up show an alpha or beta wave pattern indicative of a busy mind. Given the chance, the effects of meditation groom the mind's ability to decrease mental activity for a good night's sleep.

---

or analysis. By detaching yourself from your emotions, the process of inclusive meditation allows barriers of the ego to dissolve. In this type of meditation the eyes are usually open, but you may find that this style can best be learned with the eyes closed.

The goal of inclusive meditation is to observe the observer, meaning that you learn to step outside yourself to observe your own thought processes. In doing so, you retrain your mind to keep an even keel during times of stress in a manner that is called "domesticating the ego," not overreacting. Mindfulness is really just a name for being mindful of the present moment. Eckhart Tolle, author of the best-seller *The Power of Now* (1999), states:

> The moment you start watching the thinker, a higher level of consciousness becomes activated. You then begin to realize that there is a vast realm of intelligence beyond thought, that thought is only a tiny aspect of intelligence. You also realize that all the things that truly matter—beauty, love, creativity, joy, inner peace—arise from beyond the mind. You begin to awaken.

Zen Meditation. Zen (Zazen) meditation, or some aspects of it, can be considered inclusive meditation. Zen meditation comes from Zen Buddhism. Around 590 B.C.,

Stress with a Human Face

When Adam graduated with his degree in childhood education, he was ready to change the world, and he had every intention of doing so. An excellent student with excellent student-teaching evaluations from his supervisors, Adam believed he had everything he needed to start his teaching career. Like most college graduates, Adam believed he would take the summer off, go to Europe with a friend, and then start work in the fall. As things happened, his plans changed when he ended up graduating in January. Adam found himself looking for a teaching job immediately. His prayers were answered when he landed a job in the southeast section of the District of Columbia—or so he thought.

"You can learn all the theory you want in school, and you can do your practicum in the nicest schools around, but when it comes to working in a city school, I had to learn everything all over again. These kids need a lot of discipline and a lot more love, before they are ready to learn," he said in frustration.

As one of my former students in a stress management class, Adam took an immediate liking to meditation, and from the second semester of his sophomore year, he practiced meditation regularly every morning. He mentioned to me several times that, as a varsity soccer player (now semi-professional), meditation was what kept him grounded before, during, and after his games. He reminded me regularly how valuable meditation had become in his life. Now entering the real world, meditation took on a whole new meaning.

"I come home from work exhausted, more so than after any soccer practice. Every day, those kids zap all my energy until I am completely drained. Do you realize how attentive you have to be with kids like these?" he said one day over lunch. "And let me tell you something else," he added, "If I didn't meditate every morning before I go to work, I wouldn't have lasted the first week in that school. I can't tell you how important meditation is in my life. It's essential."

Adam proceeded to explain his daily meditation routine: a half hour of breathing exercises followed by some mental imagery. "Sometimes I even do it on the subway ride to school. In college, I used to do it for the mystical experience, which was pretty powerful in its own right, and to increase my concentration skills for soccer. I still do it for those reasons, but now more than ever, I do it to clear my mind." Meditation. It's not what you think!

a young man named Prince Gautama Siddhartha left his family, wealth, and life of foolish pleasures to become a monk, or "wanderer," living a simple life on the Ganges Plain. He became known as Sakyamuni ("Prince of the Sakyas"), and later on in life as the Buddha ("Awakened One"). Sakyamuni began a journey of profound soul searching, pondering the meaning of life and death, leading to his own enlightenment. He soon became a recognized and respected teacher with a great many followers. What separates Zen from other similar philosophies is the abandonment of the concept of dualities (good vs. bad, right vs. wrong, male vs. female), which are thought to separate rather than unite one with the universe. Thoughts expressed in either-or terms tend to be of an analytical or judgmental nature. Pure Zen thought is devoid of judgment, thus connecting rather than separating one from the world. When the word *Zen* is heard, it is often associated with deep, pensive, intellectual thought. The purpose of Zen meditation is to reach the highest level of consciousness to achieve divine enlightenment. It is believed in Eastern cultures that truth and knowledge come from within and are housed in the soul. One must be patient to receive this gift of enlightenment, however, for it will not come if one is hurried in thought or strong in emotional attachment (Dumoulin 1981).

Zen meditation has many styles. Some have a restrictive nature to them (e.g., counting your breaths from 10 down to 1), whereas others lend themselves to opening the mind (Austin 2000). Zen meditation is a very difficult and disciplined practice, often requiring several hours of motionless contemplative thought in one sitting. Moreover, Zen meditation includes the mind asking an unanswerable question, or **koan**, such as "What is the sound of one hand clapping?" or "What

Koan: An unsolvable question or riddle that aims to shift one's consciousness from analytical thoughts to profound contemplation.

did your face look like before you were conceived?" It can also include pondering riddles, such as the following: An egg is placed through the narrow opening of a glass bottle. In less than one day the egg hatches, yet the chick is too big to escape through the opening. How do you remove the chick from the glass bottle without harming the chick or destroying the bottle? Each koan invites profound contemplation. Because there are no answers, the mind acquiesces to the riddle. This submission through mental frustration is said to open the mind's door to new thought or sudden insight leading to greater awareness. The ultimate purpose of koans is to lead one up the path of enlightenment by learning, questioning, and accepting one's purpose in life. In Zen, meditation is only one step in the preparation for enlightenment.

Inclusive meditation is very difficult to practice at first. It is extremely challenging to try to divorce your emotions from your thoughts. But it is the walls of the ego that are believed to separate the mind from the soul. It is the ego (the keeper of our identity) that is vulnerable to the perceptions of stress. Initially, opening up to uncensored thoughts can be a very difficult strategy to deal with stress. Perhaps for this reason, restrictive meditation is preferred over inclusive meditation, and it is the former that is most commonly thought of when meditation is mentioned.

Everly and Rosenfeld (2002) created a meditation continuum highlighting the entire range of mental consciousness during the meditative process (**FIG. 19.5**). When one begins a meditation session, the first minute is devoted to preparation: getting comfortable, closing the eyes, perhaps even taking a few deep breaths, followed by more focused concentration. After this time, boredom may set in as the conscious mind fights the mental directive to block out all thoughts and their emotional attachments. (In many cases, people stop here in their first few encounters.) The conscious mind may then become distracted by any thoughts that will relieve the boredom. But once distracting thoughts are removed, the mind begins to enter a state of deep relaxation. In this state, a shift in dominance is said to occur from the left to the right hemisphere of the brain. This shift can be measured by a decrease in beta waves coupled with an increase in alpha waves on an electroencephalogram (EEG). With continued deep relaxation, any thoughts that appear on the mind's screen are observed objectively rather than given any emotional meaning. No judgment or analysis is associated with any thoughts (**BOX 19.3**). As the mind continues to observe, a state of supraconsciousness in which there is increased awareness of one's inner self begins to manifest. At this stage of meditation, the individual may feel almost euphoric, with sensations of enlightenment and connectedness

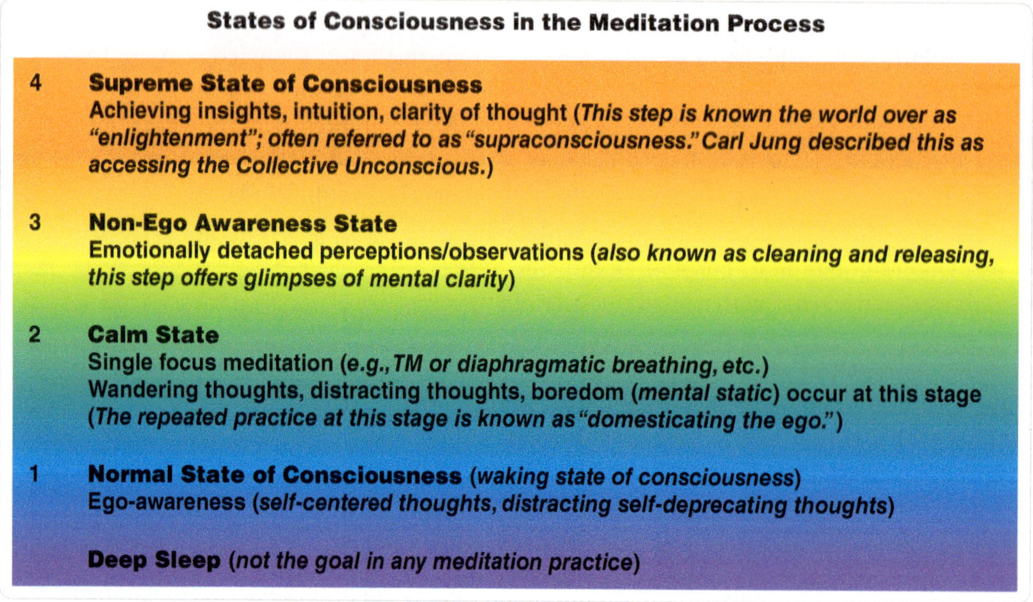

States of Consciousness in the Meditation Process

4 **Supreme State of Consciousness**
Achieving insights, intuition, clarity of thought (*This step is known the world over as "enlightenment"; often referred to as "supraconsciousness." Carl Jung described this as accessing the Collective Unconscious.*)

3 **Non-Ego Awareness State**
Emotionally detached perceptions/observations (*also known as cleaning and releasing, this step offers glimpses of mental clarity*)

2 **Calm State**
Single focus meditation (*e.g., TM or diaphragmatic breathing, etc.*)
Wandering thoughts, distracting thoughts, boredom (*mental static*) occur at this stage (*The repeated practice at this stage is known as "domesticating the ego."*)

1 **Normal State of Consciousness** (*waking state of consciousness*)
Ego-awareness (*self-centered thoughts, distracting self-deprecating thoughts*)

Deep Sleep (*not the goal in any meditation practice*)

FIGURE 19.5 The beginning of the meditation process involves "raising awareness." As a skill, one learns to "train" the mind to increase attention, and hence awareness without emotional attachment.

BOX 19.3   The Art of Mindfulness

Mindfulness is the art of living in the present moment through the eyes of nonjudgment (turning off the voice of the ego). At best, through mindfulness one learns not only to observe one's thoughts, but also to observe oneself observing one's thoughts. (This is considered the epitome of ego detachment.) Detachment is not as easy as it sounds given the ego's influence to constantly direct our thoughts toward the past (guilt) or future events or possible events (worry). Remember, it is the ego that trips the fight-or-flight response. Mindfulness helps deactivate this switch in nonthreatening times.

As a meditation practice, the roots of mindfulness date back several millennia to the beginnings of Buddhism. The introduction of mindfulness meditation in the United States during the 1970s is often credited to Thich Nhat Hanh, a Vietnamese Buddhist monk. Today mindfulness is taught and practiced by thousands of people in various demographic groups, and has become very popular in the corporate business world, all with one purpose in mind: to reduce stress through the achievement of inner peace.

Several decades ago the concept of mindfulness meditation gained a more rudimentary Western approach as a simple, nonsectarian relaxation technique for pain management through the efforts of Jon Kabat-Zinn of the University of Massachusetts Medical School, who taught mindfulness meditation to patients with chronic pain. His success with pain management quickly spread throughout the field of mind-body practitioners. This eventually led Kabat-Zinn, the author of the highly acclaimed book *Full Catastrophe Living* (1990), to create a structured, systematic program to teach other instructors his method of success. He calls it Mindfulness-Based Stress Reduction, or MBSR. Anyone who has ever taken a mindfulness meditation workshop with Kabat-Zinn knows the raisin exercise: For what seems like hours, you hold, smell, study, gaze at, and then finally taste and chew a raisin, all with the utmost awareness (some people use chocolate). The underlying premise of this mindfulness exercise is that as you become more aware of your thoughts and actions, you can control your thoughts (through detached observation) to the point where you are less stressed. Many instructors sum up mindfulness in three words: attention, intention, and attitude.

Today, MBSR is taught by certified instructors in over 250 hospitals nationwide, as well as many corporate wellness programs and the U.S. Army. Mindfulness as a relaxation technique has been well researched at Harvard, UCLA,

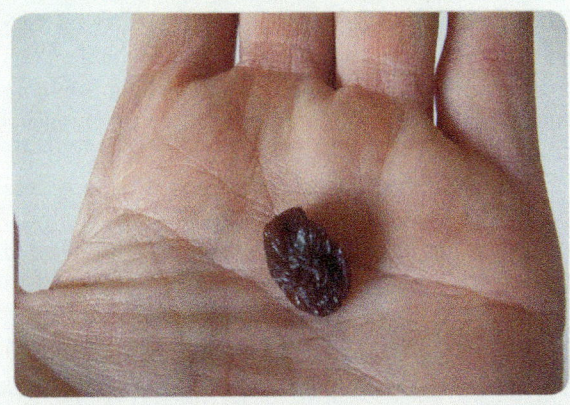

and Stanford, and perhaps is most recognized through the studies of Dr. Richard Davidson at the University of Wisconsin–Madison. Evidence-based outcomes reveal dramatic decreases in pain sensation, and through fMRI data, have led to the exploration of neuroplasticity of brain tissue. Kabat-Zinn's MBSR program is taught as a structured 10-session (31-hour) group session over an 8-week period with suggested daily home practice. Some programs, like the one at Duke Medical Center, add a 2-hour orientation program. The typical cost for this program is about $500, and it is offered on a sliding-fee scale. The basics of MBSR include the following:

1. *Sitting meditation:* Sitting still, back straight, eyes closed, with an undivided focus on your breathing.

2. *Body scan:* Moving your awareness from the top of your head, down to your neck, shoulders, torso, arms and hands, legs, and feet.

3. *Gentle yoga (stretching):* This aspect includes a series of simple hatha yoga *asanas* performed lying down.

4. *Walking meditation:* Walking (preferably outside) for a specific duration, being mindful of your foot placement, the sights, the sounds, the smells, and so on.

5. *Loving kindness meditation:* Enhancing one's sense of connection to others and the world by observing one's thoughts with an intention of loving kindness to people, events, and the like to create a more harmonious living environment. This meditation is often done by repeating an affirmation phrase such as "May you be happy."

The MBSR program offers both an informal practice and a more formal practice. The informal practice includes a free-floating awareness to be mindful in all daily activities, from breathing and eating to walking, sitting, and even washing the dishes. The formal practice invites

(continues)

BOX 19.3   The Art of Mindfulness *(continued)*

participants to maintain a specific structure to their practice (e.g., a specific time of day) by beginning with a mindful morning check-in, followed by a 5-minute mindful breathing exercise, a body scan, and a routine of mindful gentle yoga. This formal practice (a single focused effort rather than a multitasking approach) also encourages the participant to keep a journal of all the experiences through these activities to help guide and deepen the practice. Participants are encouraged to continue the formal practice until it becomes second nature.

Like all other forms of meditation, the benefits attributed to MBSR include an increased ability to relax; a decrease in physical pain; an enhanced ability to cope with physical pain; improved quality of sleep; decreased self-criticism; increased self-compassion; decreased resting blood pressure and heart rate; the ability to create and sustain an improved sense of self-esteem; and an increased ability to respond, rather than react, to stressful situations. Mindfulness is taught as an essential life skill, rather than a specific means to achieve a single result or goal.

---

with incorporeal surroundings—in essence, feeling one with the universe.

Split-Brain Theory

The idea that there is a distinct dichotomy of human thought processes (e.g., sequential versus nonlinear) is not new; it has, in fact, been suggested for centuries. Anatomical studies even seemed to support this idea when it was discovered that the human brain consists of two hemispheres. But these theories became reality when an attempt was made to find a cure for epilepsy. In the mid-1950s, researcher Roger Sperry and his colleagues conducted a series of experiments designed to alleviate the intensity of grand mal epileptic seizures in monkeys. It was hypothesized that the intensity could be halved if a seizure could be contained to only one hemisphere of the brain. To their surprise, they found that by severing the corpus callosum, the neural isthmus uniting the right and left hemispheres, seizures significantly decreased in both frequency and severity. Curious to see if similar results would occur in humans, a new series of studies was conducted on four patients who volunteered to undergo this surgical procedure. Remarkably, this operation revealed neither damaging side effects nor noticeable changes in the patient's personality or intelligence. Some minor changes in cognitive thought processes were noticed, however, and it was these subtle differences in cognition and everyday behavior that soon gave rise to a new paradigm of human consciousness (Gazzaniga 1967).

Under close observation after surgery, doctors determined that the right side of the patient's body was controlled by the left hemisphere. Conversely, the left side

was influenced by the right brain. Later these patients were asked to identify an object that was hidden from sight, placed alternately in each hand. In one study, when a pencil was placed in the right hand, it was correctly described as a pencil (**FIG. 19.6**). When the pencil was placed in the left hand, however, no description could be given at all, suggesting the absence of verbal capacity in the right hemisphere. Additional experiments were then designed to combine visual and tactile objects. In one test, a picture of a spoon was shown to the left field of vision (right hemisphere), and subjects were asked to feel around with their left hand for an

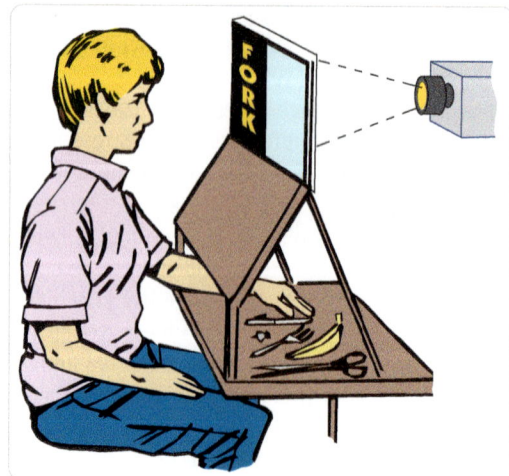

FIGURE 19.6   To test the split-brain cognitive functions of a subject, a word or object is projected onto a translucent screen. The subject is asked to retrieve the object, which is hidden from view and identifiable only by touch.

TABLE 19.1 Cognitive Functions of the Left and Right Hemispheres of the Brain	
Left-Brain Functions	**Right-Brain Functions**
Analytical skills	Synthesis skills
Judgment skills	Accepting, receptive nature
Time consciousness	Nontime consciousness
Verbal acuity	Symbolic imagery
Linear thought progression	Nonlinear thought progression
Rational thought process	Irrational thought process
Math acuity	Intuition
Sequential thought process	Imagination
Facts and detail orientation	Music appreciation
Logical thought process	Humor
	Spatial orientation

object resembling the picture. Patients had no difficulty identifying the spoon, but again could not describe the item they retrieved. Thus, it was concluded that the right brain seemed to have poor verbal acuity but was extremely proficient in spatial perception.

From these and several other studies, it was concluded that each hemisphere appears to be responsible for specific types of thinking processes. Moreover, each hemisphere can function independently as a whole brain. Additional research with stroke victims seemed to confirm these findings. As a result, we now understand that each hemisphere is responsible for different information-gathering and processing functions but work together as one unit. It should be noted that most, if not all, of the research regarding left- and right-brain lateralization has involved epilepsy and stroke patients. Whether the brain works the same way in healthy people is still left to speculation. The work of Sperry and his colleagues has prompted many other studies on the dichotomy of cognitive functions. TABLE 19.1 provides a partial list of these distinct hemispheric functions (Gazzaniga 1972).

Sperry's colleague and fellow researcher Robert Ornstein explains in his book *The Psychology of Consciousness* (1972) that right-brain cognitive functions are a foundation of intelligence yet to be explored. Intelligence is currently measured verbally; there is no standard method to evaluate nonverbal intelligence. This single approach to the duality of cognitive processes has limited

the potential for human consciousness. Perhaps it has even contributed to perceptions of stress. In the words of Ornstein, "The problem is not that our technology is leading us to a path of destruction, but that our technical innovations have outstripped our perspective and judgment. We live in a world that is often difficult for us to understand." Ornstein supports the idea that the two modes of thinking are complementary, not competitive, and that they must be integrated and balanced for the health of the mind.

Since these initial discoveries, many inferences have been drawn from split-brain research. For example, comparisons have been made between the functions of the left and right brains and dominant thinking processes of Western and Eastern cultures, respectively, and this has since been investigated with MRI brain studies (Parsons and Osherson 2001). Western culture is considered by many to be left-hemisphere dominant (strong in analytical and judgment skills, weak in intuitive abilities), whereas Eastern cultures are right-hemisphere dominant. It is also hypothesized by several sources (Borysenko 1987; Schaef 1986) that there is a strong association between left-brain thinking patterns and the frame of mind observed during the stress response. Although generalizations may cloud the understanding of both cultural differences and human cognition, comparisons of this kind may explain why meditation has been less readily accepted by industrialized nations in the Western hemisphere. It may also explain the role meditation plays in accessing right-brain functions to obtain a balance of hemispheric cognition.

Left Brain, Right Brain, Top Brain, Bottom Brain

The human brain is truly remarkable. For millennia scientists, artists, philosophers, and poets have marveled at the capacity of human thought. Scientific investigations to peer into the anatomy and physiology of the brain have revealed many of its secrets, but all of this research has barely scratched the surface of what lies behind consciousness, thought processes, memory, creativity, intuition, imagination, and so much more.

No one piece of research can explain the complexities of the brain (though many have tried). Roger Sperry won a Nobel Prize in 1981 for his research about right- and left-brain cognitive function. More recently, research has focused on understanding the "executive function" of the brain (the frontal cortex), and now with umpteen research studies using functional magnetic resonance imaging (fMRI) of the brain, many more secrets are being revealed. Some researchers are now dividing thought processes into top brain (executive function) and bottom brain (the reptilian brain associated with fight or flight).

Perhaps the greatest research finding in the past decade is that the brain and all of its neural wiring can be reprogrammed to a specific task. The ability of the brain to form and reorganize synaptic connections is called *neuroplasticity*. People who meditate regularly train the brain to stay calm during stressful events. People who engage in repetitive use of computer screens and mobile devices, which involves rapid surfing and data grazing, train their minds to be aroused and vigilant in this particular skill.

It's true that some people tend to be more judgmental (left brain) than others. Conversely, some people seem to be more intuitive (right brain) than others. It is interesting to note that the left-brain skills associated with Roger Sperry's research, when used to an extreme, tend to promote more stress-related thought processes (same with the reptilian brain). Right-brain skills are more closely associated with relaxation. No doubt, the complexities of the human brain are certainly complicated,

but the answer to all of this brain research is to use your whole brain, not just a part of it.

Altered State of Consciousness

When the results of these and other studies by Sperry and his colleagues (1964) were made public, researchers saw strong similarities between the cognitive functions of the right hemisphere and those traits associated with the altered state of consciousness produced by meditation. Studies have since shown that the act of meditation produces a different type of brain wave than that observed in either nonmeditative waking states or sleep (**FIG. 19.7**) (Murphy and Donovan 1997). In a "normal" state of consciousness, the predominant brain waves emitted are rapid and jagged beta waves (15 to 20 cycles/second). They appear to signify rapid neural conductivity. Thought processes in our typical waking state are those characteristically observed when the left hemisphere of the brain is performing its specific cognitive functions. In other words, during a normal state of consciousness, the mind leans toward censorship, analysis, judgment, and rationality. Critics theorize that this normal state of consciousness is rewarded in academic, cultural, and social practices, and that, as a result, alternative ways of thinking and processing information are frowned upon. The normal state of consciousness can be quite taxing to the brain: every now and then, for brief periods, we may catch ourselves in an altered pattern of consciousness, most likely daydreaming.

Meditation, on the other hand, tends to produce what is now called an **altered state of consciousness**. Although

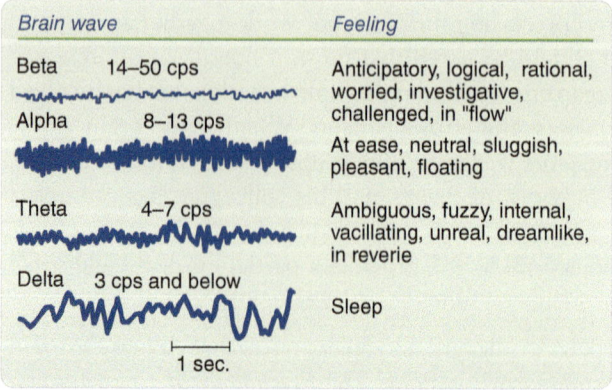

FIGURE 19.7 Neural patterns of brain activity are shown to be variable during different states of consciousness. Alpha waves are thought to suggest a relaxed yet fully alert consciousness.

> **Altered state of consciousness:** A shift in one's thought process, typically from left-brain to right-brain thinking, to become more aware and more receptive.

not advocated, alcohol and/or drugs are known to produce a similar response. An altered state of mind occurs where there is a shift in the thinking style of cognitive processes. Physiologically speaking, in an altered state the brain produces slow (7 to 10 cycles/second) and almost rhythmical oscillations called alpha waves, which represent a significant decrease in sensory input or a desensitization effect. (Sleep produces delta and some theta waves, with beta waves during periods of rapid eye movement [REM].) In many ways, an altered state of consciousness closely parallels the functions characteristically observed in the right hemisphere of the brain: The mind is open to suggestion, receptive to new ideas, and able to observe without judgment.

Characteristics that indicate the occurrence of an altered state of consciousness during meditation have been noted (Allen 1983). When these sensations are experienced, then the meditative processes are believed to have induced the desired switch from left- to right-brain dominance. These sensations are as follows:

1. **Time distortion**: Time consciousness is a left-brain function. During meditation, a distortion of time perception may result as dominant thinking shifts from the left to the right hemisphere. The usual response is a sense of time loss in which a 20-minute session appears to have been only a few minutes. The right hemisphere does not recognize the element of time; therefore, it can neither express nor judge the passage of time in the terms the left brain perceives in a normal state of consciousness.

2. **Ineffability**: Have you ever had an experience that was literally indescribable? One where you just could not find words to adequately describe the experience? Then you've experienced ineffability. The mind's verbal skills are housed in the left hemisphere. The right hemisphere "speaks" in symbols, images, and vivid colors. Many times an experience will occur during meditation that you simply will not be able to put into words. It can be appreciated in sensory (visual) form.

3. **Present-centeredness**: In a normal state of consciousness, the mind is darting at lightning speed among the past, present, and future. The past tends to be the repository for feelings of guilt, while the future harbors a wealth of worries about things that may or may not ever happen. The goal of meditation is to exist in the present moment, to be present and centered in the here and now.

4. **Perception distortion**: If you have ever felt like your arms and legs have sunk into the floor or disappeared altogether while relaxing, then you have experienced perception distortion. It is not that the mind cannot process information during an altered state of consciousness; it is just that information is processed differently by the right hemisphere of the brain. Spatial orientation is a right-brain function. When the right brain is dominant during thinking, perceptions of space appear distorted when transferred to the left brain. Perception distortions during meditation also include what is called **synesthesia**, or sensory crossover. In synesthesia, sensory stimuli are processed by neurons usually designated for other cognitive functions, thus leading to quite different interpretations. For example, you might be able to *hear* colors and *see* sounds, which is impossible to fully explain in words.

5. **Enhanced receptivity**: In a meditative state, the walls of the ego are temporarily lowered, perhaps even dissolved altogether. When this happens, thoughts from the unconscious mind enter the conscious mind freely. As consciousness expands, the mind becomes more receptive to ideas and thoughts from the unconscious mind that it might not access in a normal state of consciousness. Thus, enlightenment is self-generated. This characteristic of an altered state is similar to hypnotic

Time distortion: As an altered state, one's perception of time is changed or distorted such that a segment of time seems either longer or shorter than it actually is.

Ineffability: Experiences that cannot be expressed verbally; especially common during meditation.

Present-centeredness: An altered state in which one is fully aware of the present moment with no regard to past or future time periods.

Perception distortion: A sense during meditation (an altered state) in which, for example, one's arms and legs seem extremely heavy.

Synesthesia: A cross-wiring of one's senses (during an altered state) during which one smells sounds or sees noises.

Enhanced receptivity: In the practice of meditation, one's mind opens to become more receptive to ideas that are often censored by the ego during normal consciousness.

or subliminal suggestion; however, in meditation, the suggestions come from the inner self.

6. **Self-transcendence:** Meditation really does appear to have a mystical, spiritual quality to it. It is spiritual in the sense that it evokes the ability to experience expanded consciousness or enlightenment that is not manifested in normal consciousness (**FIG. 19.8**). This is the original premise of meditation as taught thousands of years ago to those seeking enlightenment: When the pupil is ready, the teacher will come. Self-transcendence also consists of the essence of positive thought, inner peace. Inner peace results from the realization of unity or oneness with the universe after censorship and all other barriers are removed. When a state of supraconsciousness is achieved, the lack of ego boundaries is experienced as a connectedness to virtually all things.

Physiological and Psychological Effects of Meditation

As of 2011, more than 1,200 peer-reviewed scientific studies had been conducted and published on the topic of meditation. The vast majority of these studies have observed an impressive direct influence of meditation (inclusive, exclusive, and mindfulness) on mood states

> **Self-transcendence:** A sense of becoming one with something bigger than oneself; a mystical experience that occurs in meditation.

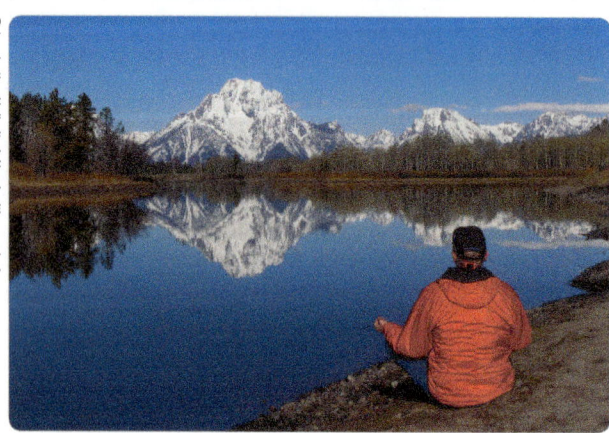

FIGURE 19.8 The abstract concept of meditation is often compared to the more tangible idea of water. When the mind is calm, like a pond, stream, or lake, it begins to reflect a bigger picture of deep-seated wisdom.

(Carlson et al. 2004; Shamini 2007), immune function (Kim et al. 2005), sleep (Bootzin and Stevens 2005), chronic pain (Morone et al. 2007), and various aspects of mental, emotional, and physical well-being (Rausch et al. 2006). Researchers Tonya Jacobs and Clifford Saron at the University of California–Davis found that resting cortisol levels decreased in 57 subjects who participated in a 3-month mindfulness meditation program, with the promise of a follow-up study with more participants (Fell 2013). The current emphasis of research is moving from outcomes toward the actual "why" with further explorations into how meditation can change the way the brain processes information (MRI studies). This section of the chapter looks at some early landmark studies as well as the contemporary focus on brain research. In reviewing the clinical studies regarding the physiological aspects of meditation, one also crosses the paths of yoga, biofeedback, and autogenic training. They all appear to be related. The first account of clinical research to measure mind control of the body occurred in 1935, when a French woman, Therese Brosse, traveled to India with a portable electrocardiogram. The yogi masters she examined had the incredible ability to decelerate their heart rates. One yogi was observed to have virtually stopped his heart from beating altogether. Brosse's (1946) pioneer research went unremarked for about two decades, perhaps because her findings contradicted all previous thought about autonomic nervous system regulation. In 1957, Bagchi and Wenger attempted to replicate Brosse's original findings with better equipment. Although no yogi meditators were observed to stop their hearts from beating, Bagchi and Wenger did observe amazing control of the autonomic nervous system in their subjects. The Swami Ramma's cooperation as a subject in several clinical case studies at the Menninger Institute by Elmer Green and Alyce Green in the early 1970s gave much credence to the earlier studies by Brosse and Bagchi and Wenger. Once again, mind control was exhibited to decrease heart rate and ventilation and alter the distribution of blood flow.

With the introduction of TM in the United States, several great claims were made regarding its effectiveness as a technique for mental calmness and relaxation. Among these were the ability to control heart rate, ventilation, and blood flow. When these claims were put under the "scientific microscope" through a battery of investigations designed by Wallace and Benson (1970, 1972), they held up. Later studies on Benson's relaxation response (Benson 1989) revealed that meditation acts to reduce the release and responsivity of norepinephrine throughout the central nervous system. Based on the original observations by Wallace and Benson and later ones by Treichel et al. (1973) and Delmonte (1984, 1985), it now appears that the practice of meditation promotes an immediate decrease in both some physical responses and learned responses. The following physiological changes have been known to occur with regular meditation practice:

1. Decreased oxygen consumption
2. Decreased blood lactate levels
3. Increased skin resistance
4. Decreased heart rate
5. Decreased blood pressure
6. Decreased muscle tension
7. Increased alpha waves

Explorations into the efficacy of meditation have investigated the effects of mindfulness meditation on everything from jet lag to cardiovascular disease. One study looked at how mindfulness meditation affected the quality of life in breast and prostate cancer patients. Findings showed favorable results, including reduced levels of pituitary-adrenal–mediated stress (Carlson et al. 2004). Bootzin and Stevens (2005) found that adolescent substance abusers who practiced mindfulness meditation showed improved sleep function. College students at Virginia Commonwealth University who were exposed to a single session of meditation (and progressive muscular relaxation) demonstrated a reduction in provoked anxiety levels (Rausch et al. 2006). Whereas mindfulness meditation may be the focus of many recent research studies, Zazen meditation was investigated by researchers in South Korea regarding its effects on several physiological factors associated with coronary heart disease, with favorable results (Kim et al. 2005).

Given the claims that meditation creates mental calmness, the psychological effects of meditation have also been investigated with great zeal. To no one's surprise, results have shown meditation to be quite effective in reducing many factors related to perceived stress and improved mental health (Baer 2003; While 2010).

In a comprehensive review of the studies investigating the psychological effects of meditation, Murphy and Donovan (1997) and Sedlmeier and colleagues (2012) concluded that, above all else, its practice did promote a greater sense of general well-being or inner peace. As a result of these and similar findings, the technique of meditation has been integrated into the practice of psychotherapy as a major tool to promote psychological well-being.

In an extensive review on the physical and psychological effects of meditation, Michael Murphy and Steven Donovan (1997) concluded that meditation, in all its many methods, unequivocally produces beneficial changes to both mind and body.

Neuroplasticity: The Neuroscience of Meditation

It is well accepted that the practice of meditation can promote relaxation, but can meditation actually change the neurobiology of the brain? The answer appears to be yes. When clinical research first began on the biological promise of meditation (e.g., in regulating heart rate, blood pressure, and muscle tension), the focus was on TM because of the specific methodology used in this relaxation practice. A conversation between the Dalai Lama and neuroscientist Richard Davidson regarding the neurophysiology of mindfulness meditation formed a new direction of research in this area: the effects of mindfulness meditation on brain physiology. The results have shattered previous "facts" about brain science.

Previously, it was commonly accepted that with the onset of adulthood the neural wiring of the brain remained unchanged. Clinical studies with Tibetan monks with this form of mental training have proved otherwise. Over the past decade, the use of fMRI has revealed a new perspective on brain physiology and the neuroscience of meditation (Davidson et al. 2003; Horrigan 2005; Rubia 2009), much of this shared by the Dalai Lama himself at the Society for Neuroscience's annual meeting in 2006. Some of the findings are as follows:

- Longtime meditators who meditate on the theme of loving kindness and compassion produce a significant level (30 times stronger) of gamma brain wave activity. (This is normally so low that it cannot be detected in people who do not meditate.)

- During meditation, the left prefrontal and limbic regions of the brain show increased activity, reflecting processes of sustained attention and emotion regulation (Rubia 2009).

- Even a short program in mindfulness meditation produces measurable effects on brain physiology and the immune system.

- Portions of the brain used in meditation practice grow in size and undergo neural rewiring (i.e., neuroplasticity).

- Meditation causes portions of the brain associated with compassion to increase in size, leading researchers to wonder whether meditation could affect the brain physiology of depression.

- Different types of meditation affect brain areas differently. "Present awareness" increased thickness of the anterior prefrontal cortex, whereas "affect meditation" corresponded with areas in the brain associated with empathy and compassion (Walton 2017).

Meditation and Brain Imaging Research

With the advent of fMRI, in which the brain can be observed as it undergoes a variety of thought processes, researchers have taken a keen interest in seeing how meditation affects different parts and layers of the brain tissue (Stein 2003). Herbert Benson and colleagues (Lazar et al. 2000) observed that during meditation there is a decrease in blood flow to the limbic system, an area associated with stress-based emotions. Research by Richard Davidson that involved Tibetan monks revealed that meditation appears to reorient the brain from a mode of stress to a sense of acceptance and contentment (Land 2003). It appears that regular meditation causes neurons to adapt to less sensory information by activating frontal lobe brain tissue that is responsible for present-moment awareness. Newberg and Iverson (2003) conclude from their research involving Tibetan monks and Franciscan nuns that, indeed, portions of the brain responsible for time and space awareness are rewired to be more receptive and less judgmental, while the hippocampus decreases neural input, thereby softening the boundaries of the self and increasing the sense of oneness. Newberg and others conducting similar research have coined the term **neurotheology** to describe the brain's circuitry for spiritual consciousness and mystical experiences. In their book *Why God Won't Go Away* (2002), Newberg, D'Aquili, and Rause suggest that the brain can be trained to decrease stressful stimuli, in essence being rewired for cerebral homeostasis. This neural reprocessing for inner peace is available to anyone who meditates.

> **Neurotheology:** The hardwiring of the brain to perceive metaphysical or mystical experiences of a divine nature.

Meditation and Chronic Pain

Many people recognize the name of Jon Kabat-Zinn as the country's greatest proponent of mindfulness meditation, but many do not know that his career in this field began by focusing on the response to pain relief through meditation (Kabat-Zinn 1982; Kabat-Zinn et al. 1987). Through this work, Kabat-Zinn found substantial evidence for nonmedical pain relief through the Zen practice of mindfulness meditation. Since then, others have replicated his findings, most recently Morone and colleagues (2007). Although pain may seem like a physical phenomenon, the mind-body-spirit paradigm suggests that by involving the mind and spirit with pain relief, the cause of the problem as well as the symptoms (pain) may be lessened, if not eradicated altogether. Whereas Kabat-Zinn's method of mindfulness utilizes association (getting in touch and comfortable with the pain), others advocate the use of meditation (exclusive) to dissociate from pain as a means of temporary relief.

Steps to Initiate Meditation

As pointed out by Benson, the elements of meditation are quite simple. All you need is a quiet space, a comfortable position, a receptive attitude, and a mental device or "meditative broom" to sweep clean the corners of your mind. One component that Benson neglected to emphasize, however, was the need to practice on a regular basis. Meditation is a state of mind, but to be effective it requires the habitual practice of employing concentration. Concentration, like so many other behaviors, is a skill. The more you practice this skill, the better it will serve you.

The following are two meditation practices I use when teaching this technique. The first is an example of exclusive meditation, which was passed on to me by a yogi master. The second is based on the concept of inclusive meditation. Read each exercise first to familiarize yourself with the technique. Then, give it a try. Start with a short duration of time (5 minutes), and then with each session add a few minutes until you build up to about 30 minutes. (It may take a few weeks to feel comfortable with this length of time.)

Grand Perspective Mental Video

The grand perspective mental video is an example of inclusive meditation. In this exercise, you invite any and all thoughts to freely enter your conscious mind. During this exercise, try not to attach any emotional responses to the images that appear on your mind's screen. See the images, but detach yourself emotionally from them. Should you find that you sense some emotional attachment, simply allow that thought to fade and invite a new thought in. This exercise is often compared to free association, and you may find your mind wandering down a trail of thoughts that all seem connected; this is fine. Try this exercise for a 3- to 5-minute period. Each time you return to this exercise, add on a few more minutes. If one issue keeps appearing on the mind's screen and you find yourself unable to be objective about it, this may be an advisory to deal with it as soon as possible. You may elect to do this exercise with some soft instrumental background music; sometimes it can help.

1. Sit or lie comfortably, keeping your back completely straight. Take a deep breath and relax.

2. Close your eyes. Imagine that your mind's eye sees all the mind's thoughts projected onto the mind's screen. The movies that play on your mind's silver screen are produced and directed by you, but now your primary role is that of an observer or audience member.

3. Separate yourself from directing your thoughts. Just let them roll, unedited and uncensored. Take a back seat in the mind's theater to get a grand perspective on these images. To do this effectively, look at whatever thoughts come onto your mind's screen objectively, without emotional attachment, ownership, or analysis. This may seem rather hard to do at first, but with time it will become easy. Just sit back in the audience and enjoy the show.

Mindfulness

Meditation does not have to be done in the confinement of your room. The underlying premise of meditation is to enjoy the present moment. And to paraphrase Buddhist monk Thich Nhat Hanh, meditation can be done anywhere (**FIG. 19.9**). This is what Eckhart Tolle means by the power of now. Mindfulness meditation means to be conscious of the present moment in all that you do, to fill your body's senses with what you are experiencing at the present moment. For example, mindfulness can be done while walking, by feeling your body's weight shift as you place each foot in front of you, and feeling every other movement of your body. Mindfulness can be done while washing dishes, by becoming aware of the feeling of the water and soap on your hands. The following

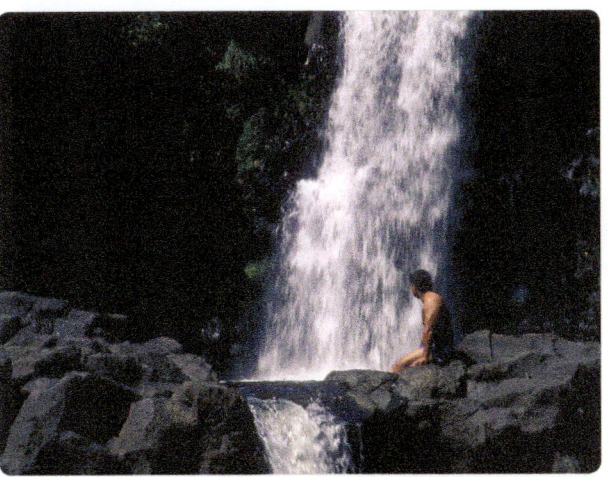

FIGURE 19.9   The practice of meditation can be done anywhere, but a quiet, peaceful place is best. Sometimes the repeated sounds of nature, such as a waterfall, help to cleanse the mind of ego-based thoughts to provide clarity of one's life and purpose.

exercise asks that you try to increase your awareness and concentration by eating an apple.

1. Pick an apple and hold it in your hand.

2. Sit comfortably, with your back straight. (You may choose to sit against a wall for support.)

3. Feel the weight of the apple in your hand. Feel the texture of the apple's skin. Feel the curves. Feel the stem (if there is one). Notice all the nuances of the apple with your fingers.

4. Look at the apple. What color is it? Look at it carefully. Study it. Know this apple so well that if it were put back into a barrel of apples, you could find it.

5. Now smell the apple. Close your eyes and focus your sense of smell on the apple. What does it smell like?

6. Bite into the apple. Savor its taste, both flavor and texture. Feel your tongue and jaws move as you chew. Feel your breathing pause as you swallow. Make each bite of the apple seem like the first.

7. Take note of any other observations about this experience.

◼ Best Application of Meditation

It has been said that in our contemporary age of sensory fulfillment, seldom if ever are we in the presence of silence for any length of time. Between the sounds made by televisions, dishwashers, radios, cell phones, refrigerators, and personal computers—not to mention air and street traffic—there is hardly an uninterrupted moment of mental calmness. As a result, the human mind becomes supersaturated with sensory stimulation. To keep one's sanity, one's mind has to unload these thoughts or it will suffer the consequences. The typical consequence for many people is heightened physical arousal, which leads to deciphering these sensory stimulations as potential threats (stress). The mind craves homeostasis just as the body does. Given the cacophony of sensory bombardment found in nearly all corners of the global village, taking time to quiet the mind is no longer a luxury but a necessity to maintain a sense of mental equilibrium (**BOX 19.4**).

Back in the days when yoga meditation was first taught, it was practiced in the early morning, between 4 and 6 A.M., because this was the time best suited to expanded awareness. Three thousand years later, early morning is still advocated as the best time to meditate. But time of day is not as important as length of time, which should be about 20 to 30 minutes per day. If you can only sit quietly for 5 minutes a day and focus on your breathing, then that is a great start. In any case, meditation necessitates a designated time period in your schedule—whatever fits into your daily routine. It is also helpful to specify a special place to meditate, any corner that you want to designate for this purpose.

However and whenever you do it, the bottom line is that we all need times of solitude to cleanse the cluttered mess from the mind. Unequivocally, meditation can be classified as a technique to help prevent the heightened, sustained arousal of stress. Rare would be the opportunity, however, to employ quality meditative skills in the face of stress, particularly during spontaneous moments of anger. It might be best used as a technique to quell the fires of fear. With practice, you will find that meditation has many layers and can create many profound effects of relaxation.

BOX 19.4   Meditation, a Culture of Distractions, and ADD

It's no secret that attention deficit disorder (ADD) has become a national epidemic in America. The inability to focus one's attention on anything for a specific period of time has become a societal norm. There are many reasons for this, ranging from poor diet (lack of omega-3s and an abundance of aspartame) to the oscillation of repeated television broadcast signals (not to mention commercial camera shots and angles with constant motion). Add to this the obsession with texts, emails, and social media, and it's a wonder anybody gets anything done at all with the proliferation of technological distractions. Despite the push for medications, we can safely assume that people do not have a Ritalin deficiency.

Zen masters laugh at the notion of ADD. Not because it's funny, but because they are of the opinion that *everybody* with an ego has some degree of ADD. They are of the opinion that meditation is the means to train the mind to focus. More specifically, meditation is the way to domesticate the ego from wandering all over the conscious map. Meditation is the age-old tool of consciousness to increase attention and sharpen one's focus.

Many people claim that because they have been diagnosed with ADD, they cannot (and perhaps never will be able to) meditate. Nothing could be further from the truth! Although it may be difficult at first (and to be honest, initially it is hard for everyone to learn to meditate), stay with it. It will get easier. It would be a good idea to learn to minimize distractions such as cell phone use and to eat healthier, too!

SUMMARY

- Meditation is thought to be the oldest form of relaxation. In simple terms, it is a mind-cleansing or emptying process. At a deeper level, meditation is focused concentration and increased awareness of one's being. When the mind has been emptied of conscious thought, unconscious thoughts can enter the conscious realm to bring enlightenment.

- Basically, there are two methods of mind cleansing: to exclude all thoughts from the mind, save the one that is used to clear the rest out, and to include all thoughts but detach oneself emotionally from these images. Transcendental Meditation (TM) and Zen meditation are examples of exclusive and inclusive meditation, respectively.

- Benson Americanized Transcendental Meditation, calling it the relaxation response. He found that all one needs to relax are four components: a quiet environment, a mental device for concentration, a passive attitude, and a comfortable position in which to meditate.

- The practice of meditation can lead to an altered state of consciousness, whereby sensory perceptions are different from those in a normal waking state of consciousness. Perceptual changes include time distortion, ineffability, present-centeredness, perception distortion, enhanced receptivity, and self-transcendence.

- These changes in perception and information processing mirror those observed by Sperry, who found that when surgically separated, the left and right hemispheres of the brain demonstrate unique and separate cognitive functions, similar to those cited under normal and altered states of consciousness, respectively.

- Research has shown that habitual meditation has extensive physiological effects on the body, among which are decreased resting heart rate, decreased resting blood pressure, and decreased resting ventilation, suggesting that there is a connection between mind and body that can profoundly influence homeostasis.

- Brain imaging studies reveal that meditation appears to rewire the brain's neurons, thereby creating the perception of inner peace.

- Research has revealed that regular meditation practice promotes neuroplasticity (i.e., new growth and a rewiring of brain tissue), leading to a deeper sense of mental well-being.

- Mindfulness meditation is known to decrease episodes of chronic pain.

- Meditation is now recommended by the American Heart Association as a means to reduce stress levels, which are thought to be a risk factor for heart disease.

- Every relaxation technique involves some aspect of meditation.

STUDY GUIDE QUESTIONS

1. Explain the difference between inclusive and exclusive meditation, and give an example of each.

2. Herbert Benson Americanized TM and called it the relaxation response. Describe his method of meditation.

3. How does the practice of meditation affect the brain?

4. What is an altered state of consciousness?

5. What effects does meditation have on the mind and the body?

6. What is neuroplasticity? How does meditation affect it?

REFERENCES AND RESOURCES

Alexander, C., E. J. Langer, R. I. Newman, H. M. Chandler, and J. L. Davies. 1989. "Transcendental Meditation, Mindfulness, and Longevity: An Experimental Study with the Elderly." *Journal of Personality and Social Psychology* 57(6): 950–964.

Allen, R. J. 1983. *Human Stress: Its Nature and Control.* Minneapolis, MN: Burgess.

Anand, B. K., G. S. China, and B. Singh. 1961. "Some Aspects of Electroencephalographic Studies in Yogis."

Electroencephalographology and Clinical Neurophysiology 13: 452–456.

Atwood, J. D., and L. Maltin. 1991. "Putting Eastern Philosophies into Western Psychotherapies." *American Journal of Psychotherapy* 45(3): 368–382.

Austin, J. 1997. "Stress Reduction Through Mindfulness Meditation." *Psychotherapy Psychosomatics* 66: 97–106.

Austin, J. 2000. "Zen and the Brain: Toward an Understanding of Meditation and Consciousness." *Philosophy East and West* 50(3): 464.

Baer, R. A. 2003. "Mindfulness Training as a Clinical Intervention." *Clinical Psychology: Science and Practice* 10(2): 125–143.

Bagchi, B. K., and M. A. Wenger. 1959. "Electrophysiological Correlates of Some Yoga Exercises." In *Electroencephalography, Clinical Neurophysiology, and Epilepsy,* International Congress of Neurological Sciences, vol. 3, edited by L. van Bogaert and J. Radermecker. London: Pergamon Press.

Baruss, I., and J. Mossbridge. 2016. *Transcendent Mind: Rethinking the Science of Consciousness*. Washington, D.C.: American Psychological Association.

Begley, S. 2001. "Religion and the Brain." *Time*, May 7, pp. 50–58.

Benson, H. 1974. "The Relaxation Response." *Psychiatry* 37: 37–46.

Benson, H. 1975. *The Relaxation Response*. New York: Morrow Press.

Benson, H. 1994. *Beyond the Relaxation Response*. Berkeley, CA: Berkeley Publications.

Benson, H. 1989. "The Relaxation Response and Norepinephrine: A New Study Illuminates Mechanisms." *Australian Journal of Clinical Hypnotherapy and Hypnosis* 10(2): 91–96.

Benson, H. 1996. *Timeless Healing*. New York: Morrow Press.

Bernardi, L., P. Sleight, G. Bandinelli, et al. 2001. "Effect of Rosary Prayer and Yoga Mantras on Autonomic Cardiovascular Rhythm: Comparative Study." *British Medical Journal* 323: 1446–1449.

Bootzin, R., and S. J. Stevens. 2005. "Adolescents, Substance Abuse, and the Treatment of Insomnia and Daytime Sleepiness." *Clinical Psychology Review* 25(5): 629–644.

Borysenko, J. 1987. *Minding the Body, Mending the Mind*. New York: Bantam Books.

Brosse, T. A. 1946. "Psychophysiological Study of Yoga." *Main Currents in Modern Thought* 4: 77–84.

Carlson, L. E., M. Speca, K. D. Patel, and E. Goodey. 2004. "Mindfulness-Based Stress Reduction in Relation to Quality of Life, Mood, Symptoms of Stress and Levels of Cortisol, Dehydroepiandrosterone Sulfate (DHEAS) and Melatonin in Breast and Prostate Cancer Outpatients." *Psychoneuroendocrinology* 29(4): 448–474.

Carroll, D., and K. Seers. 1996. "Relaxation for the Relief of Chronic Pain: A Systematic Review." *Journal of Advanced Nursing* 27: 476–487.

Castillo, R. J. 1990. "Depersonalization and Meditation." *Psychiatry* 53(2): 158–168.

Cauthen, N. R., and C. A. Prymak. 1977. "Meditation Versus Relaxation: An Examination of the Physiological Effects of Transcendental Meditation." *Journal of Consulting and Clinical Psychology* 45: 496–497.

Chalmers, D. 1995. "The Puzzle of Conscious Experience." *Scientific American*, December, pp. 80–86.

Davidson, R., J. Kabat-Zinn, J. Schumacher, et al. 2003. "Alterations in Brain and Immune Function Produced by Mindfulness Meditation." *Psychosomatic Medicine* 65: 564–570.

Delmonte, M. 1985. "An Overview of the Therapeutic Effects of Meditation." *Psychologia: An International Journal of Psychology in the Orient* 28(4): 189–202.

Delmonte, M. 1984. "Physiological Responses During Meditation and Rest." *Biofeedback and Self-Regulation* 9(2): 181–200.

Der Hovanesian, M. 2003. "Zen and the Art of Corporate Productivity." *BusinessWeek*, July 22, p. 56.

Dumoulin, H. 1981. *Zen Enlightenment*. New York: Weatherhill.

Elson, B. D., P. Hauri, and D. Cunis. 1977. "Physiological Changes in Yogi Meditation." *Psychophysiology* 14: 52–57.

Everly, G. 2002. *A Clinical Guide to the Treatment of the Human Stress Response*. New York: Plenum Press.

Everly, G. S., and R. Rosenfeld. 2002. *The Nature and Treatment of the Stress Response: A Practical Guide for Clinicians*. New York: Plenum Press.

Fell, A. 2013. *Mindfulness from Meditation Associated with Lower Stress Hormone*. UC Davis News and Information, March 27.

Ferguson, P., and J. Gowan. 1977. "TM—Some Preliminary Findings." *Journal of Humanistic Psychology* 16: 51–60.

Fosshage, J. 1978. *Healing Implications for Psychotherapy*. New York: Human Sciences Press.

Gazzaniga, M. S. 1967. "The Split Brain in Man." *Scientific American* 508: 24–29.

Gazzaniga, M. S. 1972. "One Brain, Two Minds?" *American Science* 60(3): 311–317.

Geirland, J. 2006. "Buddha and the Brain." *Wired*, February.

Gibran, K. 1981. *The Prophet*. New York: Knopf.

Goldberg, B. 1995. "Slowing Down the Aging Process Through the Use of Altered States of Consciousness: A Review of the Medical Literature." *Psychology* 32(2): 19–21.

Goleman, D. J., and G. E. Schwartz. 1976. "Meditation as an Intervention in Stress Reactivity." *Journal of Consulting and Clinical Psychology* 44: 456–466.

Green, E., and A. Green. 1977. *Beyond Biofeedback*. Topeka, KS: Knoll.

Grossman, P., L. Niemann, S. Schmidt, and H. Walach. 2004. "Mindfulness-Based Stress Reduction and Health Benefits: A Meta-Analysis." *Journal of Psychosomatic Research* 57(1): 35–43.

Hagelin, J. 2007. "Beyond Miracles—The Discovery of the Unified Field in Its Practical Applications to Prevent Crime, Terrorism and International Conflict." 17th Annual ISSSEEM Conference Keynote Address, June 22.

Holistic-Online.com. "Health Conditions That Are Benefited by Meditation." http://1stholistic.com/Meditation/hol_meditation_benefits_health_conditions.htm.

Holistic-Online.com. "Meditation May Reduce Hardening of Arteries Without Medications." https://www.yogasite.com/stroke.htm.

Horrigan, B. 2005. "Meditation and Neuroplasticity: Training Your Brain." *Explore* 1(5): 380–388.

Jaret, P. 1995. "You Don't Have to Sweat to Reduce Your Stress." *Health*, November/December, pp. 82–88.

Johnston, W. 1974. *Silent Music: The Science of Meditation*. New York: Harper & Row.

Kabat-Zinn, J. 1982. "An Outpatient Program in Behavioral Medicine for Chronic Pain Patients Based on the Practice of Mindfulness Meditation." *General Hospital Psychiatry* 4: 33–37.

Kabat-Zinn, J. 1990. *Full Catastrophe Living*. New York: Delta Books.

Kabat-Zinn, J. 1994. *Wherever You Go, There You Are: Mindfulness Living in Everyday Life*. New York: Hyperion Books.

Kabat-Zinn, J. 2011. *Mindfulness for Beginners*. Boulder, CO: Sounds True.

Kabat-Zinn, J., L. Lipworth, R. Burnery, and W. Sellers. 1987. "Four-Year Follow-up of a Meditation Based Program for the Self-Regulation of Chronic Pain." *Clinical Journal of Pain* 2: 159–173.

Kaplan, K., D. Goldenberg, and M. Galvin-Nadeau. 1993. "The Impact of a Meditation-Based Stress Reduction Program on Fibromyalgia." *General Hospital Psychiatry* 15: 284–289.

Kapleau, P. (ed.). 1980. *The Three Pillars of Zen*. New York: Doubleday.

Keys, K. 1987. *The Hundredth Monkey*. Coos Bay, OR: Visih Books.

Kim, D.-H., Y.-S. Moon, H.-S. Kim, et al. 2005. "Effect of Zen Meditation on Serum Nitric Oxide Activity and Lipid Peroxidation." *Progress in Neuro-Psychopharmacology and Biological Psychiatry* 29(2): 327–331.

King, M., and C. D'Cruz. 2002. "Transcendental Meditation, Hypertension and Heart Disease." *Australian Family Physician* 31(2): 164–166.

Kornfield, J. 1990. *Buddhist Meditation and Consciousness Research*. Sausalito, CA: Institute of Noetic Sciences.

Kuna, D. J. 1975. "Meditation and Work." *Vocational Guidance Quarterly* 23: 342–346.

Land, D. 2003. "The Dalai Lama and Scientists Unite to Study Meditation." University of Wisconsin-Madison News, August 8. https://www.news.wisc.edu/view.html?get=6205.

Larkin, M. 2000. "Meditation May Reduce Heart Attack and Stroke Risk." *Lancet* 355: 206, 812.

Lazar, S., G. Bush, R. L. Gollub, et al. 2000. "Functional Brain Mapping of the Relaxation Response and Meditation." *Neuroreport* 11(7): 1581–1585.

Levey, J., and M. Levey. 1991. *The Fine Arts of Relaxation, Concentration, and Meditation*. Boston, MA: Wisdom Books.

Levey, J., and M. Levey. 1999. *Simple Meditation & Relaxation*. Berkeley, CA: Conari Press.

Maas, J. 2001. *Power Sleep*. New York: Quill Books.

"Meditation Really Does Reduce Stress." 2007. *New Scientist* 196(2625): 21.

Merzel, G. 1991. *The Eye Never Sleeps*. London: Shambhala.

Mipham, S. 2003. *Turning the Mind into an Ally*. New York: Riverhead Books.

Morone, N., C. Greco, and D. Weiner. 2007. "Mindfulness Meditation for the Treatment of Chronic Low Back Pain in Older Adults: A Randomized Controlled Pilot Study." *Pain* 134(3): 310–319.

Motoyama, H. 1990. *Toward a Superconsciousness: Meditation Theory and Practice*. Berkeley, CA: Asian Humanities Press.

Murphy, M., and S. Donovan. 1997. *The Physical and Psychological Effects on Meditation: A Review of Contemporary Research with a Comprehensive Bibliography*. Sausalito, CA: Institute of Noetic Sciences.

Naranjo, C., and R. E. Ornstein. 1971. *On the Psychology of Meditation*. New York: Esalen Books.

Newberg, A., E. D'Aquili, and V. Rause. 2002. *Why God Won't Go Away*. New York: Ballantine Books.

Newberg, A., and J. Iversen. 2003. "The Neural Basis of the Complex Mental Task of Meditation: Neurotransmitters and Neurochemical Considerations." *Medical Hypotheses* 61(2): 282–291.

Ornish, D. 1992. *Dr. Dean Ornish's Program for Reversing Coronary Heart Disease without Drugs or Surgery*. New York: Ballantine Books.

Ornish, D. 1998. *Love and Survival*. New York: Harper Collins.

Ornish, D., L. W. Scherwitz, J. H. Billings, et al. 1998. "Intensive Lifestyle Changes for Reversal of Coronary Heart Disease." *Journal of the American Medical Association* 280(3): 2001–2007.

Ornstein, R. 1972. *The Psychology of Consciousness*. New York: Penguin Books.

Pagano, R. R., R. M. Rose, R. M. Stivers, and S. Warrenburg. 1976. "Sleep During Transcendental Meditation." *Science* 191: 308–309.

Parsons, L. M., and D. Osherson. 2001. "New Evidence for Distinct Right and Left Brain Systems for Deductive Versus Probabilistic Reasoning." *Cerebral Cortex* 11(10): 954–965.

Pritz, A. 1997. *Pocket Guide to Meditation*. Freedom, CA: Crossing Press.

Rausch, S. M., S. E. Gramling, and S. M. Auerbach. 2006. "Effects of a Single Session of Large-Group Meditation and Progressive Muscle Relaxation Training on Stress Reduction, Reactivity, and Recovery." *International Journal of Stress Management* 13(3): 273–290.

Ricard, M., A. Lutz, and R. Davidson. 2014. "Mind of the Meditator." *Scientific American* 311: 39–45.

Roth, B., and T. Stanley. 2002. "Mindfulness-Based Stress Reduction and Healthcare Utilization in the Inner City: Preliminary Findings." *Alternative Therapies* 8(1): 60–67.

Rubia, K. 2009. "The Neurobiology of Meditation and Its Clinical Effectiveness in Psychiatric Disorders." *Biological Psychology* 82(1): 1–11.

Russell, P. 2001. *The TM Technique*. Las Vegas: Elf Rock Productions.

Schaef, A. W. 1986. *Codependence: Misunderstood, Mistreated*. New York: Harper.

Seaward, B. L. 2002. *A Change of Heart: Meditations and Visualizations* (audio CD). Boulder, CO: Inspiration Unlimited.

Seaward, B. L. 2002. *Sweet Surrender: Meditations and Visualizations* (audio CD). Boulder, CO: Inspiration Unlimited.

Seaward, B. L. 2004. *A Wing and a Prayer: Meditations and Visualizations* (audio CD). Boulder, CO: Inspiration Unlimited.

Sedlmeier, P., et al., 2012. "The Psychological Effects of Meditation: A Meta-analysis." *APA PscyhNet*. 138(6) 1139–1171.

Shaffi, M. 1973. "Adaptive and Therapeutic Aspects of Meditation." *International Journal of Psychoanalytic Psychotherapy* 2: 364–382.

Shamini, J. 2007. "A Randomized Controlled Trial of Mindfulness Meditation Versus Relaxation Training: Effects on Distress, Positive States of Mind, Rumination, and Distraction." *Annals of Behavioral Medicine* 33(1): 11–21.

Shapiro, D. H., and S. M. Zifferblatt. 1976. "Zen Meditation and Behavioral Self-Control: Similarities, Differences, and Clinical Applications." *American Psychologist* 31: 519–532.

Sheldrake, R. 1995. *A New Science of Life*. Rochester, VT: Inner Traditions.

Silva, J., and P. Miele. 1975. *The Silva Mind-Control Method*. New York: Pocket Books.

Sperry, R. 1964. "The Great Cerebral Commissure." *Scientific American* 174: 44–52.

Stahl, B., and E. Goldstein. 2010. *A Mindfulness-Based Stress Reduction Workbook*. Oakland, CA: New Harbinger Press.

Stein, J. 2003. "Just Say OM." *Time* 162(5): 48–56.

Stek, R. J., and B. A. Bass. 1973. "Personal Adjustment and Perceived Locus of Control Among Students Interested in Meditation." *Psychological Reports* 32: 1019–1022.

Sudsuang, R., V. Chentanez, and K. Veluvan. 1991. "Effect of Buddhist Meditation on Serum Cortisol and Total Protein Levels, Blood Pressure, Pulse Rate, Lung Volume, and Reaction Time." *Physiology and Behavior* 50(3): 543–548.

Sun, T., C. Kuo, and J. Chiu. 2002. "Mindfulness Meditation in the Control of Severe Headache." *Chang Gung Medical Journal* 25: 538–541.

Tolle, E. 1999. *The Power of Now*. Novato, CA: New World Publishing.

Treichel, M., N. Clinch, and M. Cran. 1973. "The Metabolic Effects of Transcendental Meditation." *Physiologist* 16: 472.

Wallace, R. K. 1970. "Physiological Effects of Transcendental Meditation." *Science* 167: 1751–1754.

Wallace, R. K., and H. Benson. 1972. "The Physiology of Meditation." *Scientific American* 226: 85–90.

Walton, A. 2017. "Different Types of Meditation Change Different Areas of the Brain, Study Finds." *Forbes*, October 5.

While, A. 2010. "Mindfulness: Me-Time Counts." *British Journal of Community Nurses* 11: 570.

Winchester, E. 2007. "Pentagon Meditation Club." https://www.pentagonmeditationclub.org.

Woo, E. 2008. "Yogi, Maharishi Mahesh. Founded Transcendental Meditation Movement." *Los Angeles Times*, February 6.

Yogi, M. M. 2001. *Science of Being and Art of Living: Transcendental Meditation*. New York: Plume Publishing.

Zaichkowsky, L. D., and R. Kamen. 1978. "Biofeedback and Meditation: Effects on Muscle Tension and Locus of Control." *Perceptual and Motor Skills* 46: 955–958.

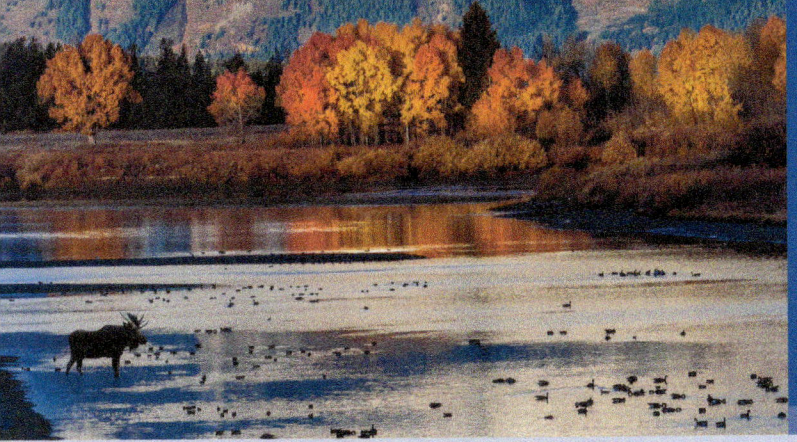

CHAPTER 20

Hatha Yoga

Yoga is the martial art of the soul, and the opponent is the strongest you've ever faced: Your ego.

—Anonymous

In the past 20 years, hatha yoga has gone from an esoteric activity people did in the privacy of their own homes to a mainstream activity—it has become fodder for late night television jokes and parody YouTube video clips. The good news is that today hatha yoga is mainstream. The bad news is that it has gone corporate, far removed from the egoless activity it started as millennia ago. Welcome to American hatha yoga, where people brag about everything from how hot the yoga studio is during a session to correctly pronouncing the sutras or attending a yoga boot camp. Today, it is quite common to see photos of U.S. Army soldiers on yoga mats doing downward dog or to read about corporate executives including hatha yoga as part of their wellness retreats. Reduced to its simplest terms, hatha yoga is a metaphor for balance: a series of physical movements that promote a sense of inner peace and tranquility. At its purest form, hatha yoga is about removing the ego from this experience in an effort to achieve inner peace. Ironically, most yoga classes in America today miss the mark. Trendy yoga instructors, posh yoga studios, expensive yoga mats, spandex yoga apparel, exclusive yoga club memberships, and high-end yoga vacations are the antithesis of this non-ego activity.

The word **yoga** comes from ancient Sanskrit. It is translated to mean "union"; specifically, the ultimate union of the mind, body, and soul. The development and practice of yoga are deeply rooted in the philosophy of spiritual enlightenment. As the practice of this technique migrated to the Western hemisphere, particularly the United States, many traditional yoga positions were assimilated into American culture. They were adopted as flexibility exercises and used both prior to and following the completion of physical activity. Currently, the *shavasana*, or Corpse Pose, is employed in many relaxation techniques, including progressive muscular relaxation and autogenic training. But many other aspects of yoga, including breathing, and the symbolism and philosophy associated with the classic positions, were abandoned. Lately, however, as Americans have acquired a thirst for additional relaxation techniques, the original concepts of yoga have not only reemerged, but also become extremely popular around the country, if not the world. They form a simple yet profound technique to promote relaxation and to unify mind, body, and spirit (Krafsow 1999).

> **Yoga:** A Sanskrit word that means union, specifically the union of mind, body, and spirit.

There are many yoga styles, and the practice of yoga can create many levels of inner peace. The **hatha yoga** style places special emphasis on physical postures, which are integrated with **pranayama**, or breathing control. The word *hatha* comes from two Sanskrit words, *ha*, meaning "sun," and *tha*, meaning "moon." The symbolic meaning of these words is the balance of universal life forces (Iyengar 1981; Rosen 2002). The more concrete meaning is the balance of mind, body, and spirit through action, emotion, and intelligence. The following is a brief introduction to several hatha yoga concepts and postures. To learn hatha yoga, you must experience it. This chapter serves only as an invitation to pursue this technique under qualified instruction.

Historical Perspective

Scholars have traced the roots of yoga as far back as the sixth century BCE, to the teachings of the Hindu philosopher Kapila. These, along with teachings attributed to the Hindu deity Krishna, laid the foundation of several concepts to promote the enhancement of life through the union of mind, body, and spirit. While ancient scriptures cite Lord Shiva, or Supreme Consciousness, as the founder of yoga, credit for its earliest postures (*raja* yoga) is given to Patanjali, who codified these *asanas* (physical postures) in a written collection called the **Yoga Sutras** (Allen 1983). Patanjali is also credited with creating the whole system of raja yoga, including raja meditation, *pranayama*, and the principles for living. Originally, *asanas* were created to cleanse the body, unlock energy paths, and raise level of consciousness. Through the ages, many variations or paths have

emerged, each with its own interpretation of the path to enlightenment. The renowned yogi master Swami Rama cites five yoga paths: *karma yoga*, the path of action; *bhakti yoga*, the path of devotion; *jnana yoga*, the path of knowledge; *kundalini yoga*, the path of spiritual awakening, an advanced form of meditation; and perhaps the most common style practiced in the United States, hatha yoga, the path of physical balance. Several yoga styles include a strong component of meditation to enhance the union of mind, body, and soul, and it is not uncommon for many people to use the terms *yoga* and *meditation* synonymously (Allen 1983).

The premise of this mind-body-spirit union, as suggested by its earliest proponents, is that humanity's most salient nature is of a divine quality. The abyss that separates the corporeal and incorporeal is the wall of conscious intellect, or ego censorship. As described in the earliest teachings, divine enlightenment is made possible when this wall is dissolved through the realization of the self, transcending the limitations of consciousness. The remnants of the dissolved wall are then constructed as a bridge to greater understanding or enlightenment.

Yoga was first formally introduced into the United States when Swami Vivekananda made a presentation to the World Parliament of Religions in Chicago in 1893. His visit to America lasted well over 2 years as he traveled to several cities around the country. By the turn of the century, two *ashrams* (yoga centers) were established in California, with many more to follow throughout the nation. In 1970, Swami Rama, a yogi master from the Himalayan Institute, was invited to the Menninger Foundation in Topeka, Kansas. There, he collaborated in several clinical investigations into yoga and physiological adaptations to meditation as measured with various biofeedback modalities. It was observed that Swami Rama demonstrated nearly incredible control over several autonomic functions (e.g., respiration, heart rate, and blood flow), indicating to clinical researchers that many of the bodily functions previously thought involuntary could in fact be controlled, in a relaxed state, by conscious thought. In what can best be described as a grassroots movement, yoga has slowly become accepted in America as a proven means to relax (Swami Rama 1979) (FIG. 20.1).

It is raja yoga, or the "royal path," that most closely resembles the practice of restrictive meditation, wherein the body must be relaxed to open the mind. Hatha yoga, by contrast, integrates components of muscular strength, endurance, flexibility, and muscle

---

Hatha yoga: One of five yogic paths; the path of physical balance.

Pranayama: A yogic term describing the concept of breath control during each of the *asanas* (yoga postures).

Yoga Sutras: The ancient yogic text attributed to Patanjali, who described each of the yoga *asanas*.

Karma yoga: One of five yogic paths; the path of action.

Bhakti yoga: One of five yogic paths; the path of devotion.

Jnana yoga: One of five yogic paths; the path of knowledge.

Kundalini yoga: One of five yogic paths; the path of spiritual awakening.

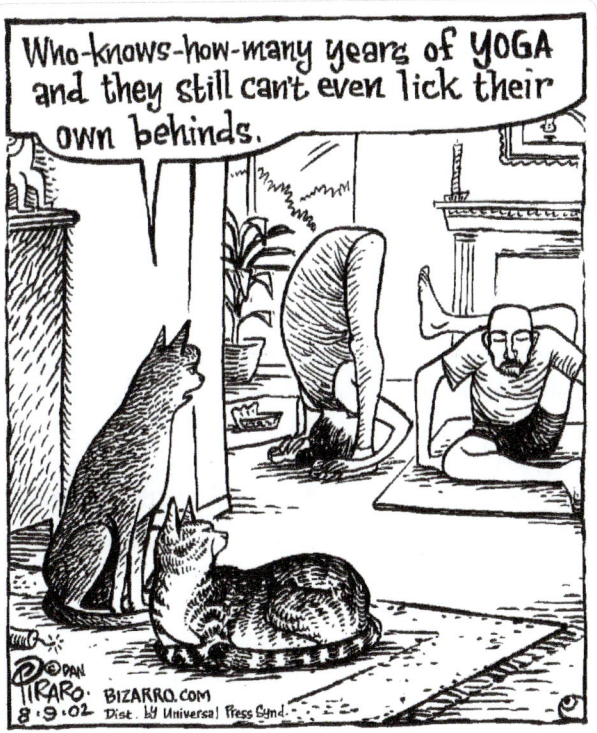

FIGURE 20.1 Yoga helps improve flexibility, but it makes no promise.

relaxation, as well as serving as a catalyst for meditation. According to statistics published by LoudCloud Health, yoga has spread across the country like wildfire, with an estimated 55 million people claiming to practice yoga regularly, 14 million of them over the age of 50 (Puac 2020). Data collected by The Good Body website (Good Body 2018) cites similar data with over 300 million practitioners worldwide. Flexibility and stress relief are cited as the most popular reasons for starting a yoga practice. As of 2018, there were 6,000 yoga studios in the United States (Good Body 2018).

"Yoga is no longer a singular pursuit but a lifestyle choice and an established part of our health and cultural landscape," said Bill Harper, publisher of *Yoga Journal* (Macy 2008).

Physiological and Psychological Benefits

Since the start of the twenty-first century, yoga (primarily hatha yoga) has been studied extensively as a means to improve one's overall health status, suggesting that age-old claims of improved vitality are indeed quite valid (Oken et al. 2006). Proponents assert that the repeated daily series of selected *asanas* promotes longevity and facilitates homeostasis of mind, body, and spirit (**BOX 20.1**). Researchers have focused on the more measurable physiological outcomes. Hatha yoga certainly has been proven to decrease stress levels (Smith et al. 2007). Claims regarding increased muscle strength and flexibility have been substantiated, and reports about increased aerobic capacity appear positive (Ray et al. 2001; Tran et al. 2001). Hatha yoga is now recognized as a suitable complementary healing modality for many chronic health-related issues as well as a multimodal approach to stress management. Here is a look at some of the most recent research.

One of the upshots of the proliferation of hatha yoga as a relaxation technique is the large number of studies that have been performed to determine its efficacy in promoting health and well-being. A Norwegian study that looked at 10 participants who engaged in a hatha yoga retreat found that in as few as four hour-long yoga sessions, 111 genes related to the body's immune function showed positively changed expression. In contrast, music and walking-based meditation were less than half as effective (Gregoire 2013). The data suggest that yoga affects the body at the molecular level and may provide long-lasting health benefits. Kiecolt-Glaser (2010) also found that the practice

BOX 20.1   Insomnia and Yoga

With its premise of promoting a union or balance between mind, body, and spirit, yoga is now touted as a skill to relieve the problems associated with repeated poor sleep quality. The spectrum of yoga styles varies from light stretching to demanding muscular endurance, all of which can groom the mind-body dynamics for a better night's sleep. Currently, the topic of hatha yoga as a bona fide treatment for insomnia is being studied through a grant from the National Institutes of Health. Conventional wisdom suggests that the combination of deep abdominal breathing and specific poses (*asanas*) evens out the mind's hemispheres to optimal consciousness (non-fear-based thinking), thereby decreasing the neural firing associated with fear-based thoughts and the subsequent fight-or-flight response. Specific poses that are used to promote a good night's sleep include the Mountain Brook Pose, Supported Child's Pose, Legs Up the Wall Pose, and *shavasana* (Corpse Pose).

of hatha yoga decreased stress levels and induced a positive endocrine/immune response, suggesting that regular yoga practice contributes to substantial health benefits. Hatha yoga is not only good for the body, but also good for the mind. An article published by the American Occupational Therapy Association (2012) showed that the practice of yoga proved extremely valuable in helping soldiers returning from the Iraq war reduce anxiety and cope with posttraumatic stress disorder (PTSD). In another study, Huang and colleagues (2013) found that hatha yoga proved to be a very beneficial technique to reduce stress in middle-aged women.

Moreover, an explosion of research studies has permeated health-related journals regarding the effects of hatha yoga on premenstrual syndrome, diabetes, clinical depression, and academic test anxiety. In studies by Booth-Laforce and colleagues (2007), Khalsa (2004), and Schell and colleagues (1994), hatha yoga proved to be an effective complementary modality to reduce menopausal symptoms (e.g., hot flashes, sleep disturbances, and reduced quality of life). Hatha yoga also appears to be a beneficial means to cope with breast cancer (Carson et al. 2007), depression (Uebelacker et al. 2010), and diabetes (Mercuri et al. 2000).

Without a doubt, hatha yoga improves flexibility (Ruiz 2000). The more difficult *asanas* require muscle endurance and even strength because these postures involve lifting the body off the ground. The practice of yoga is also thought to reduce blood pressure through the relaxation effect of these postures. But perhaps the best benefit provided by yoga is a greater sense of body awareness. It is no secret that the comforts of high-technology society and their consequent sedentary lifestyles often result in poor posture, muscle tone, flexibility, strength, balance, agility, and endurance. The progression of yoga *asanas* allows for greater awareness of all these components.

Many, if not all, yoga practitioners acknowledge a sense of mental enjoyment from the habitual physical practice of *asanas*. Now science has begun to back up these claims. Michalsen and colleagues (2005) conducted a study to determine the cognitive benefits of a 3-month intensive hatha yoga program. Results revealed that, indeed, subjects noted a dramatic decrease in anxiety levels attributed to this stress management modality. Birkel and Edgren (2000) observed that the repeated practice of hatha yoga improved the breathing (vital) capacity, considered by many to be a significant factor

for optimal health. Further empirical study of yoga in all its forms can only help to contribute to our understanding of the various paths of the mind-body connection.

Recent studies by Carneiro, Moraes, and Terra (2016) and Schuver and Lewis (2016) have confirmed previous research, finding that subjects who engaged in hatha yoga programs experienced decreased symptoms of depression and anxiety.

Hatha Yoga and Chronic Pain

Among the many videos that circulate on Facebook, one continues to be shared among all kinds of people year after year. It is the remarkable story of Arthur Boorman, a retired soldier who suffered from a disability from his years as a paratrooper. Faced with a life of severe back pain and knee problems, he was told he would never walk without the assistance of a cane or crutches and that he would never, ever run. Confronted with a bleak future of bodily decay, Arthur decided to empower himself by starting a hatha yoga practice. Over the course of several years, he not only lost weight, but now he can run without pain. Yoga has become his salvation! And he is not alone. Many people with chronic pain have found relief through the practice of yoga.

Back pain is one of the most common maladies to afflict people older than the age of 25. Poor sitting and standing posture, inadequate shoe support, weak stomach muscles, and athletic activities top the list of factors contributing to chronic lower back pain (Baxter n.d.). Many people who find little or no relief from standard medical practices are turning to hatha yoga as an alternative or complementary modality, particularly with regard to sacroiliac joint problems (Lee 1997) and lower back pain (Galantino et al. 2004; Jacobs et al. 2004). By stretching tight muscles and balancing strength and flexibility of the muscles supporting the joints where pain originates, yoga can be a positive and inexpensive means to reduce and eliminate joint pain. Yoga has also been found to be helpful for a variety of health-related problems, including carpal tunnel syndrome (Garfinkel et al. 1998).

Steps to Initiate Hatha Yoga

Chances are, you have already done some of the yoga positions before, perhaps without even knowing they were yoga postures. If you are at all familiar with hatha yoga, this will be a brief review. If you are new to these exercises, the following selection of yoga *asanas* will introduce you to the concepts and applications of hatha yoga as a relaxation technique. In the original *Yoga Sutras* text, *asanas* are described as "comfortable and steady." They are to be done slowly and gracefully. They are designed to awaken your sense of body awareness.

Each *asana* has three phases: (1) moving into the pose, (2) maintaining the pose, and (3) coming out of the pose. Always remember to come out of a pose as slowly as you enter it. At first, perhaps all you will be aware of is the physical experience of each *asana*. With time, though, you may begin to notice an internal (mental) calmness to equal the physical tranquility (muscular relaxation). As in any new learning experience, there are a couple of things to remember. First, pain and yoga *asanas* are incompatible. You should *not* push yourself to the point of pain. Some postures may seem quite easy, while others seem impossible. Move to the limit of your own physical ability. With practice, the more difficult *asanas* will become easier. Second, there are three concepts to remember when practicing yoga: breathing, conscious stretching, and counterpositions or balance.

The Art of Breathing

In the practice of hatha yoga, breathing (specifically, **the art of breathing**) plays a crucial role in the attempt to unite mind, body, and spirit. Breathing, or *pranayama*, influenced by the diaphragm, is the current that draws the flow of universal energy throughout the body. The word *prana* means "breath," and the word *yama* means "pause." Diaphragmatic breathing is the most natural style of breathing. It differs from thoracic breathing in the expansion of the stomach area as air enters the lungs (**FIG. 20.2**). The emphasis of breathing from the abdomen allows for increased relaxation throughout the body. Unlike thoracic breathing, *pranayama* invites conscious effort of the entire pulmonary system, including the nose, throat, lungs, intercostal muscles, and diaphragm.

Within each yoga posture are a contraction phase and a release phase; muscles are slowly stretched and relaxed. *Pranayama* is integrated into each posture. Breaths are comfortably slow and deep, and correspond with the contraction and relaxation phases of each movement. As muscles are stretched, air is drawn into the lungs by the diaphragm. Then when the muscles relax, air is exhaled. Inhalations are usually taken when the head is lifted up and the body is going into a position or expanding. Air is exhaled when the head is down and the body is coming out of a position. Usually a breath is held for

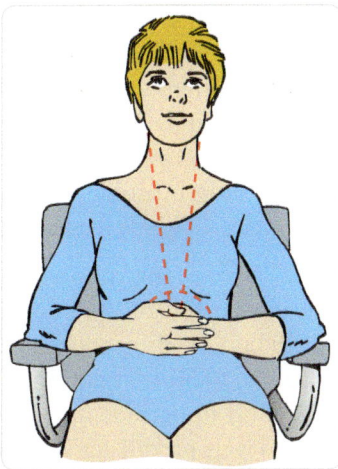

FIGURE 20.2   The art of breathing means becoming conscious of your breathing and allowing your abdominal area to expand as you inhale.

approximately 10 seconds. When first learning these positions, you may find breathing sequences difficult to coordinate with movements. Over time, coordination will become easier.

The Art of Conscious Stretching

Have you ever noticed a cat or dog stretch after taking a nap? Animals do this to prepare the body for motion. Stretching is a natural reflex. In a sleeping or fetal position, the body coils up, and several muscles, specifically those on the back of the body, contract and shorten. To move efficiently upon awakening, these muscles must be stretched and elongated (**FIG. 20.3**). But the fetal position is not the only posture that allows muscles to constrict in this manner. Desk work, computer work, prolonged

> **The art of breathing:** A term in hatha yoga that honors the importance of the pause of the breath (*pranayama*).

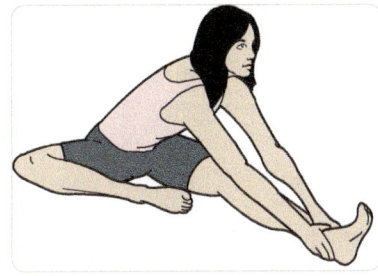

FIGURE 20.3   The art of conscious stretching means becoming aware of the flexibility of your muscles as you move a specific joint through a range of motion.

driving, even walking in high-heeled shoes cause muscles, tendons, and ligaments to shorten. Eventually, the body adapts to these positions and muscles remain contracted. The result is a significant loss in flexibility and restricted movements of certain joints. With time, loss of flexibility may result in muscular stiffness and joint pain as body alignment is slightly distorted.

Exercise physiologists have long known that chronically tight muscles are less capable of a full range of motion. Decreases in flexibility are also related to decreases in strength. Extremely tight muscles during a resting state may actually clamp off or occlude the blood supply at the microcapillary level, producing a vicious cycle of tension. Furthermore, as we mature physically (particularly after the age of 30), the body gradually loses its ability to produce elastin, a protein that gives muscle fibers stretching capabilities. Thus, the need to maintain flexibility becomes more important throughout the aging process. For these—and perhaps some cultural—reasons, the yoga postures may seem difficult at first. However, with continued practice, the body will adapt and they will become easier.

It is important to remember that in all yoga postures, one should not go to the point of pain; this may result in tears to muscle, tendon, and ligament fibers. Body awareness is a kinesthetic skill: being fully conscious of each body movement and what each body part is experiencing—specifically, the contraction and relaxation of each set of muscles. This is the **art of conscious stretching**. Don't push yourself. Hatha yoga is meant to be enjoyable.

The Art of Balance

The art of balance refers to counterpositions. Yoga philosophy asserts that balance is the key to life. To find harmony in life, there must be balance. Thus, the practice of *asanas* is a reminder to seek balance in all thoughts and actions, and the progression of *asanas* is a subtle lesson in its meaning. As you try the *asanas*, you

> **The art of conscious stretching:** An expression that suggests to yoga participants to be fully mindful as they assume and maintain an *asana*.
>
> **The art of balance:** A term in hatha yoga that requires a balance of *asanas* on both the right and left sides of the body.
>
> **Salute to the Sun (*Surya Namaskar*):** One of the most classic and symbolic series of hatha yoga postures, often performed at the beginning and/or end of each yoga session.

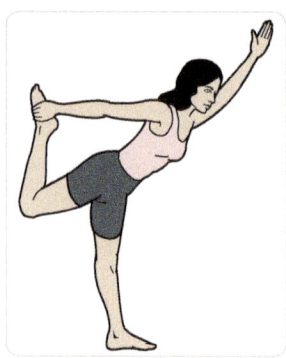

FIGURE 20.4   The art of balance means following the natural laws of balance as the body moves into each position. Once one muscle group has been stretched, the body is balanced by performing the same posture on the opposite side.

will soon notice that there is a progressive pattern to the series of positions. For example, a position that stretches the lower back muscles should be followed by a posture that relaxes muscles in that same area (**FIG. 20.4**). When the body can maintain a balanced position, as well as balance the tension and relaxation of muscles through a series of postures, then greater unity will be experienced between body, mind, and soul. Regardless of the philosophical underpinnings involved, the concept of balance demonstrated in the *asanas* will provide a better range of motion and potentially reduce the risk of injury with advanced postures (**BOX 20.2**).

The following is a series of simple yoga *asanas*. As you try these, slowly integrate the concepts of breathing, body awareness, and balance.

Salute to the Sun (*Surya Namaskar*)

The **Salute to the Sun** is a very symbolic series of *asanas*. It is traditionally performed at the beginning and end of each yoga session. *Surya Namaskar* began as a form of meditation worship wherein one would start the day by facing east and performing the series of movements to maintain harmony throughout the day. Today it is recognized as an excellent exercise to stretch and limber muscles throughout the entire body, but particularly the spine and legs. Runners and joggers may recognize a few of these stretches because they are excellent flexibility exercises for hamstrings and calf muscles. The Salute to the Sun should be performed slowly, and every effort should be made to maintain balance through each posture. Once the movements become more natural, the exercise can be done more rapidly. Each posture is counterbalanced in the next *asana*. A complete Salute to

BOX 20.2   Desk/Cubicle Yoga *Asanas*

Getting away to your favorite yoga studio is a great escape from one's home office or work routine, but you don't have to head off to the nearest yoga center each day to practice hatha yoga. Several *asanas* can (and should) be adapted to one's desk or workstation for ideal posture in the course of each day. Prolonged sitting (with poor posture) will cause a lot of tension in the muscles of the neck, shoulders, and back.

Keeping in mind that many of the yoga *asanas* are based on assuming correct spinal posture and balance, the adaptation of several yoga positions are ideal for those in a sitting position. Here are a few simple exercises to try and incorporate into your daily work routine.

1. *Trunk-Rotation:* Sitting in your chair, lift your hands to shoulder height and twist your body from the waist up toward your right side. Hold for 5 to 10 seconds. Relax and return to a straightforward sitting position. Then, with hands at shoulder height, twist toward your left side. Hold for 5 to 10 seconds. Repeat two to three times on each side.

2. *Lower Back Arch:* Sitting straight, head over shoulders, arch your lower back, pushing your abdominal area toward your desk. Hold for 5 to 10 seconds. Relax. Repeat two to three times.

3. *Shoulders to Ear Stretch:* Sitting straight up and facing your desk, slowly lower your right ear to your right shoulder without moving your shoulder. Hold for 5 to 10 seconds. Relax and return to resting position. Next, slowly lower your left ear to your left shoulder without moving your shoulder. Hold for 5 to 10 seconds. Repeat each side twice.

4. *Sitting Mountain Pose:* Sitting with your spine straight, extend your hands over your head, reaching for the ceiling. Hold for 5 to 10 seconds. Grasp hands and lean toward your right side (from your shoulders to your hands, keeping your torso straight). Hold for 5 to 10 seconds and then relax, bringing arms/hands overhead. Then reach/lean toward your left side, hold for 5 to 10 seconds, and then relax, arms down by your side. Repeat one to three more times.

5. *Cat Back Arch:* Push your chair away from your desk about 12 inches. Lower your chin to your chest, and then your head to your desk, stretching your arms in front of you (or off to the sides), arching your back (like a cat). Hold for 5 to 10 seconds. Sit back up straight. Repeat one to three times.

6. *Chest Expansion:* Sitting up straight, grasp your hands (interlocking fingers) behind your lower back. Straighten your arms and pull your shoulders back. Hold for 5 to 10 seconds. Relax. Repeat one to three times.

7. *Eye Yoga:* Sitting straight up, with your chin up, keep your head still, but look in the upper-right corner of your field of vision and hold for 5 to 10 seconds. Then, keeping your head still, moving only your eyes, shift your focus to your lower-left corner of your field of vision. Hold for 5 to 10 seconds. Next shift your field of vision to your upper left and hold for 5 to 10 seconds. Then shift the focus of your field of vision to the lower right. Hold/stare for 5 to 10 seconds. Relax and return to a forward gaze. Repeat all four corners of your field of vision in a random order, occasionally looking at the tip of your nose in between corners.

the Sun consists of two sequences. In the first cycle, lead with the right foot in position 4; in the second, lead with the left. It makes no difference what direction you face when doing this exercise; however, facing east marks symbolic awareness of the beginning of the life of each new day.

Pre-position: Stand with your feet shoulder-width apart, spine completely aligned, and weight evenly distributed on both feet. Hold hands straight above head, palms facing out, with arms fully extended.

Position 1 (**FIGs. 20.5** and **20.6**): Raise your arms in a wide circular motion over the head and then slowly

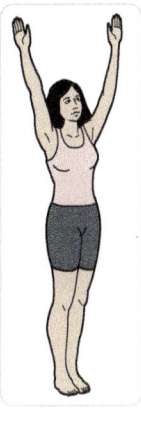

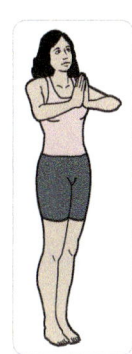

FIGURE 20.5   **FIGURE 20.6**

bring them down in front of the face to the midpoint of the chest. Hold palms together and exhale.

Position 2 (**FIG. 20.7**): Raise your arms directly over your head, pushing from the waist, keeping legs straight and back slightly arched. As you do this, slowly inhale and look up to the sky.

Position 3 (**FIG. 20.8**): Leading with your hands, reach to your toes, exhaling as you lower your head to your knees. Keep your back comfortably straight and knees slightly bent. (Tight hamstrings will decrease the length of your reach. Reach only as far as is comfortably possible.)

Position 4 (**FIG. 20.9**): Place your palms on the floor, and then bring your right foot between your hands. Extend the left leg behind you, and lower your knee to the floor. Inhale as you extend the leg, arch your back, and look up to the sky.

Position 5 (**FIG. 20.10**): Bring the right foot back to meet the left, and exhale. Raise your hips and buttocks high, keeping your head down and eyes directed toward your feet. Arms should be fully extended.

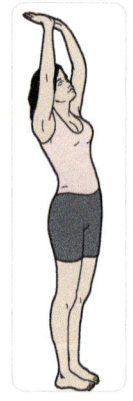
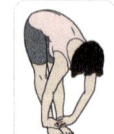

FIGURE 20.7   **FIGURE 20.8**

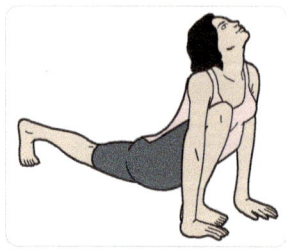
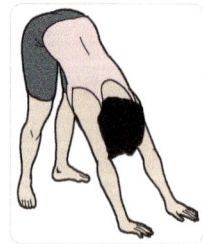

FIGURE 20.9   **FIGURE 20.10**

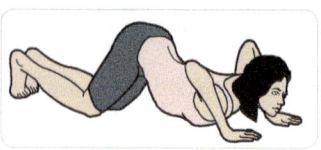
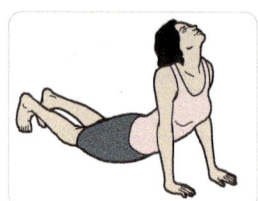

FIGURE 20.11   **FIGURE 20.12**

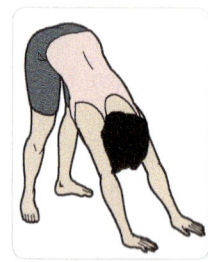
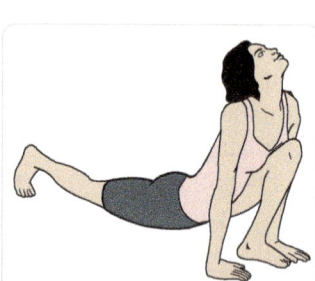

FIGURE 20.13   **FIGURE 20.14**

Position 6 (**FIG. 20.11**): Lower your knees to the floor, followed by your chest and then your forehead. Hips should be slightly bent and raised off the floor. Breath is slowly exhaled throughout.

Position 7 (**FIG. 20.12**): Bring your hips to the floor, fully extending your legs behind you. Then, inhale while placing your hands directly beneath your shoulders and raising your chest. Look up to the sky, and arch the head and back slightly.

Position 8 (**FIG. 20.13**): Raise hips and buttocks high off the floor, keeping your palms and feet flat on the floor. As you do so, exhale. Keep your head down, eyes directed toward your feet, and your arms fully extended.

Position 9 (**FIG. 20.14**): Place your left foot between your hands, extend your right leg back, and place the knee on the floor as you inhale. Arch your back and head slightly, looking up to the sky.

Position 10 (**FIG. 20.15**): Bring your feet together, shoulder-width apart, with arms extended and hands reaching toward feet. Keep your back straight, and knees slightly bent. As you bring your head to your knees, exhale.

Position 11 (**FIG. 20.16**): Reach with your hands overhead, and slowly inhale. Extend your head back to look up to the sky, arching the back slightly.

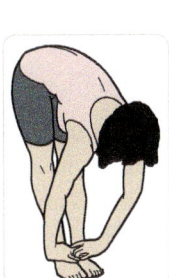
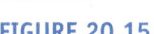

FIGURE 20.15

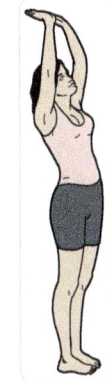

FIGURE 20.16

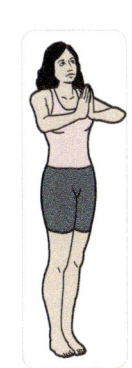

FIGURE 20.17

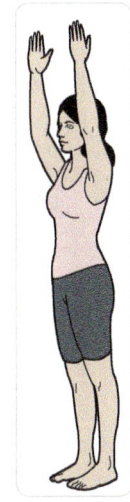

FIGURE 20.18   Mountain Pose (*Tadasana*).

Position 12 (**FIG. 20.17**): Lower your arms to mid-chest height, palms facing together, and exhale.

Now repeat the entire exercise, this time leading with the left foot in position 4. Upon completion, turn your attention inward to observe physical sensations.

Hatha Yoga Asanas

The following *asanas* are arranged in order from standing, to sitting, to lying down. It is important to remember, however, that every posture should be counterbalanced with one that works the opposite muscle groups. Positions should be done slowly and held for about 10 seconds. These 13 *asanas* are but a few (the simplest) of the many hatha yoga postures. Even in hatha yoga, nuances in each position vary from instructor to instructor, so you may notice slight differences between these *asanas* and previous or future experiences. A sample workout of exercises is listed after the descriptions of the *asanas*. Remember that your yoga workout should end with the Corpse Pose for a few minutes of quiet time. This time period can also include body awareness, with specific attention to relaxing all body parts (and self-reflection).

1. **Mountain Pose (*Tadasana*) (FIG. 20.18):** Stand with your feet about shoulder-width apart, spine completely straight, and eyes straight ahead. Raise your arms completely over your head, palms

> **Mountain Pose (*Tadasana*):** A classic yoga *asana* intended to promote balance and stability.
>
> **Head of Cow (*Gomukhasana*):** A classic yoga *asana* intended to promote balance with arms and shoulders.
>
> **Fist over Head (*Araha Chakrasana*):** A classic yoga *asana* intended to promote balance with arms and shoulders.

facing inward, and inhale. Hold comfortably for 10 seconds, and exhale as you return your arms slowly to your sides.

2. **Head of Cow (*Gomukhasana*) (FIG. 20.19):** Stand with feet shoulder-width apart and spine straight. Reach under and behind your back with your left arm as if to scratch between the shoulder blades. Reach over and behind with your right arm. Try to touch hands behind your shoulders, and hold for 10 seconds. (If hands cannot touch, you may use a hand towel.) Relax. Then, reverse arm positions and try to touch hands; hold for 10 seconds. Breathe normally throughout this exercise.

3. **Fist over Head (*Araha Chakrasana*) (FIG. 20.20):** Begin with the Mountain Pose. Place arms behind the waist, grasping hands (fist) together. Lean forward while slowly raising hands over head. Hold for 10 seconds, and then slowly release

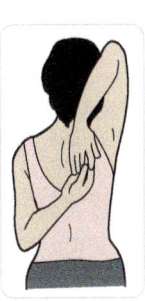

FIGURE 20.19   Head of Cow (*Gomukhasana*).

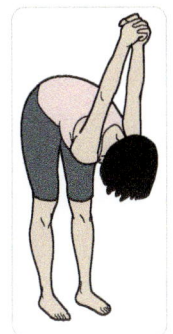

FIGURE 20.20   Fist over Head (*Araha Chakrasana*).

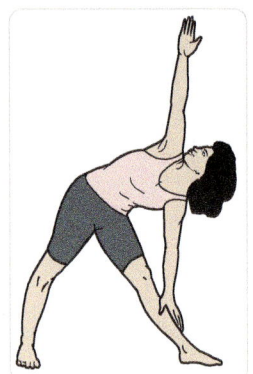

FIGURE 20.21 Human Triangle (*Trikonasana*).

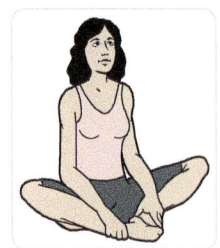

FIGURE 20.22 Thigh Stretch (*Bandha Konasana*).

hands, letting them hang toward floor. Slowly straighten spine to fully erect position. Exhale as you raise fist over your head, and inhale as you release and return to the Mountain Pose.

4. **Human Triangle (*Trikonasana*) (FIG. 20.21):** Beginning in the Mountain Pose, slowly move legs to 3 feet apart. Raise right arm and hand straight above head. Rotate head to look at right hand. Bend slightly at the waist and extend left arm and hand down to left ankle, palm open and facing in. As you reach down, rotate left foot out to protect knee joint. Hold for 10 seconds. Inhale as your right hand reaches up, and then exhale. Inhale as you return to the Mountain Pose. Exhale upon completion.

> **Human Triangle (*Trikonasana*):** A classic yoga *asana* intended to promote balance with the upper torso.
>
> **Thigh Stretch (*Bandha Konasana*):** A classic yoga *asana* intended to promote balance with the leg muscles.
>
> **One Knee to Chest (*Pawan Muktasana*):** A classic yoga *asana* intended to promote balance with the lower back.
>
> **Two Knees to Chest (*Apanasana*):** A classic yoga *asana* intended to promote balance with the lower back.
>
> **Cobra (*Bhujanghasana*):** A classic yoga *asana* intended to promote balance with the lower back.
>
> **Sit and Reach (*Paschimottasana*):** A classic yoga *asana* intended to promote balance with the hamstrings and lower back.

5. **Thigh Stretch (*Bandha Konasana*) (FIG. 20.22):** Sit in a comfortable position with knees bent and soles of the feet touching each other. Gently press knees toward the floor until tension is felt, and hold for 10 seconds. Allow thighs to relax, and repeat. Breathe normally throughout.

6. **One Knee to Chest (*Pawan Muktasana*) (FIG. 20.23):** Lying on your back and keeping the back flat, bring the right knee to the chest by clasping your hands around the right calf. Hold for 10 seconds. Relax by extending the right leg back onto the floor. Then, bring the left leg to the chest and hold for 10 seconds. Exhale as each leg is brought to the chest; inhale as the leg is returned to full extension.

7. **Two Knees to Chest (*Apanasana*) (FIG. 20.24):** Lying on your back and keeping the back flat, bring both legs to the chest by holding the legs with your hands behind the knees. Hug the knees to the chest for 10 seconds. Breathe normally throughout.

8. **Cobra (*Bhujanghasana*) (FIG. 20.25):** Lie on your stomach with legs fully extended and feet curled. Placing your hands directly under your shoulders, slowly raise your chest and head off the floor by contracting the lower back muscles. Try not to push with your hands. Hold for 10 seconds, and then slowly return chest to the floor. Inhale as the chest rises off the floor, and exhale as you return to starting position.

9. **Sit and Reach (*Paschimottasana*) (FIG. 20.26):** In a sitting position, extend legs straight in front of the hips, keeping spine straight. Lean chest comfortably toward the knees, ankles, or feet, reaching forward also with the hands. Keep back straight; hold for 10 seconds. Then, relax by slightly bending the knees and sitting upright. Exhale as you

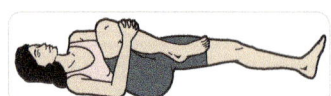

FIGURE 20.23 One Knee to Chest (*Pawan Muktasana*).

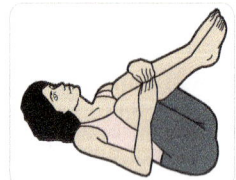

FIGURE 20.24 Two Knees to Chest (*Apanasana*).

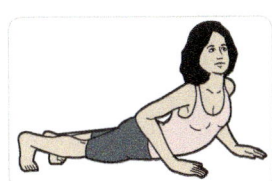

FIGURE 20.25 Cobra (*Bhujanghasana*).

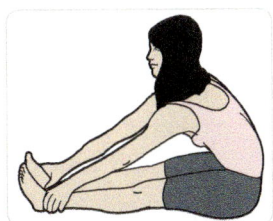

FIGURE 20.26 Sit and Reach (*Paschimottasana*).

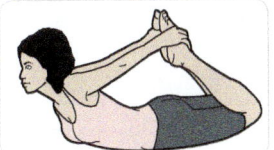

FIGURE 20.29 Bow Pose (*Dhanurasana*).

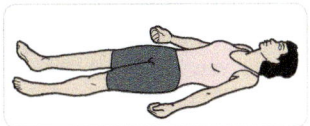

FIGURE 20.30 Corpse Pose (*Shavasana*).

lean toward the feet, and inhale as you relax. Repeat three more times. If having both legs extended is uncomfortable, try one leg at a time.

10. **Spinal Twist (*Ardha Matsyendrasana*)** (**FIG. 20.27**): In a sitting position, with spine erect, place left leg over right knee and position the foot flat on the floor. Extend right arm and place hand on left ankle. Extend left arm behind waist and place the palm on floor for balance. Turn head and trunk to the left side, keeping the chin up. Hold for 10 seconds. Breathe normally throughout.

11. **Fish (*Matsyasana*)** (**FIG. 20.28**): Lying on your back with legs fully extended, place hands palm down beneath the lower back. Raise chest by arching lower back and neck. Hold for 10 seconds. Relax and then repeat three times. Breathe normally throughout.

12. **Bow Pose (*Dhanurasana*)** (**FIG. 20.29**): Lying on stomach, grab either the left or right foot with the opposite hand. Slowly arch back by pulling feet over buttocks. Hold for 10 seconds. Relax with hands on floor by shoulders and legs fully extended. Repeat with each leg three times. Inhale as back is arched; exhale as body comes to full extension. (**Note:** This exercise should be avoided if you have lower back problems.)

13. **Corpse Pose (*Shavasana*)** (**FIG. 20.30**): Lie on your back, shifting your legs back and forth to find a comfortable position. Rotate your arms from the shoulders and rest comfortably, palms facing up. Next, rotate your spine, turning your head side to side. Then, return spine to resting alignment. Breathe from the diaphragm.

If you wish, you can start your workout with the Corpse Pose and return to this position intermittently or after each *asana*. A yoga session should always conclude with this position.

Sample Workout

The following is a sample yoga practice:

1. Salute to the Sun
2. Mountain Pose
3. Head of Cow
4. Fist over Head
5. Human Triangle
6. Cobra
7. Two Knees to Chest
8. Mountain Pose
9. Salute to the Sun
10. Corpse (relaxation) Pose

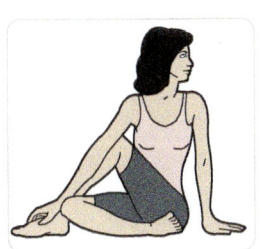

FIGURE 20.27 Spinal Twist (*Ardha Matsyendrasana*).

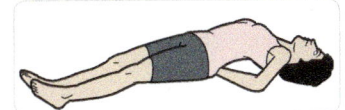

FIGURE 20.28 Fish (*Matsyasana*).

Spinal Twist (*Ardha Matsyendrasana*): A classic yoga *asana* intended to promote balance with the upper and lower back and hips.

Fish (*Matsyasana*): A classic yoga *asana* intended to promote balance with the lower back.

Bow Pose (*Dhanurasana*): A classic yoga *asana* intended to promote balance with the muscles of the lower back and stomach, as well as neck and shoulders.

Corpse Pose (*Shavasana*): This is the typical position assumed at the close of each yoga session to restore energy.

■ Additional Thoughts on Hatha Yoga

The following guidelines may add to the enjoyment of yoga:

1. It is best not to perform *asanas* on a full stomach. Allow 1 to 2 hours between eating and yoga practice.

2. Wear loose-fitting clothing and avoid heavy jewelry. Bare feet are recommended to make better floor contact.

3. Find a quiet place to practice; a well-lit and well-ventilated room is ideal. A thin rug is also suggested to perform the positions in greater comfort.

4. Early morning is the preferred practice time for conscious awareness. But evening is the time when the body is more limber, and yoga postures tend to have a greater relaxation effect after a busy day. Find a time that is best suited to your own schedule.

5. Concentrate on the postures, sensing each move and your body's response to it.

6. There are no nutritional guidelines accompanying this relaxation technique, but if you pursue yoga further, you will find that a healthy, well-balanced diet is considered an important part of the art-of-balance concept.

7. The ultimate goal of all aspects of yoga is to lower the walls of the conscious mind—the ego. If you approach it with a competitive attitude, there is no chance for the union of mind, body, and spirit to occur. Beginning yoga students often push themselves to match the postures of the instructor or fellow classmates. This can result in physical pain as well as a deeper abyss to enlightenment. In the words of yogi master Swami Rama, "This is absolutely not the way to practice yoga."

8. Meditation is not a requirement of hatha yoga, but it is a nice complement to it. After you finish your selection of *asanas*, ending with the Corpse Pose (*shavasana*) is the perfect time to collect your thoughts and perhaps do some internal awareness or soul searching.

The popularity of hatha yoga has now fully exploded in the American culture, to the point where the various styles and more than 70,000 instructors (Hodge 2005) have become very territorial (e.g., certifications, trademarks, patents, precision in postures), making hatha yoga more technical (and ego based) than it needs to be. The upshot of all this is that finding a quality yoga instructor is quite easy. However, not all hatha yoga classes are created equal (**TABLE 20.1**). If possible, it would be a good idea to sample a class (a 1-day pass) to determine if you find the instructor's teaching style and health philosophy compatible with your own. Most instructors will agree to an introductory class where you can either participate or observe. Classes are often offered at community recreation centers, yoga centers, and YMCAs and YWCAs, as

TABLE 20.1   Types of Hatha Yoga

Type	Method	Advantages	Website
Ashtanga yoga	Intense classes that synchronize breath work with speed series of *asanas*	Considered a serious workout for muscles and cardio work	www.ashtanga.com
Power yoga	Hatha yoga with intense muscle power *asanas*	Americanized yoga, very demanding for muscular strength	www.power-yoga.com
Bikram yoga	Yoga practiced in 105°F heat to replicate Indian climate	Heat brings its own challenge; said to provide a cleansing feeling	https://www.shape .com/fitness/workouts /things-you-need-know -about-bikram-yoga
Iyengar yoga	Focus is placed on the specifics of each *asana* with each posture held for more time	Good for beginners who are not flexible; props (blocks) are often used	https://iynaus.org iyengar-yoga/about

Stress with a Human Face

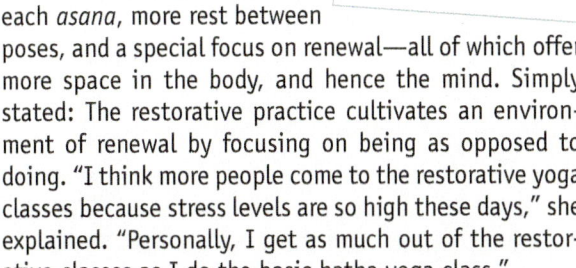

Courtesy of Kelly Andrews.

As the Assistant Dean of Wellness at Florida Southern College in Lakeland, Florida, Kelly Andrew's position entails administering the entire campus wellness program for more than 3,000 faculty, staff, and students. Her position allows her to teach a weekly yoga class, which she embraces with great passion. She has also opened her own yoga studio, which holds weekly classes and workshops. Although Kelly had been practicing yoga on and off over the past decade, it was the heart-wrenching breakup of a serious relationship in 2000 that propelled her into making yoga a regular practice, one that allowed her to regain and maintain balance in her life. It worked! Once committed to a regular yoga practice, she decided to become certified with the Southern Institute of Yoga Instructors. Hatha yoga has provided an unparalleled stability in her life ever since.

Kelly teaches a variety of beginning and intermediate yoga sessions in her new yoga studio, The Yoga Place, but has found that over the years, more and more people are coming to her restorative yoga classes, which offer a greater emphasis on breath work, longer time with each *asana*, more rest between poses, and a special focus on renewal—all of which offer more space in the body, and hence the mind. Simply stated: The restorative practice cultivates an environment of renewal by focusing on being as opposed to doing. "I think more people come to the restorative yoga classes because stress levels are so high these days," she explained. "Personally, I get as much out of the restorative classes as I do the basic hatha yoga class."

Like many yoga instructors, Kelly is concerned about the dogmatic approach some instructors are now taking with yoga instruction, as highlighted in a 2011 *Newsweek* article entitled "Bow Down to the Yoga Teacher" (Schwartz 2011). "First and foremost we are there for people's health and safety. Hatha yoga is not about ego! When a teacher forgets they are also a student, it's trouble for everyone; they have lost the essence of teaching." You can visit Kelly's website at www.kellyandrewstoday.com

well as through private instruction. One book on yoga stands far above the rest in its detailed explanations and wonderful photographs: *The Sivananda Companion to Yoga* (1983) by Lidell et al. I recommend it for further reading on yoga as a special relaxation technique.

Best Application of Hatha Yoga

As previously mentioned, hatha yoga can be practiced at the start of each day or at the conclusion of each day. Even if you do only a few *asanas* each morning before you begin your working day, this would be a good start, and many *asanas* can be done (briefly) in the course of a day (e.g., stepping away from the computer,

before or after exercise). As a relaxation technique, it is best employed to unleash the stress and frustration that for whatever reason have to be resolved. The use of individual *asanas* to stretch various muscle groups during waking hours might be the best course of action when you feel muscles begin to tense. Research indicates that yoga helps decrease anxiety and maintain a sense of emotional balance, reinforcing the mind-body connection that the promise of yoga (union) promotes. Those who teach hatha yoga recognize that the union of mind, body, and spirit is solidified by self-acceptance, self-love, and the absence of anger and fear in one's life. The inner peace derived from practicing yoga is credited with keeping people emotionally well balanced during unexpected encounters of the stressful kind.

SUMMARY

- *Yoga* is a Sanskrit word meaning "union," which is accomplished through meditation. More specifically, it refers to the union of mind, body, and spirit. Hatha yoga is one of five types of meditation, and it emphasizes physical balance. *Hatha* actually translates to (a balance of) the sun (*ha*) and the moon (*tha*). Hatha yoga is the most commonly practiced form of yoga meditation in the United States.

- Hatha yoga, first and foremost, is a non-ego-based exercise. The American culture has added layers of ego with various certifications, clothing fashions, mats, posh studios, and even a competitive nature regarding precision in the *asanas*. There is no room for ego with true hatha yoga.

- Hatha yoga is known to decrease episodes of chronic pain, particularly lower back pain.

- Hatha yoga is built on three concepts: the art of breathing, the art of conscious stretching, and the art of balance.

- In most cases, a hatha yoga session will begin with the *Surya Namaskar* (Salute to the Sun), which is a series of movements or postures initiating integration of the mind, body, and spirit. It also serves as a warm-up for the other postures, or *asanas*.

- There are literally hundreds of *asanas*. This chapter highlighted some of the more popular ones that can easily be incorporated into a yoga session.

- Although not meant solely as a series of flexibility exercises, hatha yoga increases flexibility. It has also been shown to improve muscle tone and create inner calmness, which yoga instructors attribute to improved self-esteem.

STUDY GUIDE QUESTIONS

1. Why is hatha yoga thought to be an effective relaxation technique?

2. Explain both the physiological and the psychological effects of yoga.

3. Hatha yoga involves three aspects (arts); name and explain each.

4. How does one's ego affect one's yoga practice?

REFERENCES AND RESOURCES

Allen, R. J. 1983. *Human Stress: Its Nature and Control.* Minneapolis, MN: Burgess Press.

American Occupational Therapy Association. 2012. "Iraq Study Shows Yoga Warriors Method Reduces Symptoms of Combat Stress & Potentially PTSD." AOTA.com, January 15. http://www.aota.org/news/media/pr/2012 -press-releases/yoga.aspx.

Arpita, B. 1990. "Physiological Effects of Hatha Yoga: A Review of the Literature." *International Journal of Yoga Therapy* 1: 1–28.

Ballantyne, J. 1963. *Sankhya Aphorisms of Kapila.* Varanasi, India: Chowkhamba Sanskrit Series.

Baxter, C. n.d. "Chronic Pain Release Through Yoga." The Yoga Site. https://www.yogasite.com/chronicpain.htm.

Bell, B. n.d. "Insomnia and Hatha Yoga." https://www .couplescompany.com/Advice/Jayson/yoga/insomnia.htm.

Bender, B. 2001. "Power Yoga for Better Health: More Strength and Flexibility, Less Pain and Stress." *Bottom Line/Health* 15(3): 14.

Birkel, D. 1991. *Hatha Yoga.* Dubuque, IA: Eddie Bowers.

Birkel, D. A., and L. Edgren. 2000. "Hatha Yoga: Improved Vital Capacity of College Students." *Alternative Therapies* 6(6): 55–63.

Booth-LaForce, C., R. Thurston, and M. Taylor. 2007. "A Pilot Study of a Hatha Yoga Treatment for Menopausal Symptoms." *Maturitas* 57(3): 286–295.

Carneiro, E. M., G. V. Moraes, and G. A. Terra. 2016. "Effects of Isha Hatha Yoga on Core Stability and Standing Balance." *Advances in Mind Body Medicine* 30(3): 4–10.

Carson, J., K. M. Carson, L. S. Porter, et al. 2007. "Yoga for Women with Metastatic Breast Cancer: Results from a Pilot Study." *Journal of Pain and Symptom Management* 33(3): 331–341.

Chaudhuri, H. 1975. "Yoga Psychology." In *Transpersonal Psychologies*, edited by C. T. Tart. New York: Harper & Row.

Chopra, A., and V. Doiphode. 2002. "Ayurvedic Medicine: Core Concept, Therapeutic Principles and Current Relevance." *Medical Clinics of North America* 86(1): 75–89.

Coulter, A. 1998. "Yoga and Cancer: A Move Toward Relaxation." *Alternative and Complementary Therapies* 4(3): 150–155.

Desai, Yogi Amrit. 1984. *Kripalu Yoga: Meditation in Motion*. Lenox, MA: Kripalu Publications.

Etsten, D. 2002. "The Benefits of Yoga: Treating Mind and Body Helps Clients Recover from Addictions." *Journal of Addiction and Mental Health* 5(20): 9.

Feuestein, G. 1998. *The Yoga Tradition: Its History, Literature, Philosophy and Practice*. Prescott, AZ: Holm Press.

Feuestein, G. 2000. "Yoga and Stress: A Bibliography." *International Journal of Yoga Therapy* 10: 11–16.

Folan, L. 1981. *Lilias, Yoga, & Your Life*. New York: Macmillan.

Galantino, M. L., T. M. Bzdewka, J. L. Eissler-Russo, et al. 2004. "The Impact of Modified Hatha Yoga on Chronic Low Back Pain: A Pilot Study." *Alternative Therapies in Health and Medicine* 10(2): 56–59.

Garfinkel, M., A. Singhal, W. A. Katz, et al. 1998. "Yoga-Based Intervention for Carpal Tunnel Syndrome." *Journal of the American Medical Association* 280(18): 1601–1603.

Good Body. 2018. "Yoga Statistics: Staggering Growth Shows Ever-Increasing Popularity." TheGoodBody.com, November 16. https://www.thegoodbody.com/yoga -statistics/.

Gregoire, C. 2013. "Yoga Associated with Gene Expression in Immune Cells, Study Finds." *Huffington Post*, April 24. https://www.huffingtonpost.com/2013/04/24/yoga-immune -system-genetic-_n_3141008.html.

Greuel, J. 2012. "Iraq Study Shows Yoga Warriors Method Reduces Symptoms of Combat Stress and Potentially PTSD." Yoga Warriors International, January 26. http:// www.yogawarriors.com/about-yoga-warriors/news /iraq-study-shows-yoga-warriors-method-reduces-symptoms -combat-stress.

Haich, E., and S. Yesudian. 1966. *Self-Healing, Yoga, and Destiny*. New York: Aurora Press.

Hodge, J. 2005. "Yoga Teaching Profession Grows Along with Interests in Yoga." Yoga, May 5. https://www.yogayoga .com/press/YYTTmove.

Huang, F. J., D. K. Chien, and U. L. Chung. 2013. "Effects of Hatha Yoga on Stress in Middle-Aged Women." *Journal of Nurse Research* 21(1): 59–66.

Iyengar, B. K. 1981. *Light on Pranayama*. New York: Crossroad.

Jacobs, B. P., W. Mehling, A. L. Avins, et al. 2004. "Feasibility of Conducting a Clinical Trial on Hatha Yoga for Chronic Low Back Pain: Methodological Lessons." *Alternative Therapies in Health and Medicine* 10(3): 80–83.

Kant, S., S. Bhattacharya, U. S. Pandey, et al. 2000. "Evaluation of Effect of Yogic Breathing and Exercises on Pulmonary Function, Free Radicals and Antioxidant Status Among Healthy Individuals." *Chest* 118(4): 204S.

Kelly, A. L. 2003. "Team up to Fight Pain." *Yoga International*, September/October, p. 98.

Khalsa, H. K. 2004. "How Yoga, Meditation, and a Yogic Lifestyle Can Help Women Meet the Challenges of Perimenopause and Menopause." *Sexuality, Reproduction and Menopause* 2(3): 169–175.

Kiecolt-Glaser, J. K. 2010. "Stress, Inflammation, and Yoga Practice." *Psychosomatic Medicine* 72(2): 113–121.

Krafsow, G. 1999. *Yoga for Wellness with the Timeless Teachings of Viniyoga*. New York: Penguin.

Krishna, G. 1971. *The Kundalini: The Evolutionary in Man*. Berkeley, CA: Shambhala.

Lasater, J. 1995. "Down in the Back: Poses for Lower Back Pain." *Alternative Therapies for Health and Medicine* 1(5): 72–82.

Lasater, J. 1995. *Relax and Renew*. Berkeley, CA: Rodmell Press.

Lee, M. 1997. *Phoenix Rising*. Deerfield Beach, FL: Health Communication.

Lidell, L., with N. Rabinovitch and G. Rabinovitch. 1983. *The Sivananda Companion to Yoga*. New York: Simon and Schuster.

Macy, D. 2008. "Yoga Journal Releases 2008 'Yoga in America' Market Study." *Yoga Journal*, February 26. https://www .yogajournal.com/advertise/press_releases/10.

Mercuri, N., E. Olivera, et al. 2000. "Yoga Practice in People with Diabetes." *Diabetes Research and Clinical Practice* 50(suppl. 1): 234–235.

Michalsen, A., P. Grossman, A. Acil, et al. 2005. "Rapid Stress Reduction and Anxiolysis Among Distressed Women as a Consequence of a Three-Month Intensive Yoga Program." *Medical Science Monitor* 11(12): CR555–561.

Mishra, R. 1959. *Fundamentals of Yoga*. New York: Julian Press.

Oken, B. S., D. Zajdel, S. Kishiyama, et al. 2006. "Randomized, Controlled, Six-Month Trial of Yoga in Healthy Seniors: Effects on Cognition and Quality of Life." *Alternative Therapies in Health and Medicine* 12(1): 40–47.

Ott, M. J. 2002. "Yoga as a Clinical Intervention." *Advance for Nurse Practitioners,* January, pp. 81–90.

Oz, M. 2003. "Say 'Om' Before Surgery." *Time*, January 20, pp. 71–73.

Pettinati, P. 2001. "Meditation, Yoga and Guided Imagery." *Holistic Nursing Care* 16(1): 47–55.

Puac, D. 2020. "20 Fresh Yoga Statistics and Facts You Should Know in 2020." LoudCloud Health, January 6. https:// loudcloudhealth.com/resources/yoga-statistics/.

Qu, S., S. Mjelstad Oalfsrud, L. A. Meza-Zepeda, and F. Saaticioglu. 2013. "Rapid Gene Expression Changes in Peripheral Blood Lymphocytes upon Practice of a Comprehensive Yoga Program." *PLoS One* 8(4): e61910.

Ray, U. S., B. Sinha, O. S. Tomer, et al. 2001. "Aerobic Capacity and Perceived Exertion after Practice of Hatha Yogic Exercises." *Indian Journal of Medical Research* 114: 215–221.

Rosen, R. 2002. *The Yoga of Breathing: A Step-by-Step Guide to Pranayama.* Boston, MA: Shambhala Books.

Ruiz, F. 2000. "What Science Can Teach Us about Flexibility." *Yoga Journal*, March/April, pp. 92–101.

Schaffer, R. 2002. "Calm Digestive Upset with Yoga." *Natural Health* 32: 38–40.

Schell, F. J., B. Allolio, and O. W. Schonecke. 1994. "Physiological and Psychological Effects of Hatha-Yoga Exercise in Healthy Women." *International Journal of Psychosomatic Medicine* 41(1–4): 46–52.

Schuver, K. J., and B. A. Lewis. 2016. "Mindfulness-Based Yoga Intervention for Women with Depression." *Complementary Therapies in Medicine* 26: 85–79.

Schwartz, C. 2011. "Bow Down to the Yoga Teacher." *Newsweek*, February 20.

Serber, E. 2000. "Stress Management Through Yoga." *International Journal of Yoga Therapy* 10: 11–16.

Sivananda, S. 1950. *Raja Yoga.* Rishikesh, India: Yoga Vendanta Forest University.

Smith, B. 1982. *Yoga for a New Age: A Modern Approach to Hatha Yoga.* Englewood Cliffs, NJ: Prentice Hall.

Smith, C., H. Hancock, J. Blake-Mortimer, and K. Eckert. 2007. "A Randomized Comparative Trial of Yoga and Relaxation to Reduce Stress and Anxiety." *Complementary Therapies in Medicine* 15(2): 77–83.

Stoller, C., J. J. Greuel, L. S. Cimini, M. S. Fowler, and J. A. Koomer. 2012. "Effects of Sensory-Enhanced Yoga on Symptoms of Combat Stress in Deployed Military Personnel." *American Journal of Occupational Therapy* 66(1): 59-68.

Swami Karmananda. 1976. "Relaxation Through Yoga." In *Relax,* edited by J. White and J. Fadiman. New York: Dell.

Swami Rama. 1979. *Lectures on Yoga.* Honesdale, PA: Himalayan International Institute of Yoga Science and Philosophy.

Swami Satyananda Saraswati. 1973. *Asana, Pranayama, Mudra, Bandha.* Monghyr, Bihar, India: Bihar School of Yoga.

Taylor, M. 2007. "Good Grief: Use Yoga and Meditation to Make Sense of Loss." *Alternative Medicine*, October, 73–76.

Tran, M. D., R. G. Holly, J. Lashbrook, and E. A. Amsterdam. 2001. "Effects of Hatha Yoga Practice on the Health-Related Aspects of Physical Fitness." *Prevention Cardiology* 4(4): 165–170.

Uebelacker, L. A., G. Epstein-Lubow, B. A. Gaudiano, et al. 2010. "Hatha Yoga for Depression: Critical Review of the Evidence for Efficacy, Plausible Mechanisms of Action, and Directions for Future Research." *Journal of Psychiatric Practice* 16(1): 22–33.

Walton, A. 2016. "How Yoga Is Spreading in the US." *Forbes*, March 15. https://www.forbes.com/sites/alicegwalton /2016/03/15/how-yoga-is-spreading-in-the-u-s/#42911 e02449f.

Weintraub, A. 2000. "Yoga: It's Not Just an Exercise." *Psychology Today* 33(6): 22.

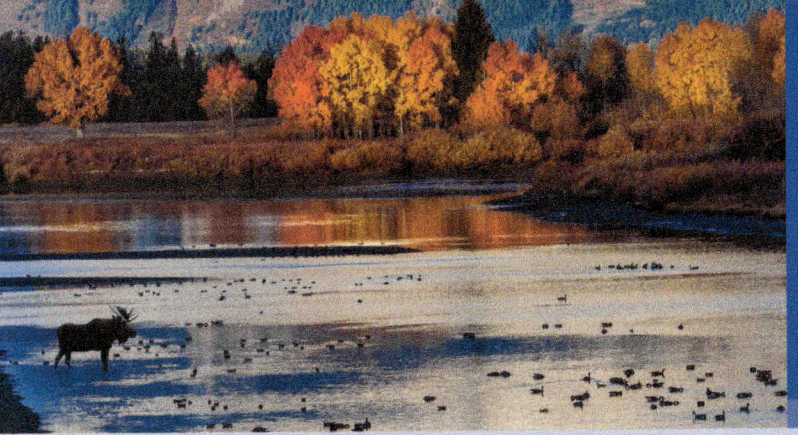

Mental Imagery and Visualization

*I saw the angel in the marble and carved until
I set him free.*

—Michelangelo

Close your eyes for a moment and listen to the gentle, rolling waves of the ocean. See the clear, aqua-blue water break as it approaches the shore. Feel the white sand between your toes, the warm sun on your hair, and the soft wind as it caresses your face and continues on to sway the branches of a royal palm tree behind you. The salt air fills your senses, and as you exhale, you feel completely relaxed.

Imagination is a powerful gift. It is one of the characteristics that makes humans unique creatures on Earth. As a cognitive skill, imagination is the first step of the creative process. Yet imagination is a skill we do not use to our full advantage or potential. When Einstein said that imagination was more powerful than knowledge, he meant that our wealth of knowledge is based on the framework of the depths of human imagination. Knowledge without imagination is like a car without fuel: It is not functional; it won't go anywhere. It would be inaccurate to say that imagination isn't used in times

of stress. It is. More often than not, though, it is used in the wrong way. Our imagination creates worst-case scenarios from our frustrations and fears. We imagine the most drastic consequences of stressful situations by making mountains out of molehills. Why do we do this? Have we been socialized to think this way? Is it a defense mechanism? One can only guess the real reason. It is fair to say, however, that when imagination is used in this negative way it feeds behaviors that somehow reward the ego, or humanity would have discontinued this mode of thinking generations ago. Stress management therapists have concluded that in the face of stress, imagination can be an asset as well as a liability. As the saying goes, "If it was your mind that got you into this mess, then use your mind to get you out of it." Employed in a positive way, imagination can be a very valuable asset as a tool to conquer stress. The rewards produced through positive imagery range from slain metaphorical dragons, to attained goals and answered dreams, to an improved overall state of health.

The technique of **mental imagery** goes by several names based on its purpose and how it is performed. For example, the word **visualization** often is used synonymously with mental imagery, but it can also mean additional aspects of mental imagery not directly related to the relaxation effect. Psychophysiologist and biofeedback specialist Patricia Norris (1992) describes visualization as "a conscious choice with intentional instructions," whereas "imagery is a spontaneous flow of thoughts originating from the unconscious mind."

Mental training and mental rehearsal are also part of the mental imagery process. These terms are used primarily in sports psychology and behavioral medicine to express a more elaborate type of imagery for behavioral change. The purpose in these two disciplines is to promote positive behavioral changes such as, for example, the refinement of motor skills for improved athletic performance or positive changes in health behaviors, such as smoking cessation.

In cases where suggestions are given by an instructor, therapist, or counselor to enhance imagination, the technique is referred to as **guided mental imagery**. In his book *Visualization for Change* (1988), Patrick Fanning defined visualization as "the conscious, volitional creation of mental sense impressions for the purpose of changing yourself." The skill of visualization involves the creation of images, scenes, or impressions by engaging one's imagination of the body's physical senses of sight, sound, feel, smell, and even taste for an overall pleasurable desired effect.

Mental imagery goes by another name altogether in psychological circles: **predictive encoding**—a mental

> **Mental imagery:** Using the imagination to observe, in the first person, images created by the unconscious mind to promote relaxation, to substitute a less desirable behavior with a healthier one, or to help heal damaged body tissue.
>
> **Visualization:** A directed exercise in mental imagery that involves the conscious creation of images of success, healing, or relaxation for the purpose of self-improvement.
>
> **Guided mental imagery:** An exercise in which one is guided through a series of suggestions provided by an instructor, therapist, or counselor to enhance one's imagination.
>
> **Predictive encoding:** A mental training strategy to utilize the unconscious mind for better performance; an academic term for mental imagery.

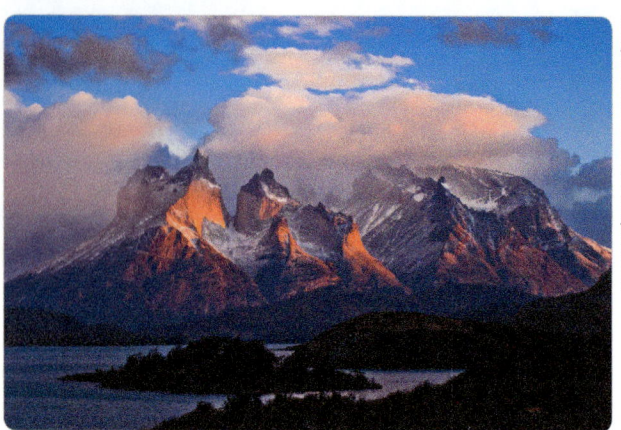

FIGURE 21.1   Either viewing a beautiful sunrise or creating an image of one in your mind can help to relax mind, body, and spirit.

training strategy to utilize the unconscious mind for better performance. The relationship between mental training and personal performance continues to be studied around the world, from elite athletes to cancer patients and everyone in between.

Mental imagery and visualization, when used to promote physical calmness, involve several components of meditation—specifically, increased concentration and expanded awareness of consciousness of the scene created in the mind's eye. Perhaps the greatest strength lies in the ability to turn down the volume and intensity of information received by the five senses, and in many cases to replace threatening stimuli with pleasurable ones from the depths of the imagination. The net result is an overall calming effect and, in some cases, even a healing effect (**FIG. 21.1**).

■ Historical Perspective

The use of mental imagery as a healing technique can be traced back to the origins of virtually every culture on nearly every continent. In one form or another, mental imagery and visualization have been used by Australian Aborigines, Native American shamans, Hindu yogis, and the ancient Greeks as a supplemental tool to fight disease and promote health. For example, in the book *Black Elk Speaks*, a semi-autobiographical account of a Sioux medicine man, Black Elk describes the use of "visions" in his treatment of several sick people (Neihardt 1988). Other cultures have their stories as well. Too sophisticated for cures of the mystical type, Western culture abandoned such practices centuries ago. During the Renaissance, the Cartesian principle separated the study of the mind (philosophy) and body (medicine), weakening the authority of mental imagery as a healing practice. Although visualization in its many forms was still practiced by various cultures throughout the world, it failed to gain approval of the influential medical community in the West until the turn of the twentieth century. As the field of modern psychology began to unfold, however, the concepts of mental imagery and visualization reemerged as viable means to connect mental and physical aspects of well-being.

In the early works of Joseph Breuer, Sigmund Freud, and Carl Jung, the elements of imagination were introduced into psychoanalysis. Each therapist documented cases in which patients' ability to tap into their imagination helped cure them of specific ailments. Whereas Freud theorized that imagination was insight into basic human drives, Jung believed that it was the wealth of knowledge in the unconscious mind surfacing as images to consciousness. Jung formulated a hypothesis that many images have an "archetypal nature," a term he used to describe symbols common to all people of all races. These include trees, circular objects (mandalas), and winged creatures. As early as 1940, Jung encouraged his patients to use **active imagination**, a creative exercise to complete the final scenes of recurring dreams, in an effort to find a peaceful resolution. In many cases, it helped to cure them of their physical ailments.

From Jung's lead, several other psychologists, including Robert Assaglioli, Erik Peper, and Paul Eckman, demonstrated the power of imagination to influence cognitive processing as well as physiological changes produced by creative thoughts. With time, mental imagery became well accepted in the practice of clinical psychology, with the Rorschach ink-blot test becoming one of the most renowned applications of this technique. Joseph Wolpe suggested the use of imagination when he advised that systematic desensitization be employed as a coping technique when known stressors would be encountered. Systematic desensitization is a process of progressive tolerance to stress through the replacement of stressful stimuli with more comfortable images created in the mind. (This will be described in more detail later in this chapter.) In the 1970s, O. Carl Simonton and his wife, Stephanie, resurrected the use of active imagination, applying this technique to help fight cancer in patients who were terminally ill. It is largely their inspiring work that has prompted much research on the use of mental imagery in clinical settings.

One of the most respected names in the field of guided imagery today is Belleruth Naparstek. As a practicing psychotherapist, Naparstek sees three kinds of people in her practice: trauma victims, people with self-defeating behaviors, and the chronically ill. Guided imagery, she states, works for people in all three categories. "Guided imagery," she says, "is a kind of directed daydreaming, a way of using imagination very specifically to help mind and body heal, stay strong, and even perform as needed" (Naparstek 1995). She has dedicated her life work to helping scores of people suffering from trauma, including Vietnam vets, Iraq War vets, Columbine high school teachers and students, and those who survived the horrors of September 11 in New York City. The author of several books and more than 100 audio recordings, she now makes her audios available as CDs or MP3 files to people who have suffered from traumatic events (https://www.healthjourneys.com).

Neurophysiologists now understand that of the hundreds of billions of cells in the human brain, only a fraction (approximately 2 billion, or 10 percent) are used for conscious thought. The remaining cells may actually constitute the tangible network associated with the unconscious mind. Work inspired by Sperry to gain a greater understanding of the cognitive functions of the right and left hemispheres of the brain has deduced that imagination, like intuition, music appreciation, and spatial awareness, is a right-brain function. And the ability to access and employ right-brain functions is considered an asset in dealing with perceived stress.

■ Mental Imagery Research

The practices of mental imagery and visualization as healing modalities are relatively new to Western medicine and are not universally accepted among healthcare professionals. Two scientific journals are devoted to research on this topic: *The Journal of Mental Imagery* (Marquette University) and *Imagination, Cognition, and Personality* (Yale University). Studies involving mental imagery can be found in several other journals as well.

Researchers have examined the use of visualization as a complementary tool for improved health status in the

> **Active imagination:** A term coined by Carl Jung describing a mental imagery process where, in a lucid dream state or relaxed state, one consciously imagines (and resolves) the end of a recurring dream. It is a form of visualization.

treatment of cancer, elevated blood pressure, chronic pain, asthma, obesity, bone fractures, and headaches. The promising results of these studies have added substance to the emerging field of psychoneuroimmunology. Other studies have observed positive changes in various behaviors through the use of mental imagery, including sports performance and recovery from chemical dependencies. The following are examples of the type of research that has been conducted in this field.

To examine the effects of mental imagery as a relaxation technique on various biochemical reactions, Jasnoski and Kugler (1987) measured the response of salivary immunoglobulin A (SIgA), cortisol, and mood states when under the influence of mental images specific to enhancement of the immune system. Results supported the hypothesis that when cognition is directed toward these biochemical factors, there is a subsequent change in neuroimmunomodulation.

Ievleva and Orlick (1991) studied the effects of mental imagery, positive self-talk, and goal setting on subjects diagnosed with knee and ankle injuries, compared to subjects with the same types of injuries who had no such treatment. Those subjects who practiced these relaxation techniques demonstrated more rapid healing of their injuries than the control subjects.

The stories emerging regarding the use of mental imagery for cancer are mostly anecdotal, but Epstein (1989) believes they must be regarded with as much validity as controlled studies. Jeanne Achterberg (1978, 1984, 1985), who is renowned for her use of mental imagery in the treatment of cancer, is also of the opinion that this type of treatment is as essential as radiation and chemotherapy and must not be thought of as "a last alternative." She believes that mental imagery plays both a reactive and a causative role in the biochemical healing process.

Despite claims of remission of cancerous tumors, note that mental imagery has never been touted as a panacea for all ailments and diseases. Furthermore, not all studies of mental imagery have shown promising results. For example, Barrie Cassileth (1990) found no relationship between psychosocial factors (mental imagery and sheer will) and physiological effects in 359 cancer patients. These results confirmed her hypothesis that mental imagery falls in the realm of "fraudulent quackery." A caveat to findings such as these is explained by health psychologist Shelly Taylor (2005), who, in an attempt to explain the placebo effect, indicates that the *attitude* of the physician is sometimes more important than the medicine he or she administers. Citing several clinical studies, Taylor notes that healthcare practitioners who show confidence in the treatment they administer, as well as professional bonding with the patient, always observe a stronger effect than those who are skeptical of the treatment. This occurs whether the medication is "real" (Feldman 1956) or a placebo (Miller 1989). Thus, Taylor considers the placebo effect neither a "medical trick" nor a purely psychological side effect, but rather a very real aspect of the healing process.

More recent research involving guided imagery has examined the use of various suggestive images with bulimics (Tuschen-Caffier et al. 2003), people with clinical depression (Chou and Lin 2006), nursing home patients (Crow and Banks 2004), kidney dialysis patients (Matthews et al. 2001), and cancer patients (Freeman and Dirks 2006; Wyatt et al. 2007), as well as the use of imagery as a means to improve memory (Paddock et al. 2000), all with favorable results. This suggests that the power of the mind is a force to be reckoned with when used to promote our highest potential. If there is any doubt about how the mind can affect the body's stress physiology, researchers in Japan found that the use of guided imagery relaxation resulted in a significant decrease in salivary cortisol (Watanabe et al. 2006), suggesting one more link in the mind-body equation.

The U.S. military brass has taken note regarding the promising effects of mind-body skills in helping to regulate the autonomic nervous system, particularly for returning soldiers with posttraumatic stress disorder (PTSD) and traumatic brain injury (TBI). In a white paper (summarized research findings) drafted by the Defense Center of Excellence for Psychological Health and Traumatic Brain Injury, mental imagery (along with diaphragmatic breathing, meditation, and biofeedback) was highlighted for its ability to positively influence nervous system regulation, specifically referred to as "balanced autonomic functioning." The white paper stated that brain scans indicate that imagery can stimulate the same areas of the brain and nervous system as an equivalent experience can.

In terms of evidence supporting the use of guided imagery, a meta-analytic review of 46 studies suggests that guided imagery may be helpful for managing stress, anxiety, depression, and pain management (Naparstek 2011). Simply stated, the combined power of symbolic creativity and imaginary sensory stimulation holds great promise for optimal (improved) health and performance for people of all walks of life.

As the former director of biofeedback research at the Menninger Clinic in Topeka, Kansas, Dr. Patricia Norris documented several case studies in which mental imagery and visualization were used successfully to complement traditional medical treatment. She lists eight characteristics that help to make mental imagery effective as a healing tool, especially with regard to cancer:

1. *Visualization needs to be idiosyncratic.* An **idiosyncratic** image is one that is self-generated. Images that are created by the practitioner and not the patient appear to be ineffective in the healing process.

2. *The imagery must be egosyntonic.* For an image to be **egosyntonic**, it must fit with the person's values and ideals. If, for example, the individual is a pacifist, then combative or warlike imagery will undermine the effectiveness of this type of treatment. Norris notes that typically there is emotional involvement with the imagery. Many patients actually protected their cancer in their imagery, even during disposal (e.g., in packing it out in garbage bags, or viewing cancer cells longing to be released).

3. *The imagery must have a positive connotation.* Imagery that is negative reinforces negative thoughts, which are not conducive to healing. As an example, Norris notes that sharks, as a healing image, are not a good idea. Imagery must be what she calls "restorative and preparative."

4. *The imagery must be kinesthetic and somatic.* Rather than watching the imagery on a movie screen, the patient should experience sensations of the imagery "in the first person." They should sense that what they are seeing is happening inside their body, not "out there somewhere." The imagery must be **kinesthetic**, involving all the senses.

5. *The imagery must be anatomically correct and accurate.* Knowing exactly what body region and physiological system is diseased and what the nature of the disease truly is should dictate the type of imagery used. In other words, one needs to know whether to access the central nervous system or the immune system. Certain diseases and illnesses fall under specific categories. Norris suggests accessing one's body wisdom as well as clinical data and test results. She also states that more than one image can be used in the healing process. In her work with children, she noted that kids used both a symbolic (figurative) image and a literal (representational) one.

6. *Maintain constancy and dialogue.* Constancy means regularity in one's imagery. Norris suggests three 15-minute sessions per day, with brief intermittent thought messages at other times. Through a dialogue of self-talk, Norris suggests thanking the pain for raising awareness of the problem so that it can be fixed. Finally, she suggests destroying a tumor with its permission and with love. The afflicted part of the body should be treated as a child to be protected and nurtured. The goal is to make peace with one's body.

7. *Employ a blueprint visualization.* A blueprint is a strategy. A **blueprint visualization** is like a time-lapse photograph where a flower (symbolizing a tumor) is shown to bloom within seconds and then close back up and fade away. Visualize a formula and see it through to completion. An example would be to see the construction of a building, from the hole in the ground to opening day when you are cutting the ribbon at the entrance.

8. *Include the treatment in the imagery.* Norris has found that patients who use mental imagery incorporating chemotherapy treatment and radiation do better than those who "fight" these medical procedures. She notes that it helps to have benevolent feelings (versus ambivalent feelings) toward the treatment. She suggests mentally "welcoming the treatment into the body." From her patients, she offers these examples:

   - *Chemotherapy*: A gold-colored fluid that healthy cells, acting as a bucket brigade, pass along to cancer cells, who drink it up.

Idiosyncratic: A term meaning "self-generated," such as images used in visualization that are created by the person performing the visualization.

Egosyntonic: A visualization expression meaning that the images created/suggested in the visualization process must fit with the values and ideals that are most beneficial.

Kinesthetic: A visualization expression that refers to the involvement of all five senses in the practice of this technique.

Blueprint visualization: A term to suggest that a visualization has a goal to complete or accomplish; thus, the blueprint is the template for completion (e.g., a healed wound).

■ *Radiation treatment*: A stream of silver energy aimed at the cancerous tumor(s). Ask the white blood cells to move out of the way—or shield themselves—and act like mirrors to reflect the radiation toward the cancer cells; then watch the cancer cells go belly-up.

Norris, like other researchers (Krippner 2000; Rossman 2002), admits that just exactly how visualization promotes healing is still a mystery and that the answers to this mystery can be learned as we further explore human consciousness and the human energy field. Achterberg (1984) hypothesizes that the function of imagination, housed in the right brain, converts thoughts to biochemical messages and intentionally directs them toward target body regions. Although mental imagery and visualization have been hailed as wonderful adjuncts to clinical medicine, their benefits can be obtained by anyone in any state of health, especially to promote and enjoy a deep sense of relaxation.

■ Mental Imagery as a Relaxation Technique

Daydreaming may be the most common type of mental imagery used to relax (**FIG. 21.2**). Researchers have come to understand that the conscious mind needs to break away periodically and "download" sensory information for "reprocessing." (Computer software screensavers are loosely based on this concept.) Many people are aware that they daydream, yet when asked to recall the images, they are hard-pressed to give an answer. Mental imagery as a form of relaxation has taken the concept of daydreaming and organized it to give it a sense of legitimacy. People rarely daydream spontaneously during a bout of stress. Instead, as noted earlier, the mind conjures up worst-case scenarios that seem more real than the actual event. So, to alter this mind frame, the daydreaming concept has been adapted to intercept the stress response and give the body a chance to unwind. It does this by replacing negative thoughts and perceptions with peaceful scenes. Just as real or imaginary thoughts can trigger the stress response, relaxing thoughts can promote the relaxation response. This is the primary goal and purpose of mental imagery. When imagination is used to promote relaxation, the body's five senses are in effect deactivated or desensitized to stressful stimuli. The body is allowed to recharge so that upon return to the physical environment the perceptions of stress can be dealt with more effectively (**BOX 21.1**).

In many ways, the creation of mental imagery is like making a motion picture in which characters wear a

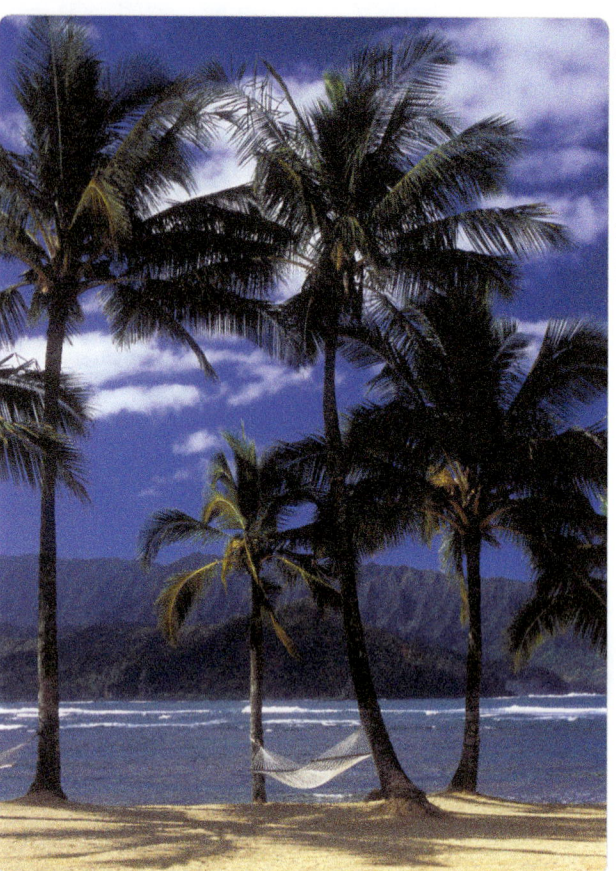

FIGURE 21.2   A beach scene such as this, reminiscent of some vacation areas, is often used by people to promote relaxation.

number of hats. In this case, you take on all the roles: producer (selecting the sets and scenery), director (organizing the sensory cues), actor, and audience (experiencing the effects of the production). All the roles are equally significant to making the images as powerful as possible. With practice, the use of this technique will enhance your skills in all these roles, and great satisfaction will be derived from participation in your own creation.

Over time, as the concept of mental imagery developed, it was divided into three distinct categories. However, as more and more people have begun to share this technique, many variations and combinations have emerged. The original three categories are discussed here.

Tranquil Natural Scenes

The use of guided mental imagery gained popularity and clinical approval in the late 1960s and early 1970s when therapists and psychologists began to explore variations

---

BOX 21.1   Peaceful Scenes to Promote Relaxation

As a class assignment, I ask my students to create five mental images that promote a sense of deep relaxation specifically for them. Some are long, some are short, but each conveys an image that promotes calmness in the person who created it. I never cease to be amazed at what they come up with. The following is a "best-of" collection of mental imagery scenes as seen through the creative eyes of my students. Close your eyes for a moment after reading each one and decide whether it brings you a sense of tranquility.

■ Stretched between two trees is a hammock, and I am lying in that hammock swinging slowly in the breeze. There are a few trees around, and in front of me is a large meadow. The grass is lush green and spotted with hundreds of multicolored flowers that seem to stretch forever. The sky is blue and clear, with only a few small white clouds moving slowly across the sky. The breeze caresses my face in syncopation with the hammock's motion.

■ I am in the wilderness, staring into a clear, star-filled sky. There is a campfire nearby, which is slowly losing its zest, but is still throwing off intense amounts of heat. I'm lying on my sleeping bag, my face is looking straight up. The fire occasionally crackles and a spark is seen shooting in the air. As I examine the sky, a shooting star lights up the darkness and throws a brilliant white light for what appears to be miles. My body snuggles into the sleeping bag as I dream of the wish I just made.

■ With my legs I can feel the sides of my horse expand as he breathes. We have stopped in the middle of a clearing. We have been riding through a woods blanketed with snow. The snow is no longer falling, and the air is cool and crisp. The horse's breath can be seen as mist rising from his nose. We remain still for a moment, listening to the sounds of the other animals in the woods. I give my horse a nudge and he responds, moving forward through this winter wonderland.

■ The water is turquoise, even at a depth of 30 feet, with perfect visibility. I am weightless. The rays of the sun pierce through the water, but seem to soften as they reach to touch the sand below. The coral varies in shape and color; I can't begin to describe its beauty. Schools of small fish surround my body and then disappear in the blink of an eye. With each kick, my body is caressed by the warmth of the water; the bubbles tickle as they pass my face headed for the surface.

■ I am soaring through the crisp blue air. I am flying as if I have wings. I do; I am hang gliding. The sky is a deep blue with white puffy clouds. As I float through one, it is silent. I am completely alone. I see Earth below me. It is far away. I feel weightless. I hear the soft hush of the breeze. My hands make waves in the air. I can see the sun. I can almost touch it as I glide effortlessly through the air.

---

on meditative thought. With this type of visualization, patients are instructed to close their eyes and follow a series of suggested scenes during which they access and utilize the cognitive skills of imagination. In essence, through the creative process, individuals mentally place themselves in the peaceful and relaxing scenes. These **tranquil natural scenes** are selected because they simulate locations where people typically vacation to escape the stress of home or office environments. Images such as a tropical island beach, a mountain vista, or a path through an evergreen forest are often used.

Once introduced to this technique, participants who repeatedly engage in the practice of visualization find that, like actually being at a vacation site, the re-creation of these settings provides an equal, if not more profound, sense of relaxation. These natural scenes, full of vivid color, fresh air, nature sounds, and other elements of nature, allow participants to put their thoughts in perspective. Natural scenes, like the real ones they imitate, have the ability to place perceptions and the people who harbor them in proportion to the rest of the natural world, turning distorted perceptions back into manageable thoughts. Moreover, with repeated practice of visualization, physical changes indicating a return to homeostasis begin to occur. Consequently, to gaze at a wide ocean horizon at sunrise or sunset, to stare at a deep blue sky filled with stars close enough to touch, or to reflect before a backdrop of jagged mountain peaks covered with snow tends to momentarily dwarf

---

Tranquil natural scenes: One of three categories used in mental imagery (e.g., ocean beach, mountain vista, old-growth forest, lavender gardens).

any problem, no matter how big or stressful. Although the visualization of these scenes will not make personal problems go away, it appears to help shrink them down to tolerable size, which then makes them manageable to deal with and resolve. And the acknowledgment of stressors in the presence of any one of these scenes makes the concern less threatening, if not insignificant altogether.

Of all the natural settings used to promote relaxation, the most common include water, such as ocean beaches, mountain lakes, or waterfalls and streams. It is commonly believed that scenes of water are reminiscent of the earliest sensations experienced in the womb. Any scene perceived to be relaxing, however, can have the same effect. The power of this type of imagery lies in using not just visual imagination sense but other senses as well. Seeing the image, hearing the sounds, smelling the fragrances or freshness of the air, sensing the air temperature, and feeling the wind and the sun on your skin all coalesce into a very powerful scene. By accessing the imagination of these sensations, you go from being a passive observer to an active participant in your own image. Furthermore, by acknowledging all sensations, you experience the calming effects of this technique firsthand rather than observing them from a vicarious or "third-person" viewpoint.

There is no dearth of images that can help produce the relaxation response, nor is there one image that will have the same effect on everyone. Perhaps the greatest positive influence on the visualization of natural scenes is the perception that it promotes tranquility. A disturbing association with a natural image may actually promote stress rather than decrease it. For instance, an image of a mountain vista may not be considered relaxing to someone with a fear of heights. When introducing guided mental imagery, a good instructor will suggest that participants take the liberty to augment or change the suggestions so that the tailored image promotes a

personal sense of relaxation. For example, because of my Colorado roots, I often use a mountain lake as a peaceful image when I teach mental imagery. But once I had a student who had never experienced a view of a mountain lake. As a former lifeguard, he instead took the concept of a body of water and envisioned looking at reflections from an undisturbed indoor pool. It was a scene he could relate to; it worked for him.

Some guided mental imagery invites individuals to compare the visualized image with their own state of physical relaxation. Such comparison tends to promote a deeper sense of calmness throughout the body.

Behavioral Changes

For years, many psychologists have held strongly to the belief that the key to addressing negative health habits is to change behavior. This, more than values and attitudes, is the part of personality that is easiest to change. Ingestive habits such as smoking, drinking, various eating behaviors, and substance addictions are the most common health concerns targeted for behavioral changes. Process-addiction behaviors (workaholism, shopaholism, and the like) fall into this category as well. Mental imagery combined with power of suggestion was taken up as the premise of behavioral medicine to help people change negative health behaviors into positive ones. Although this technique alone will not produce changes, when used in conjunction with other behavior modification tactics and coping strategies, **behavioral changes** have proved effective for some people. What mental imagery does is reinforce a new desired behavior. Repeated use of images reinforces the desired behavior more strongly over time.

Mental imagery used to influence behavioral changes is a specific style of cognitive restructuring. As mentioned earlier, in his work to help people overcome their fears, Wolpe created a process of mental imagery called **systematic desensitization**. In this process, a person uses his or her imagination to help overcome anxiety related to a specific situation by building up a tolerance to the stressor through progressive exposures to it. The first step is for the subject to create the exposures in his or her own mind while in a relaxed state. For example, let's say that you have a fear of public speaking and you are slated to give a presentation to 300 people next month. In the process of systematic desensitization, you would create a scene in your mind where you are standing at a podium in an empty

Behavioral changes: One of three categories used in mental imagery to change negative behaviors into positive ones (e.g., quitting smoking, improved athletic performance, weight loss programming).

Systematic desensitization: A term coined by psychologist Joseph Wolpe to describe a process of progressive tolerance to stress by gaining a greater sense of comfort with the unknown through repeated exposure and visualization.

auditorium giving a flawless speech. Along with this image you might also practice some diaphragmatic breathing and mental imagery of tranquil natural scenes to calm down before you start talking. After repeating this image several times, you then imagine one or two people (very close friends) in the audience who applaud vigorously when you are done. After repeating this image enough to feel comfortable, you then imagine that you give your successful speech to half an audience, followed by the same great speech to a full house, both to thunderous applause. With practice, the strength of this calm image overrides the intensity of the stressor so that your stress response is minimal, if triggered at all. The second phase of systematic desensitization would be to actually rehearse your speech at a podium while recalling the images (either relaxing scenes or your image of success) to help re-create the feeling of calmness you attained earlier. Again the stress response is minimal and disappears seconds after the speech starts.

Another example of someone who made behavioral changes through mental imagery is Allison, who tried numerous times to quit smoking. She cut down from two packs to six cigarettes per day, but still felt the need to smoke when she was driving to and from work. Attempting to quit smoking altogether, Allison practiced mental imagery wherein she visualized herself in her car driving to work. She imagined that she opened the window a little and played soft music on the radio. At traffic lights—a point of frustration and impatience—she looked for birds until the light changed. After having found a parking space, she got out of her car and imagined herself walking into the office without feeling the need for a cigarette. By taking herself through the drive to work in her imagination, Allison was able to envision herself accomplishing the goal she set. The repeated use of her image laid the groundwork—the reinforcement of the desired behavioral change—enabling her to accomplish her task when she encountered the problematic situation directly.

At about the same time that mental imagery and visualization started being used in the clinical setting to promote positive behavioral health changes, the discipline of sports psychology took root and was also introduced into the world of athletics. The sport that first received publicity for its use of mental imagery was tennis. In the book *The Inner Game of Tennis* (1974), Timothy Gallwey described his theory that by rehearsing the game in

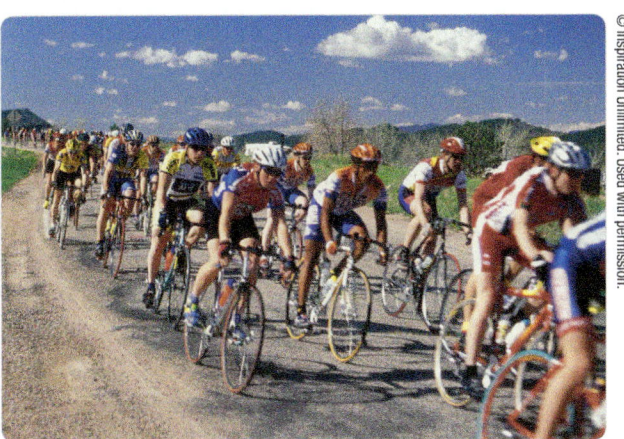

FIGURE 21.3 Many athletes use mental imagery (mental training, mental rehearsal) to complement their physical training. For amateurs and professionals alike, the mental skills of competition are extremely important for peak performance.

one's mind, one could improve one's game on the court. Studies employing this technique began to show support for the theory, concluding that when the mind rehearses a motor skill, the neural tract through which impulses are sent from the brain to the muscles is better defined (Harris and Robinson 1986). An example is imagining practicing the serve into the service box. When repeated over and over again, the result is improved coordination during actual play. Thus, the technique of mental training became very popular in amateur and professional sports when athletes were sidelined with injuries, and it was soon incorporated into rehabilitation programs. In addition, athletes began to use visualization (**FIG. 21.3**) in their mental training programs to decrease competitive anxiety and to improve motivation and self-esteem through the use of positive affirmations.

Integrated into the technique of mental imagery to influence behavioral change is the use of verbal messages (positive affirmations) to reinforce the strength of the image. Positive affirmations are positive thoughts that the conscious mind sends to itself as well as to the unconscious mind to build confidence, assertiveness, and self-esteem. These positive thoughts, expressed in words, phrases, or sentences, are repeated through one's inner voice while in a relaxed state. Often they are used in conjunction with diaphragmatic breathing, and are repeated silently during the exhalation phase, when the body is most relaxed. The mind is most receptive to the message it hears in a relaxed state. For example, the famous coffee mug slogan "Damn, I'm Good" is a wonderful positive affirmation that can be combined with an image of personal success to reinforce its message. Members of Alcoholics Anonymous also use a number of these statements as mental reminders or *mantras* in their recovery program, the most common being "One day at a time."

The rationale behind positive affirmation statements goes something like this. Either through learned behaviors or as an innate characteristic common to all humans, we tend to feed our minds a preponderance of negative thoughts. The cumulative effect of these thoughts is to erode the foundations of self-esteem. And low self-esteem makes us vulnerable to stress. The advertising industry employs this concept through ads that target our insecurities. They repeatedly suggest that we buy the products to improve our self-image. The underlying message is that we are not good enough unless we do. Research reveals that we are bombarded with an average of over 3,000 media messages per day (MortarBlog 2006). Although not all advertisers exploit our insecurities, so many slant their messages in a negative direction that they reinforce our tendency toward negative self-feedback, making the cycle even harder to break. We become our own worst critic. The voice inside our head, the sentry guard of the ego, constantly tells us that we are doing something wrong or that we fail to meet our own expectations. By contrast, the use of positive affirmations helps to balance the emotional scales, disarm the internal critic, and reinforce the foundations of positive self-esteem. Any positive thought or phrase will do. Take a moment to think of a phrase you can say to yourself to make you feel good inside. Once you have one, repeat it to yourself when you practice your relaxation techniques. When you are feeling low or stressed out, close your eyes for a moment and try to recall the phrase. Repeat it to yourself along with a supporting mental image and feel the strength it gives you. It may take a few tries, but this technique has proved effective for a great many athletes in their games—and in the game of life. It can work for you, too!

> **Internal body images:** One of three categories used in mental imagery for the purpose of healing disease or illness (e.g., shrinkage of cancerous tumors, mending broken bones) by involving direct changes in one's physiological state, using the power of imagination to see a particular body region in a healthy state.

For example, I once worked with an Olympic athlete who years previously had defected from the (then) Soviet Union. Although he enjoyed his newfound freedom, at times he felt that he had lost his "European" competitive edge. He never took hold of the idea of positive affirmations, perhaps because he didn't believe this internal feedback would work. At the 1987 World Championships in Lake Placid, he once again found himself competing face to face against his former Soviet teammates. During the final competition, in a sudden burst of energy, he pulled ahead to win. After his victory, he told me about his new positive affirmation statement. With an undeniable accent coming through a smile, he said, "I still got the goods."

Remember, not only can positive affirmation statements combined with mental images augment a message during a relaxed state, but this same technique can be used during stressful encounters such as traffic jams, public speeches, or staff meetings. Many times negative behaviors or stress-prone behaviors are manifestations of low self-esteem, feelings of failure, or rejection we place on ourselves. Positive visualization can often be used to boost and maintain high self-esteem.

Internal Body Images

The third type of mental imagery, **internal body image,** involves direct changes in physiological functions by using imagination to see a particular body region in a healthy state. Signs and symptoms of the stress response manifested throughout the body are by far the greatest concern to people. The major question posed by health practitioners is this: If stress-related thoughts produce physical ailments, can the mind repair the body with healing thoughts? This type of mental imagery was springboarded into the realm of progressive medicine in 1971 when Simonton and Simonton taught a group of cancer patients several relaxation techniques, including the use of mental imagery. Specifically, patients were invited to imagine the white blood cells of their immune systems fighting the cancerous tumor cells. By employing their sense of imagination and assuming responsibility for their treatment and recovery, many patients saw their tumors go into remission. Their book, *Getting Well Again* (1971), which described the protocol used to develop this landmark program, served as a catalyst for similar programs across the United States. As the cofounder of the Academy for Guided Imagery, Marty Rossman, M.D., is currently championing the cause of mental imagery and the healing powers of guided visualization for everything from asthma to cancer, as described in his book, *Fighting Cancer from Within* (2003).

Over the past 10 years, there have been many documented cases of people using mental imagery to rejuvenate and restore their bodies to health, from spontaneous remissions of cancerous tumors and dysfunctional organs, to mended bones and connective tissue. These cases have predominantly involved cancer patients, but other illnesses have been targeted as well, including hypertension, migraines, and low back pain. Although these cases are anecdotal in nature, and mental imagery was not the sole intervention, but rather one of many therapies used, they do imply that there is indeed potential benefit when mental imagery and other related therapies are used in conjunction with conventional medicine. The key is that the patient must begin to assume responsibility for his or her own health status.

As mentioned earlier, the healing mechanism of mental imagery is not fully understood scientifically. Achterberg (1984) hypothesized that the images produced in the mind, specifically in the right brain, appear to send, or are converted to, biochemical messages, most likely through neuropeptides, and affix themselves to receptor sites on lymphocytes and perhaps other targeted cells to promote the healing process. This process somehow initiates a path of cancer-cell destruction or organ-cell reconstruction. Quite possibly this healing process employs the integration of several body systems, including the inhibition or suppression of the nervous and endocrine systems from secreting stress hormones. Keep in mind that mental imagery is not meant to be a replacement for standard medical practices. However, the use of this technique as a complement to medical treatment appears, for some people, to be more effective than pharmacological medicine alone. The stories of those who survive their ordeals with cancer are remarkable testimonials. It would be inaccurate and misleading, however, to imply that every case of mental imagery ended in successful spontaneous remission of cancerous tumors or healed organic tissue.

Among the group of characteristics that affect the success of mental imagery, several factors seemed crucial to Achterberg, Simonton, and Norris. These include willpower, or the desire to take responsibility for health status, and faith, the belief that self-generated thoughts will bear fruit and are not an exercise in futility. In addition, it has been shown that suggestive imagery is more effective when individuals have a detailed understanding of their body's physiological functions, the nature and location of the disease, and the specific physiological mechanisms involved.

In an autobiographical case study reported in the book *Why Me?* (1985) by Garrett Porter and Dr. Patricia Norris, a young boy describes his fatal diagnosis of a malignant inoperable brain tumor and his fight to live. Through the use of mental imagery, biofeedback, and art therapy, Garrett was able to "think" or visualize the cancerous tumor away by imagining the tumor being destroyed and eaten away by friendly yet hungry white blood cells (**FIG. 21.4**). Having an incredible sense of imagination and body awareness, and knowing exactly where the tumor was located, he visualized shrinkage of the tumor successfully. Within several months a CT scan revealed that the cancerous tumor had indeed vanished.

In her acclaimed book *It's Always Something* (1989), comedienne Gilda Radner described her use of mental imagery with her ovarian cancer, which eventually claimed her life. She created the image that her body was like a big, fluffy pink towel. Washing and drying the towel was symbolic of the chemotherapy. In her mind, Gilda saw the cancer cells as pieces of lint on the towel when it was pulled from the dryer. To rid her body of the unwanted cancer cells, she imagined that she

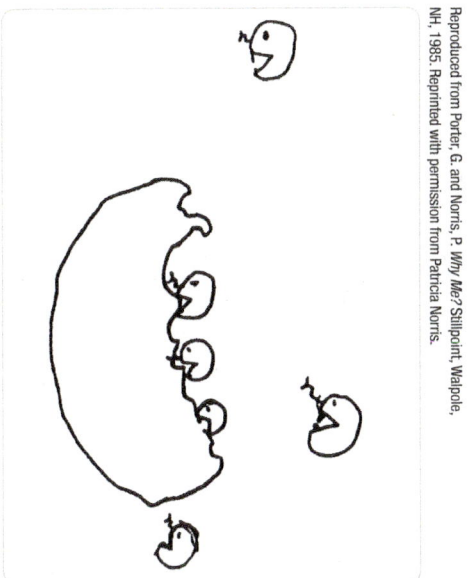

FIGURE 21.4 A sketch made by Garrett Porter to help him visualize the healing process in his body. The small "Pac-Man" creatures (white blood cells) are destroying and eating the tumor, which he named "planet meatball."

would pull the lint off the towel and make it completely clean.

Healing images can be as specific as one ailment or illness (e.g., cancer or thyroid dysfunction) or general in scope, depending on the desired effect. It appears that images, whether direct or indirect (symbolic), can have the same effect on the healing process. Ulcers have been "healed" through images of darning the heels of socks as well as repairing spider webs. Elevated blood pressure has been decreased through images of the release of bottle-neck traffic jams as well as dilating blood vessels to reduce pressure and resistance. There are many examples of a more symbolic approach to imagery as an aid in the physical healing process. They can be adapted to a host of specific physical manifestations.

■ Color Therapy

Exposure to colored light and color imagery is another technique to promote relaxation. In a series of landmark studies to determine emotional and physiological responses to color stimulation, Faber Birren (1961, 1978) learned of differences between the colors red and blue. Red was associated with the heightened emotional responses of love, fear, and anger. Corresponding neural activity of the autonomic nervous system included increased heart rate, blood pressure, respiration, muscle tension, and perspiration. When subjects were in a state of emotional arousal, exposure to red light was perceived to be more "disturbing." Blue showed the opposite effect, a return to physiological homeostasis. Blue light was described as a calming color. In situations where babies are exposed to blue light, they tend to show a calm response, whereas the colors yellow and green give a neutral response. If you feel tense or frustrated, close your eyes and feel yourself surrounded by the color blue—aqua-blue, sky blue, indigo, any shade of blue you can imagine. Perhaps even imagine yourself floating in aqua-blue water. Then take a deep breath and feel your body relax all over.

> **Color therapy:** A type of mental imagery exercise for which color is imagined as an agent for tranquility (e.g., green) or healing (e.g., blue).
>
> **Light therapy:** An extension of color therapy for which full-spectrum lighting or one color from the light spectrum is used to promote homeostasis and healing.

Since Birren's initial work in **color therapy**, the ability to heal with colors has attracted new interest, particularly in the concept of vibrational medicine. Light, as expressed in colors, it seems, is energy made visible. Colors are actually vibrations of energy particle waves at different rates. In his book *Light: Medicine of the Future* (1991), Dr. Jacob Liberman points out some interesting facts about light and **light therapy**. Artificial indoor lighting (incandescent and fluorescent) is not full-spectrum lighting; it is missing some wave particles, including the color blue. People denied exposure to full-spectrum lighting (which Liberman calls "mallillumination") are more prone to bouts of stress and depression, more prone to dental decay, and more likely to have higher levels of serum cholesterol. Studies conducted on plants grown under full-spectrum and different colors of light reveal that the health of the plant is dependent on full-spectrum lighting (Ott 1985). According to Liberman, the same may be true for people. He suggests that when proper lighting is not available, one should use the imagination to see one's body as a prism that captures and splinters light into the colors of the rainbow (red, orange, yellow, green, blue, indigo, and violet). Colors that are pale or hard to imagine require more attention to bring them into detail. Furthermore, some specialists (Gardner 1990) hypothesize that light therapy and color therapy may add yet another dimension to the healing process. According to Gardner, this theory, in conjunction with the vibrations of human chakras, has been studied at MIT and UCLA.

■ Mental Imagery and Chronic Pain

Since the publication of Carl O. Simonton's classic book *Getting Well Again*, mental imagery and visualization have been used extensively for pain management—initially with cancer patients, but now with a wide variety of chronic pain problems, from low back pain to fibromyalgia. Seldom are mental imagery and visualization used alone as therapies. Rather, these techniques are used in combination with diaphragmatic breathing, biofeedback, art therapy, meditation, and other modalities. Rossman (2002) states that a symptom of pain is a signal; mental imagery is used to answer the question, "What does this signal mean?" Chronic pain, resulting from causes ranging from sports injuries and low back pain to gastrointestinal problems and cancer, is just one of the many types of pain that this modality is used to treat.

■ Steps to Initiate Mental Imagery

The steps to initiate mental imagery are as follows:

1. *Assume a comfortable position.* Mental imagery, like diaphragmatic breathing, can be done anywhere you can close your eyes momentarily to your current surroundings and allow your imagination to replace it with a setting more conducive to relaxation. When starting out, either sit or lie comfortably with your eyes closed and loosen any constrictive clothing around your neck and waist. You may even want to kick your shoes off. Sometimes it helps if you dedicate a special place to the practice of mental imagery.

2. *Concentrate and maintain a positive attitude.* As with other relaxation techniques, mental imagery requires sound concentration. It is important to find a quiet place and try to reduce interrupting noises that may compete with the sensory images you create (**FIG. 21.5**). Concentration, like imagination, is a skill, and the two are very compatible in their development. A mental image can last anywhere from seconds to minutes. Initial exposure to this technique may be short, while allowing powers of concentration to build. When employing mental imagery, tap into the imaginative powers of all your senses to place yourself at the scene you have created. Focus your attention on the vividness of colors, shapes, textures, sounds, noises, silence, smells, and the entire feel

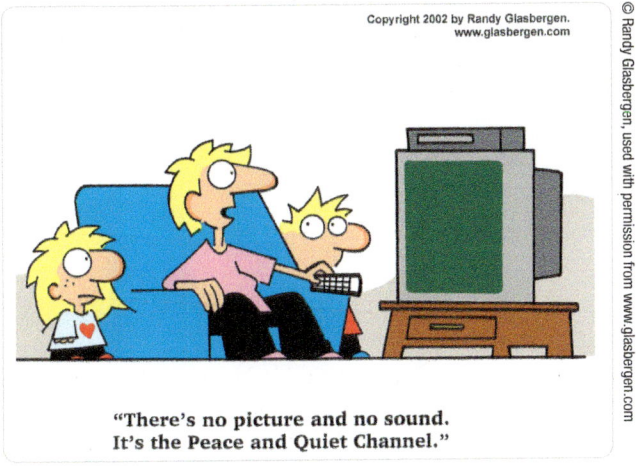

Copyright 2002 by Randy Glasbergen.
www.glasbergen.com

© Randy Glasbergen, used with permission from www.glasbergen.com

"There's no picture and no sound.
It's the Peace and Quiet Channel."

FIGURE 21.5 Sometimes mental imagery begins without an image or picture, it begins simply by clearing the mind.

of the environment you have created. At first it is common to visualize a third-person image of yourself in a scene. But the real power of imagery is delivered when you experience the image in the first person, as you normally do in life. Focus your attention on the image in your mind's eye (the image you see with your eyes closed). Over time you will be able to focus for longer periods of time and in greater detail with each image you work with. As with all relaxation techniques, remind yourself to breathe comfortably, deeply, and regularly. If your mind begins to wander to other thoughts while you initiate an image, try to steer your attention back to the details of the image and allow it to hold you captive.

A positive attitude is crucial to the effectiveness of mental imagery. The cornerstone of a positive attitude is the faith that your imagination can deliver the goods. As was noted by Simonton and colleagues (1980), *belief* in the power of the image is as important as the image itself. Whether it is called hope, faith, or confidence, this is the element that dreams, and more important, images, are made of.

3. *Choose visual themes.* The choice of mental images is unlimited. Begin by deciding the purpose of your visualization. Is it a momentary escape to clear your thoughts? Will it help promote a healthier lifestyle through adaptations of current health behaviors? Is it a healing image to restore and rejuvenate your body? Once you have decided, build on your purpose and tailor a vision to answer it. This chapter has offered several images you can start with, but eventually you may want to use these to create your own special image. The use of imagination and creativity is a skill: The more it is employed, the stronger it becomes, and the better it is as a stress management resource. Sometimes on journeys travel guides are used to lead the way. In her therapy, Norris uses questions to help guide her patients through their mental imagery experience. For instance, with an image of a house or castle, she may ask, "What does your castle look like? What is it made of? What colors are the materials? Walk up to the entrance. What does the door look like? What do the doorknob and knocker look like? Push the door open and walk inside. What do you see?" Norris states that by asking questions

such as these, individuals are encouraged to create images from the depths of their own unconscious minds, the place where healing takes place.

Best Application of Mental Imagery

Mental imagery is very portable. Although it is best to learn mental imagery in a quiet environment, once you are proficient, the technique can be used right in the middle of a stressful situation. It can be employed minutes before a public speech, at the start of an exam, waiting in line at the post office, sitting in the dentist's chair, during a boring staff meeting, or in any circumstance where you can close your eyes for a moment to regain composure. With practice, some people can even recall an image with their eyes open. Unlike other techniques, which need a minimum amount of time to be effective, mental imagery can be effective even when used for a short period. Thus, this is considered an optimal intervention technique to use in the face of stress. As a preventive technique, the art of visualization can be a powerful meditation practice for training the body to lower stress. Mental imagery is effective in both dispelling the thunderheads of fear and defusing the powder kegs of anger.

SUMMARY

- Mental imagery describes the ability of the unconscious mind to generate images that have a calming, healing effect on the body. Visualization is one aspect of mental imagery, wherein there is conscious direction of self-generated images. Guided mental imagery is a variation wherein images are suggested by another person (either live or via an audio recording).

- Mental imagery in some form has been used for thousands of years as a means to access the power of the mind to heal the body, mind, and soul.

- Freud and Jung reintroduced mental imagery in the twentieth century. Jung coined the term *active imagination* to mean the powers of the unconscious mind to help resolve issues associated with recurring dreams.

- Several studies have been conducted using mental imagery and visualization as a complementary healing tool, specifically with cancer patients. Norris outlined several criteria necessary for mental imagery to prove effective.

- Mental imagery can be divided into three types: (1) peaceful natural scenes, or images that place one in a natural environment; (2) behavioral changes, or images that allow one to see and feel oneself performing a different, more health-conscious behavior; and (3) internal body images, or images of trips inside the body to observe damaged, diseased, or dysfunctional tissue being healed or repaired.

- Systematic desensitization is a technique that breaks down a stressor into small parts and allows one to slowly gain control of feelings and perceptions about a stressor through progressive exposures to it. Mental imagery is used to augment this process.

- Color therapy and light therapy, which are loosely associated with mental imagery, have been shown to have a healing quality. Colors of light have specific vibrations that may augment the healing abilities of the mind. Red is said to generate feelings of arousal, whereas blue is believed to have a calming quality to it.

- Certain criteria contribute to profound experiences with mental imagery: a quiet environment, a comfortable position, and a passive attitude.

- Mental imagery is commonly used as a modality to decrease episodes of chronic pain and is often used in combination with other stress management modalities for an optimal effect.

STUDY GUIDE QUESTIONS

1. What is mental imagery, and how does it differ from visualization?

2. List three ways that imagery and visualization can be used for relaxation.

3. What is color therapy, and how can it be used to promote relaxation?

4. List three steps that, when followed, help promote relaxation.

REFERENCES AND RESOURCES

Academy of Guided Imagery. 10780 Santa Monica Blvd., Suite 290, Los Angeles, CA 90025. (800) 726-2070. http://acadgi.com.

Achterberg, J. 1978. *Imagery and Cancer*. Champaign, IL: Institute for Personality and Ability Testing.

Achterberg, J. 1984. "Imagery and Medicine: Psychophysiological Speculations." *Journal of Mental Imagery* 8(4): 1–14.

Achterberg, J. 1985. *Imagery in Healing: Shamanism and Modern Medicine*. Boston, MA: Shambhala Publications.

Araoz, D. L. 1983. "Use of Hypnotic Technique with Oncology Patients." *Journal of Psychosocial Oncology* 1(4): 47–54.

Arnheim, R. 1972. *Visual Thinking*. Berkeley, CA: University of California Press.

Atamaniuk, M. 2020. "How Many Ads Do You Actually See Daily?" Clario, April 21. https://clario.co/blog/live-secured/ads-seen-daily/.

Becker, W. 1990. *Cross Currents*. Los Angeles: Tarcher Press.

Birren, F. 1961. *Color Psychology and Color Therapy*. Secaucus, NJ: Citadel Press.

Birren, F. 1969. *Light, Color, and Environment*. New York: Van Nostrand Reinhold.

Birren, F. 1978. *Color and Human Response*. New York: Van Nostrand Reinhold.

Bry, A. 1979. *Visualization: Directing the Movies of Your Mind*. New York: Harper.

Bryant, L., and A. G. Harvy. 1996. "Visual Imagery in Post-Traumatic Stress Disorder." *Journal of Traumatic Stress* 9(3): 613–619.

Cassileth, B. R. 1990. "Mental-Health Quackery in Cancer Treatment." *International Journal of Mental Health* 19(3): 81–84.

Chou, M. H., and M. F. Lin. 2006. "Exploring the Listening Experiences During Guided Imagery and Music Therapy of Outpatients with Depression." *Journal of Nursing Research* 14(2): 93–102.

Clark, L. 1974. *The Ancient Art of Color Therapy*. Old Greenwich, CT: Devon-Adair.

Coue, E. 1922. *Self-Mastery Through Conscious Auto-Suggestion*. London: Allen & Unwin.

Crow, S., and D. Banks. 2004. "Guided Imagery: A Tool to Guide the Way for the Nursing Home Patient." *Advances in Mind Body Medicine* 20(4): 4–7.

Einstein, A. 1979. *Living Philosophies*. New York: AMS Press.

Epstein, G. 1989. *Healing Visualizations: Creating Health Through Imagery*. New York: Bantam Books.

Fanning, P. 1988. *Visualization for Change*. Oakland, CA: New Harbinger Publications.

Feldman, P. E. 1956. "The Personal Element in Psychiatric Research." *American Journal of Psychiatry* 113: 52–54.

Fisher, S. 1970. *Body Experience in Fantasy and Behavior*. New York: Appleton-Century-Crofts.

Freeman, L., and L. Dirks. 2006. "Mind-Body Imagery Practice Among Alaska Breast Cancer Patients: A Case Study." *Alaska Medicine* 48(3): 74–84.

Gallwey, W. T. 1974. *The Inner Game of Tennis*. New York: Random House.

Gardner, K. 1990. *Sounding the Inner Landscape*. Stonington, ME: Caduceus Publications.

Garfield, P. 1975. *Creative Daydreaming*. New York: Simon & Schuster.

Gawain, S. 1978. *Creative Visualization*. San Rafael, CA: New World Library.

Gawain, S., with D. Grimshaw. 1978. *Reflections in the Light: Daily Thoughts and Affirmations*. Mill Valley, CA: Whatever Publishing.

Gebhardt, P. 2000. "Helping Veterans Overcome Their Fears." *The Washington Post*, January 11.

George, L. 1986. "Mental Imagery—Enhancement Training in Behavior Therapy: Current Status and Future Prospects." *Psychotherapy* 23: 81–92.

Giusto, E., and N. Bond. 1979. "Imagery and the Autonomic Nervous System: Some Methodological Issues." *Perceptual and Motor Skills* 48: 427–438.

Harris, D. V., and W. J. Robinson. 1986. "The Effects of Skill Level on EMG Activity During Internal and External Imagery." *Journal of Sport Psychology* 8(2): 105–111.

Holt, R. 1964. "Imagery, the Return of the Ostracized." *American Psychologist* 19: 254–264.

Hope, A., and M. Walch. 1990. *The Color Compendium*. New York: Van Nostrand Reinhold.

Ievleva, L., and T. Orlick. 1991. "Mental Links to Enhanced Healing: An Exploratory Study." *Sport Psychologist* 5(1): 25–40.

Isaacs, N. 2005. "Good Health Could Be All in Your Imagination." *Alternative Medicine*, October, pp. 78–82.

Jasnoski, M., and J. Kugler. 1987. "Relaxation, Imagery, and Neuroimmunomodulation." *Annals of the New York Academy of Sciences* 496: 722–730.

Jung, C. 1964. *Man and His Symbols*. New York: Anchor Press.

Katra, J., and R. Tang. 1999. *The Heart of Mind*. Novatno, CA: New World Library.

Klisch, M. 1980. "The Simonton Method of Visualization: Nursing Implications and a Patient's Perspective." *Cancer Nursing* 33: 295–300.

Krippner, S. 1985. "The Role of Imagery in Health and Healing: A Review." *Saybrook Review* 5(1): 32–41

Krippner, S. 2000. "Healing and the Mind." International Conference on Science and Consciousness, Albuquerque, NM, April 28–May 3.

Lang, P. J. 1977. "Imagery and Therapy: An Information-Processing Analysis of Fear." *Behavior Therapy* 8: 862–886.

Leland, N. 1985. *Exploring Color*. Cincinnati, OH: North Light.

Liberman, J. 1991. *Light: Medicine of the Future*. Santa Fe, NM: Bear & Company.

Matthews, W. J., J. M. Conti, and S. G. Sireci. 2001. "The Effects of Intercessory Prayer, Positive Visualization, and Expectancy on the Well-Being of Kidney Dialysis Patients." *Alternative Therapies in Health and Medicine* 7(5): 42–52.

McKim, R. 1972. *Experiences in Visual Thinking*. Monterey, CA: Brooks/Cole.

Menzies, V., and A. Gill Taylor. 2004. "The Idea of Imagination: An Analysis of 'Imagery.'" *Advances in Mind-Body Medicine* 20(2): 4–10.

Miller, N. E. 1989. "Placebo Factors in Types of Treatment: View of a Psychologist." In *Nonspecific Aspects of Treatment*, edited by M. Shepherd and N. Sartorious. Lewiston, NY: Hans, Hubur.

Murphy, S. 1990. "Models of Imagery in Sport Psychology: A Review." *Journal of Mental Imagery* 14: 153–172.

Murphy, S., and M. Jowdy. 1991. "Imagery and Mental Rehearsal." In *Advances in Sport Psychology*, edited by T. Horn. Champaign, IL: Human Kinetics.

Naparstek, B. 1995. *Staying Well with Guided Imagery*. New York: Warner Books.

Naptarstek, B. 1998. *Your Sixth Sense*. New York: Harper One.

Naparstek, B. 2004. *Invisible Heroes*. New York: Bantam Books.

Naparstek, B. 2005. "Entering Our Broken Hearts: Guided Imagery for Posttraumatic Stress—An Interview with Belleruth Naparstek." Interview by Sheldon Lewis. *Advances in Mind Body Medicine* 21(1): 29–32.

Naparstek, B. 2011. "DCoE Releases 'Promising Practices.'" White paper, June 6. https://www.healthjourneys.com/blog/promising-practices-paper-is-out-fort-sill-effort-kicks-up-a-notch.

Neihardt, J. G. 1988. *Black Elk Speaks*. Lincoln: University of Nebraska Press.

Norris, P. 1992. "Psychoneuroimmunology: Visualization and Imagery." Paper presented to the Association for Applied Psychophysiology and Biofeedback, Colorado Springs, CO, March 19.

Ornstein, R., and D. Sobel. 1987. *The Healing Brain: Breakthrough Discoveries About How the Brain Keeps Us Healthy*. New York: Simon & Schuster.

Ott, J. N. 1985. "Color and Light: Their Effects on Plants, Animals, and People." *Journal of Biosocial Research* 7: 1.

Paddock J. R., S. Terranova, R. Kwok, and D. V. Halpern. 2000. "When Knowing Becomes Remembering: Individual Differences in Susceptibility to Suggestion." *Journal of Genetic Psychology* 161(4): 453–468.

Parnes, S. 1988. *Visionizing*. East Aurora, NY: D. O. K. Publishers.

Peale, N. 1956. *The Power of Positive Thinking*. Englewood Cliffs, NJ: Prentice Hall.

Pelletier, K. 1977. *Mind as Healer, Mind as Slayer*. New York: Dell.

Pettinati, P. 2001. "Meditation, Yoga and Guided Imagery." *Holistic Nursing Care* (16)1: 47–55.

Phillips, C. 2004. *Color for Life*. London: Ryland, Peters & Small.

Porter, G., and P. Norris. 1985. *Why Me? Harnessing the Healing Power of the Human Spirit*. Walpole, NH: Stillpoint.

Radner, G. 1989. *It's Always Something*. New York: Simon & Schuster.

Richardson, A. 1969. *Mental Imagery*. New York: Springer.

Richardson, M., J. Post-White, E. A. Grimm, L. A. Moye, S. E. Singletary, and B. Justice. 1997. "Coping, Life Attitudes and Immune Response to Imagery and Group Support After Breast Cancer Treatment." *Alternative Therapies* 3(5): 62–70.

Rossman, M. 2000. *Guided Imagery for Self-Healing* (2nd ed.). Tiburon, CA: HJ Kramer.

Rossman, M. 2002. "Imagery: The Body's Natural Language for Healing (An Interview)." *Alternative Therapies* 8(1): 80–89.

Rossman, M. 2003. *Fighting Cancer from Within*. New York: Owl Books.

Samuels, M. 1975. *Seeing with the Mind's Eye*. New York: Random House.

Scarf, M. 1980. "Images That Heal: A Doubtful Idea Whose Time Has Come." *Psychology Today* 14: 33–46.

Seaward, B. L. 2002. *A Change of Heart: Meditations and Visualizations* (audio CD). Boulder, CO: Inspiration Unlimited.

Seaward, B. L. 2002. *Sweet Surrender: Meditations and Visualizations* (audio CD). Boulder, CO: Inspiration Unlimited.

Seaward, B. L. 2004. *A Wing and a Prayer: Meditations and Visualizations* (audio CD). Boulder, CO: Inspiration Unlimited.

Simonton, O. C., S. Matthews-Simonton, and J. L. Creighton. 1980. *Getting Well Again*. New York: Bantam Books.

Singer, J. 1966. *Daydreaming*. New York: Random House.

Singer, J. 1974. *Imagery and Daydream Methods in Psychotherapy and Behavior Modification*. New York: Academic Press.

Singer, J., and K. Pope. 1978. *The Power of Human Imagination*. New York: Plenum Press.

Sokel, B., S. Devane, and A. Bentovim. 1991. "Getting Better with Honor: Individualized Relaxation/Self-Hypnosis Techniques for Control of Recalcitrant Abdominal Pain in Children." *Family Systems Medicine* 9(1): 83–91.

Taylor, S. 2005. *Health Psychology* (6th ed.). Englewood, NJ: McGraw-Hill.

Tuschen-Caffier, B., C. Vogele, S. Bracht, and A. Hilbert. 2003. "Psychological Responses to Body Shape Exposure in Patients with Bulimia Nervosa." *Behavior Research Therapy* 41(5): 573–586.

Tusek, D., J. Church, and V. Fazio. 1997. "Guided Imagery: A Significant Advance in the Care of Patients Undergoing Elective Colorectal Surgery." *Diseases of the Colon and Rectum* 40: 172–178.

Vines, S. 1988. "The Therapeutics of Guided Imagery." *Holistic Nursing Practice* 2: 34–44.

Watanabe, E., S. Fukuda, H. Hara, Y. Maeda, H. Ohira, and T. Shirakawa. 2006. "Differences in Relaxation by Means of Guided Imagery in a Healthy Community Sample." *Alternative Therapies in Health and Medicine* 12(2): 60–66.

Wilkinson, J. B. 1990. "Use of Hypnotherapy in Anxiety Management in the Terminally Ill." *British Journal of Experimental and Clinical Hypnosis* 7(1): 34–36.

Winger, W. 1977. *Voyages of Discovery*. Gaithersburg, MD: Psychogenics Press.

Wolpe, J. 1969. *The Practice of Behavioral Therapy*. New York: Pergamon Press.

Wyatt, G., A. Sikorskii, A. Siddiqi, and C. W. Given. 2007. "Feasibility of a Reflexology and Guided Imagery Intervention During Chemotherapy: Results of a Quasi-experimental Study." *Oncology Nursing Forum* 34(3): 635–642.

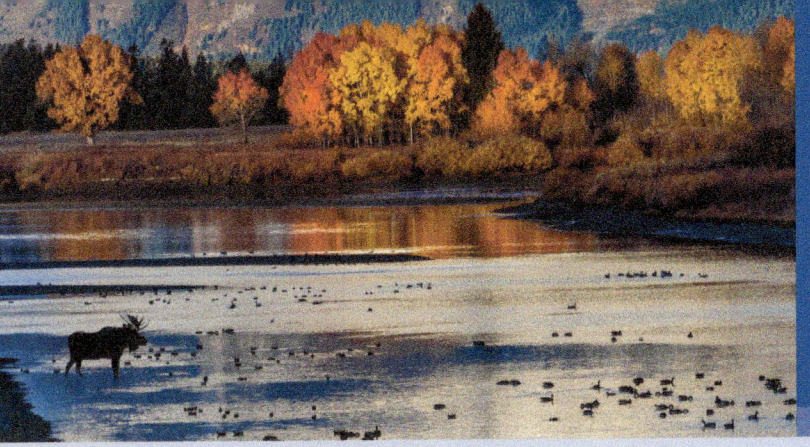

CHAPTER 22

Music Therapy

Music is a moral law. It gives soul to the universe,
wings to the mind, flight to the imagination,
and charm and gaiety to life and to everything.
It is the essence of order, and leads to all that is
good, just, and beautiful.

—Plato

When the coronavirus struck Italy in 2020 and quarantine measures were put in place, the Italians adapted very quickly to this new social mandate. In a country renowned for the likes of Puccini, Vivaldi, Albinoni, Scarlatti, Corelli, Pavarotti, Caruso, and Andrea Bocelli, COVID-19 could not stop the music, nor Italians' love of it. Soon videos appeared on social media of people singing opera arias on their balconies to their neighbors. People pulled out their keyboards and gave mini concerts to their friends and neighbors for weeks. As the coronavirus spread around the world, so, too, did videos of people in countries under lockdown playing music and singing songs to people within earshot as a means to join in solidarity under times of tremendous stress. People in the United States pulled out their guitars, keyboards, and fiddles and also played to their neighbors under quarantine. One of the best videos to hit social media were two American physicians playing/singing John Lennon's "Imagine" in the hospital lobby of the Mayo Clinic.

Perhaps since the first melodic birdsong was recognized by the human ear for its beautiful sound, music has been perceived to hold a special property of subtle mystical influence. Close your eyes for a moment and think of your current favorite song. Let the music linger in your mind, consciously savor it, and then sense how your body responds to the tones and rhythm of the melody. Various sounds, as a sensory stimulus, can provoke what is known as **stimulus generalization**, a type of conditioned response. For example, the sound of a car backfiring may elicit anxiety among combat veterans who have posttraumatic stress disorder (PTSD), just as a favorite love song can immediately retrieve memories of

Stimulus generalization: A conditioned response to a sound.

a former courtship. Without a doubt, the auditory stimulation called music can strongly influence our physical and emotional states. Music has the ability to motivate: For centuries it was utilized in the call to war with fife and drum. More recently, it has been used for a similar purpose during sports events with pep bands. But music can equally pacify or sedate: One need only think of a lullaby to help send a crying baby off to sleep.

For this reason, music in all its many styles can be considered a way to profoundly affect the human condition and a positive influence on relaxation. Although this seems to have been known intuitively for ages, music is now finally being recognized scientifically as possessing a strong therapeutic quality. There are two schools of thought regarding **music therapy**. The first advocates music making through singing and/or instrumentation for a therapeutic effect. This school of thought, clinically based on and shaped by specialists in the field, defines music therapy as the systematic application of music by the music therapist to bring about helpful changes in the emotional or physical health of the client. The second approach to music therapy seeks to achieve relaxation by listening to music. In this sense, music therapy can be defined as the ability to experience an altered state of physical arousal and mood through processing a progression of musical notes of varying tone, rhythm, and instrumentation of pleasing effect. It is this approach to music therapy that receives the greater attention in this chapter.

Music is a formidable part of the American (and world) culture, as evidenced by the popularity of streaming music services such as Spotify, Pandora, and Apple Music. Music as a means to promote tranquility has proven itself many times over as a very popular relaxation technique for all age groups, though the types of music used certainly vary. Although music therapy is considered, for the most part, a treatment to promote relaxation, it has characteristics of a coping technique as well, the main one being to increase conscious awareness of the inner self. Listening to certain types of music is believed by several musicologists to enhance the mind's receptivity to new ideas by accessing the less dominant right-brain thought processes. More specifically, music is thought to enhance creativity through spontaneous mental imagery. In many ways, music soothes the

> **Music therapy:** The use of music—listening to, singing, or performing—as a means to promote relaxation and homeostasis.

"savage beast" of us all. Those who play video games will tell you how important music is to the experience.

Although investigations of this type of relaxation technique are young, and the physiological dynamics affected are not fully understood, the benefits of music therapy are unequivocal. So popular is this relaxation technique that it has become an area of great research interest in the past several years. Today, the focus of research into the benefits of music therapy is wide and far-reaching, including the effects of music on postoperative pain (Bradt 2010; Whitaker 2010), Alzheimer's patients (Zare et al. 2010), and pediatric health care (Treurnicht Naylor et al. 2011), all of which reveal the healing powers of music as a powerful agent for stress reduction. To best understand how music is currently used as a therapy, it is helpful to see how this tool has been used through the ages.

■ Historical Perspective

The earliest humans about which we have any knowledge believed that music could exorcise evil spirits and heal wounds. The ancient Greeks, including Aristotle, Plato, and Pythagoras, possessed an intuitive understanding of the healing power of music, suggesting that daily exposure could contribute to health. Aristotle held the notion that flute music offered a cathartic release of emotions. Plato indicated that music restored the harmony and contentment in one's soul as well as the moral welfare of the nation at large. "Music is the moral law," he wrote. "It is the essence of order and leads to all that is good, just, and beautiful, passionate and eternal form." Pythagoras credited the rhythm of music with special healing qualities. "All things are constructed of harmonic patterns. It is only when we are out of step with the natural harmonic that disharmony arises," he wrote (Merritt 1990).

Medieval monarchs employed court minstrels, as well as jesters, to bring the comfort of peaceful melodies to their castles to relieve their melancholy, depression, and fevers. Later, many classical musicians, including Bach, Pachelbel, and Mozart, were commissioned by royalty and nobility to compose pieces of music for this very reason. But the power of music was enjoyed not only by the upper classes. For centuries, long before radios, videos, and streaming music services, family members of all social classes gathered together regularly for words and melody. It was not uncommon for both parents and children to learn to play instruments for the purpose of soothing entertainment. The ability to play together harmoniously was a metaphor for attempts to live together in peace.

Native American medicine men or shamans often used music in their healing rituals as a powerful medicine for the sick and dying, as well as for peace and prosperity. The musical incantations and accompanying drumbeats served as a vehicle of divine communication to heal or strengthen the will of the human spirit. Likewise, across the ocean, Africans have been known for centuries to employ percussion rhythms as healing tools to lower heart rates and fever in the sick (Assagioli 1999). Music, including Gospel spirituals, was a saving grace to Africans brought to the New World as slaves, who lived under the most austere and brutal conditions. In fact, all music was a relief to those subjected to the institution of slavery, and the influence of African music and percussion on American music gave birth to jazz, Delta blues, soul, and hip hop.

With the invention of the phonograph in 1877, music became more easily accessible to people in all corners of the globe. In the late nineteenth and early twentieth centuries, it became a respected therapeutic practice in Europe for the treatment of mental disorders. Not until 1926, however, was music recognized by the established medical community as a form of therapy for the treatment of several clinical disorders, most notably depression. And although music in its many forms and styles, and in nearly every culture around the world, has been accepted by the masses as a tool to promote relaxation and healing, it was not until 1946 that it was formally acknowledged in the United States as a bona fide therapy and legitimate discipline worthy of investigation. The introduction of music in several Veterans Administration hospitals serving World War II veterans with battle fatigue (now called PTSD) demonstrated that this type of stimulation could boost morale and improve patients' mental state by decreasing symptoms associated with depression. The National Association for Music Therapy (NAMT) was founded in 1950. Through the work of several pioneer researchers, by the 1970s and 1980s music therapy was advocated as a viable tool to deal with the clinical symptoms of stress.

Norman Cousins is most well known for introducing and legitimizing the healing power of humor and laughter, but in his acclaimed book *Anatomy of an Illness as Perceived by the Patient* (1979) he dedicated a whole chapter to the healing properties of music. Recounting stories of when he met cello virtuoso Pablo Casals and famed physician Albert Schweitzer, Cousins described how both men took creative refuge in playing the piano. Cousins once observed Casals, at the age of 90, get painfully out of bed, and then become youthfully transformed when he sat down at the piano to play Brahms's B-flat Quartet. Similarly, Schweitzer, in his eighth decade of life, would balance his work in medicine with a nightly rendition of Bach's Toccata in D minor. Cousins saw in both men a regeneration and restoration in their savoring of music, hinting that it may have contributed to their health and longevity. Renowned neurologist and author Oliver Sacks discovered the use of music as therapy for his patients with severe Parkinson's disease. His insights were made famous in the movie *Awakenings* (1990) starring Robin Williams. In his book *Musicophilia* (2007), Sacks noted that people suffering from Alzheimer's, strokes, and severe depression can all benefit from the use of music therapy. "Music is full of mysterious powers," he stated.

In the late 1970s and early 1980s, about the same time that stress entered the consciousness of the American public and became a household word, there began to emerge a new type of relaxing composition now commonly referred to as New Age music. Markedly different from rock, pop, blues, classical, and jazz, New Age music consists of slow-tempo, instrumental, often synthesized, and occasionally acoustic collaboration of melodies and chord progressions to alter mood and increase conscious awareness. Musicologists Andrew Watson and Nevill Drury trace the beginnings of New Age music to the counterculture period of the 1960s, when elements of rock, jazz, folk, Indian *ragas*, and meditative music were integrated to create repeated cycles of gentle undulating sounds for a relaxing effect. The band Pink Floyd is given credit for making this style of music popular with its *Meddle* album in which the entire second side, "Echoes," is a single instrumental composition played on a synthesizer. The lineage of New Age musicians unfolded from Pink Floyd's inspirational work to include a collaborative effort by King Crimson's Robert Fripp and Roxy Music's Brian Eno entitled "Evening Star." Eno went on to record several albums, including "Music for Airports" and "Ambient Two," becoming a dominant force in the New Age genre (Watson and Drury 1987). This style of music has now spread to all continents, giving rise to many other New Age and environmental musicians, including Kitaro (Japan); Andreas Vollenweider (Germany); Jean-Michel Jarre (France); Vangelis (Greece); Enya (Ireland); and Paul Horn, Philip Glass, Steven Halpern, David Lanz, and William Ackerman (North America), to name a few. Although the methods of distribution of music have changed over the years from record stores to streaming music services, the popularity of various types of music has not changed. Perhaps this is most obvious with the plethora of music programming on satellite radio (SiriusXM) and various online broadcasts. Although New Age music is no longer "new," the ambient relaxing style of this genre remains quite popular for many adults. However, New Age music is just one of many styles that can promote relaxation. Classical, jazz, and acoustic folk are thought to be equally successful in effecting or enhancing the relaxation response. Today, music of all styles is used in many different clinical and professional settings as a therapeutic tool.

From Sound to Noise to Music

Sound is energy made audible. It is created through random or periodic vibrations that are represented as waves. Sounds can be perceived as either pleasant or unpleasant, the latter commonly referred to as "noise." Sound waves or oscillations are measured in **hertz (Hz)**—cycles or vibrations per second. These oscillations are perceived as **pitch** by the human ear (**FIG. 22.1**). The audible frequency or sonic range detectable to the

> **Hertz (Hz):** A measure of sound frequency. It is the number of oscillations or vibrations produced per second.
>
> **Pitch:** The detection of sound by the human ear as higher or lower based on the frequency of vibration.
>
> **Decibel (dB):** A unit of measurement (named in honor of Alexander Graham Bell) to denote the level of sound/noise measured as pressure through air.

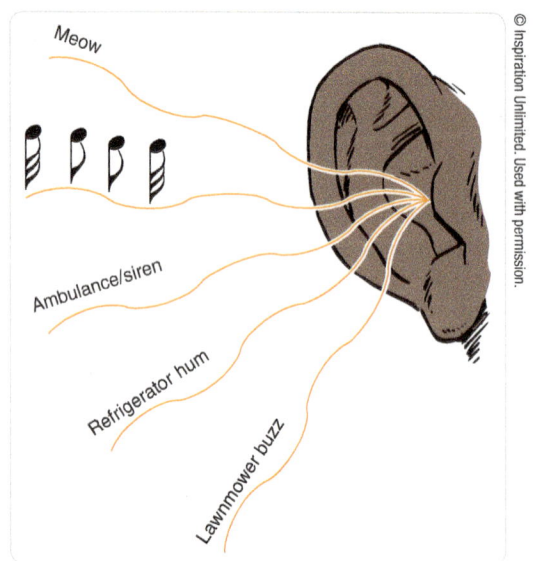

FIGURE 22.1   Sound waves enter the ear and pass through the eardrum to be processed by the brain.

human ear is 20 to 20,000 Hz, depending on the health and training of the auditory nerve tissue. Sound waves can also be detected by means of different neural pathways through the conduction of skin and bone tissue.

Whereas vibrations are measured in hertz, or frequencies representing a number of oscillations per second, sounds are recorded in units of measurement called **decibels (dB)**, in honor of inventor Alexander Graham Bell. Decibels signify the air pressure that specific sounds produce as detected by the human ear. One decibel is said to be the softest sound that can be detected by humans. In the days of horse-drawn carriages, calls for help could be yelled from windows and heard across town. With the advancement of modern technology, however, average ambient noise levels in metropolitan cities are currently measured at 122 dB, 2 decibels above the demarcation inducing pain. Today, a yell would not be heard over the cacophony of sounds two city blocks away. Repeated exposure to high-decibel noise can not only trigger the body's stress response, but also cause damage to the human ear (Halpern 1985) (**FIG. 22.2**). Noise-induced hearing impairment

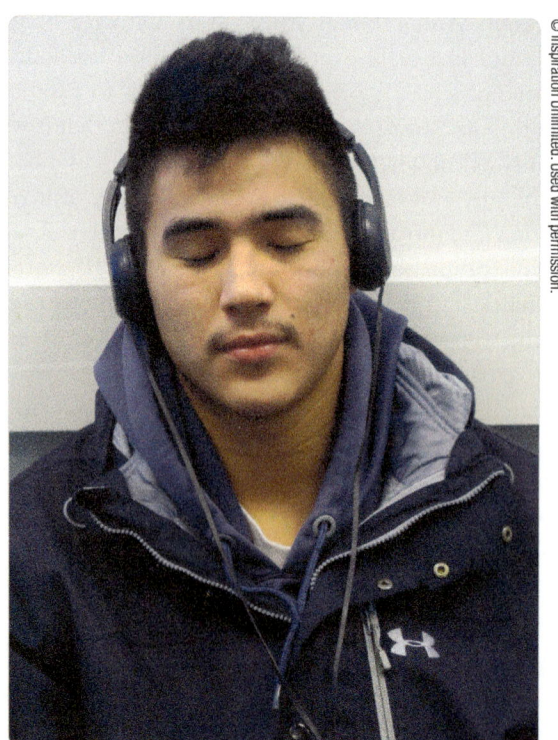

FIGURE 22.2   Headphones can provide a sense of solitude when listening to music. Repeated exposure to high volumes with headsets, however, can impair hearing and result in early onset deafness.

or loss is both cumulative and permanent. **Tinnitus** is the clinical name given to constant buzzing, hissing, or ringing in the ear that can arise from repeated exposure to loud noise. A concern exists today among the nation's audiologists that the onset of hearing impairment from ambient noise levels, combined with use of portable headphones, will occur at an increasingly younger age. It has been speculated that not only can noise be perceived as stressful, but hearing dysfunction may also become a low-intensity chronic stressor. Like hypertension, the early stages of hearing loss go undetected without a diagnostic test. TABLE 22.1 contains a list of outdoor locations and various noise producers and their respective decibel levels.

Perhaps in reaction to noise pollution, sound stimulation, called white noise, has been used to mask, balance, or neutralize stressful, noisy environments. Technically speaking, white noise is composed of broadband sounds that include all frequencies of the audible spectrum. This is the concept behind the noise-canceling headphones you see advertised in airports and various magazines. Although some music can serve as white noise, its greatest potential is in enhancing tranquility. In his acclaimed book *This Is Your Brain on Music* (2007), former rock musician turned neuroscientist Daniel Levitin explores exactly how music coordinates the hemispheres

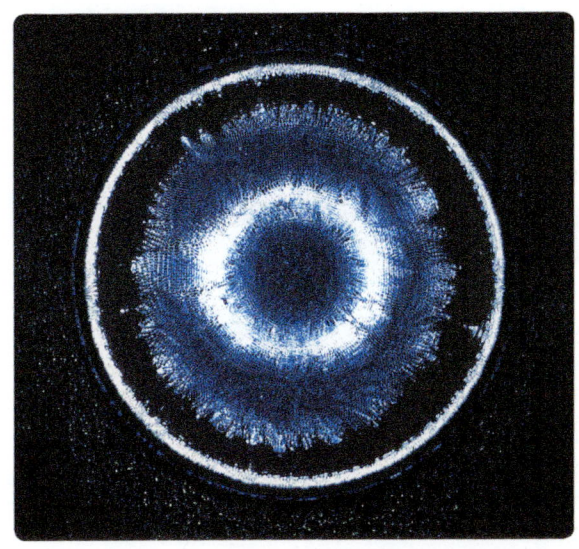

Photographs from Water Sound Images by Alexander Lauterwasser. © 2006 MACROmedia Publishing, Eliot, ME, USA. www.cymaticsource.com. Used by Permission.

FIGURE 22.3 Sound waves produced by the didgeridoo, an Australian Aboriginal instrument, are captured in a small sample of water revealing this beautiful harmonic pattern and showing the entraining effect of sonic vibration on water.

of the brain in ways previously unknown before the use of magnetic resonance imaging (MRI). From Mozart to U2, Levitin concludes that music, more so than language, is fundamental to the development of human nature.

Music in its entirety is greater than the sum of its parts. In the words of music scholar Randall McClellan (1988), "Music is a dynamic multilayered matrix of constantly shifting tonal relationships unfolding within time." It is this dynamic matrix that induces a profound sense of relaxation (FIG. 22.3).

■ Music as a Relaxation Technique

There are several schools of thought, developed by both the hard and soft sciences, regarding the relationship between music and relaxation. Each can make a contribution to the understanding of music's role in the relaxation response. Regardless of the theory invoked, the frequencies transmitted as the sounds of music and received by the body significantly affect human physiology. But exactly how these frequencies are received is still in the speculation stage. Maybe the answer is a combination of two or more theories (BOX 22.1).

TABLE 22.1	Loudness of Some Everyday Sounds
Sound	**Loudness (dB)**
Rustling leaves	10
Normal conversation	50
Suburban neighborhood noise	52
Vacuum cleaner	70
City noise; busy traffic	80
Inside a passenger jet (take-off)	78–83
Heavy trucks at 50 feet	76–88
Home shop tools	65–110
Subway noise	80–114
Nearby jet airplane	150
Shooting a gun	150–170

Reproduced from S. Alters and W. Schiff. 2011. *Essential Concepts for Healthy Living*, 5th ed. update. Sudbury, MA: Jones & Bartlett Learning, p. 470.

Tinnitus: The clinical name given to the symptom of ringing, hissing, or buzzing in the ears.

BOX 22.1   The Distinctive Qualities of Music

Music consists of many qualities that combine for an aesthetic auditory experience:

Tone: An initial sound or vibration.

Pitch: The frequency of oscillations or vibrations. The higher the pitch, the more rapid the vibrations. A high pitch is thought to produce sympathetic nervous arousal, whereas a low pitch is thought to be conducive to relaxation.

Intensity: Relative loudness or amplitude of vibrations. High intensity has the effects of emotional domination and coerciveness, whereas low intensity is considered more tranquil and serene.

Timbre: "Tone color." Timbre is what makes the same notes played on different instruments sound very different.

Harmony: The ratio and relationship between tones (sounds) and their rhythmic patterns.

Interval: The units of the musical scale and the vertical distance between notes, giving rise to the structure of melodies and harmonies.

Rhythm: The most dynamic of musical qualities. Rhythm is described as the time pattern (horizontal distance) of music that seems to elicit such strong emotional responses. The bass frequencies most influence the rhythm of music.

Perceptual quality: The intellectual processing of sounds with the attachment of subjective attitudes to each sound.

Modified from A. Watson and N. Drury. 1987. *Healing Music: The Harmonic Path to Wholeness*. Dorset, UK: Prism Press.

Biochemical Theory

Music appears to affect human physiology directly through the cerebral cortex and autonomic nervous system. Through the ear's complicated structure, sound stimuli are received by the brain via special nervous tissue of the ear (organ of Corti, or hair cells), where vibrations are converted to electrical nerve impulses. (It is interesting to note that these hair cells are only a membrane away from the lymph fluid of the inner ear, suggesting a link to

Essentic forms: Musical patterns (vibrations) that are thought to influence neuropeptide activity and thus metabolic activity in the body.

the immune system. In addition, the eardrum appears to have a liaison with the parasympathetic nervous system via the vagus nerve.) In a very complex network of neurons, these impulses are thought to be first decoded by the cerebral cortex, then deciphered by the subcortex, and subsequently directed from the limbic system through the autonomic nervous system, potentially throughout the entire body. Elements involved with these auditory sensations include pitch, rhythm, tone, tempo, volume, and, perhaps most important, perceptual quality, or the emotional effects of deciphered sounds. Depending on interpretation (like or dislike), either the sympathetic or parasympathetic nervous system may be activated.

One theory proposed by neuropsychologist and composer Dr. Manfred Clynes (1982) suggests that humans have a dominant rhythm style (DRS), a pulse indirectly controlled by the heart, directed by neural and hormonal chemical processes. This DRS, like a thermostat, has a set point specific to these internal influences. The body's rhythm, however, can be additionally influenced by external rhythms, from the repetitive pulsations of a jackhammer to the symphonic rhythm of Mozart's Piano Concerto in C minor. The body's DRS is thought to be subject to the influences of musical resonance or sympathetic vibrations. Clynes hypothesizes that the nervous system contains several codes capable of influencing the body's responses to musical rhythm, melody, and tone. Clynes's theory implies that these codes comprise **essentic forms** that influence neuropeptide activity, and thus the metabolic functions of body organs, most notably the heart muscle.

Although many organs are involved in producing the DRS, the most obvious window to the body's rhythm is heart rate. Although there are variations from person to person, the average human heart rate has a rhythm of between 60 and 80 beats per minute. Music therapists have found that most Western music is paced at this same tempo, and some believe that music with this rhythm has the greatest influence on physiological homeostasis. Several studies have investigated the effects of music on electrical stimulation of the heart, with inconclusive results (Knight 2001; Shaw 2000). Although some suggest that slow-paced music lowers heart rate, others find no significant effect. This may be related to the perceptual quality of the music, because other studies indicate the relaxation response is most pronounced when subjects select their own music.

A neurological study involving subjects connected to an electroencephalograph (EEG device) while listening to slow-tempo music revealed that the musical rhythm quickly synchronized brain rhythms to its beat, and even more so with musicians than nonmusicians (Bhattacharya and Petsce 2005).

Researchers have examined other physiological effects of musical stimulation, including muscle tension and corticosteroid levels. In these cases, music was used in conjunction with other relaxation techniques such as guided mental imagery and biofeedback. In one study conducted by Mark Rider and his colleagues at Eastern Montana College in 1985, subjects listened to audiotapes of two orchestral pieces for a 3-week period. Progressive relaxation techniques were dubbed over the music track. Results revealed decreases in cortisol levels much more pronounced than those observed when listening to relaxation techniques without a music track. Similarly, when music was integrated with biofeedback, the combined effect was even greater in reducing muscle tension than by biofeedback alone. The use of relaxing music as a sedative has also been shown to be effective in reducing stress and muscular tension associated with the process of childbirth, especially when subjects have had numerous positive exposures to a piece of music prior to delivery.

If a slow musical rhythm is conducive to relaxation, is there a rhythm or beat that is unhealthy? A theory called switching, postulated by Dr. John Diamond (1983), hints of the validity of this notion. Measuring electrical conduction and strength in muscle fibers, Diamond found that the "stop anapestic beat" common in rock music (i.e., short, short, long, pause, or da-da-DAA-pause) decreased the force of muscle contractions. Diamond hypothesized that this "weak" beat distorts or switches the communication of neural messages from the right and left hemispheres of the brain. Diamond also believes this beat decreases several cognitive functions, including judgment and perception. In addition, Diamond suggests that music with this beat has an addictive quality and that repeated exposure may, in fact, be harmful. That is, music of this kind may be associated with the inability to return to a homeostatic baseline, as measured by higher resting heart rate and blood pressure values.

Music appreciation is thought to be a right-brain function; it is the right hemisphere of the brain that recognizes and processes auditory stimulation in the form of musical note and chord progressions. This appears especially true when music is instrumental, or without lyrics. The left cerebral hemisphere, proficient in verbal acuity, is thought to intercept auditory stimulation of music *with* lyrics, if analysis of musical composition and instrumentation is initiated. For this reason, instrumentals are thought to promote a greater sense of relaxation than music combined with lyrics. (Note: Lyrics sung in a foreign language—such as Enya singing in Latin or Celtic—can be relaxing because the brain merely interprets the singer's voice as a calming instrument.) In addition, music that consists of a series of repetitive notes or beats may act much like a mantra, inducing a meditative state of relaxation. Although yet unproven, it has been speculated by some that music may release endorphins (neuropeptides and chemical opiates) from the brain and other body tissues, which create a sensation of euphoria or inspirational high. Another neurotransmitter, melanin, has been researched to determine its effects as an electrical semiconductor. According to Dr. Frank Barr, melanin is capable of converting light energy to sound energy through neurochemical messages. Further research on these and other functions of special neurotransmitters may support the **biochemical theory** (Barr 1983).

Entrainment Theory

Scientists are in agreement that cell metabolism operates on chemical energy—the breakdown of carbohydrates, fats, and proteins for energy metabolism at the biochemical level. There is also agreement that the human body is a channel for electrical energy that can be measured through various types of biofeedback, including EKGs, EEGs, and EMGs, which record the electrical impulses given off by various organ tissues. You have probably experienced this type of energy when getting a shock from walking across a carpeted and then touching something. A new theory, which parallels and possibly integrates with the biochemical theory, suggests that sounds are received through a sixth sense, the human energy field (Campbell 1991; Halpern 1985).

Virtually all objects produce oscillations, including living organisms. Any object that produces vibrations creates its own field of energy, and the movement of subatomic particles is typically called an electromagnetic field. In terms of human beings, this may be referred to

> **Biochemical theory:** A theory suggesting that music is received internally through the eardrum with sounds converted into neurochemicals that are registered by the brain, which one then finds either pleasant or unpleasant.

as an energy field or aura. In quantum physics, research has shown that the smallest subatomic particles create vibrations. The human body contains many organs that produce biorhythmic oscillations (e.g., brain waves, heart rate, and those produced through muscle tension). But the body as a whole, composed of jillions of atoms, also produces oscillations. As suggested by Itzhak Bentov in *Stalking the Wild Pendulum* (1988), in a natural, relaxed state, the body itself produces a single unified series of oscillations at 7.8 Hz; this is the frequency of human homeostasis. **Schumann's resonance** is a term used to describe the planet Earth's own vibration, which is a function of its circumference and electromagnetic radiation calculated at a frequency of approximately 7.8 cycles per second. Remarkably, this frequency is identical to both the frequency of alpha waves produced by the human brain at rest and the sounds produced by dolphins. In the words of music therapist Steve Halpern (Halpern, with Savary, 1985), "Being in harmony with oneself and the universe is more than a poetic concept."

In 1665, a Dutch physicist named Christian Huygens discovered that when he placed two clocks side by side, eventually their pendulums would swing together in a unified rhythm (**FIG. 22.4**). This matched rhythm is called **entrainment** and is defined as: mutual phase-locking oscillations of like frequencies in the same environment. When two or more objects produce oscillations in close proximity, the dominant frequency will prevail. Eventually, they will "entrain" together in a unified frequency. The entrainment of oscillation is thought to be nature's own attempt to conserve energy.

Like a tuning fork that begins to resonate when another tuning fork producing sound waves is brought in close proximity, entrainment theory suggests that if one organ—the heart, say—increases its oscillations as a result of heightened metabolic activity, adjacent organs will entrain to that frequency. If several body organs are influenced to entrain at a higher frequency, over time the result is a decreased ability to return to a homeostatic condition. The same phenomenon occurs in response to external oscillations. Like a radio receiver, the body is a

> **Schumann's resonance:** The vibration of planet Earth: 7.8 Hertz.
>
> **Entrainment:** The mutual phase locking of like oscillations; in human physiology, organs or organisms giving off strong vibrations influencing organs or organisms with weaker vibrations to match the stronger rate of oscillation; thought to conserve energy.

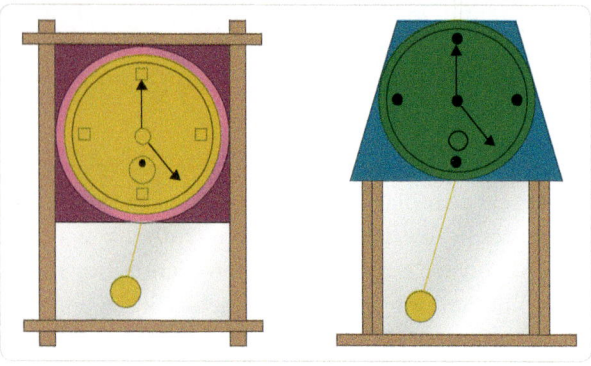

FIGURE 22.4 The concept of entrainment was first observed in the motion of two pendulum clocks. This energy pattern has since been detected in both inanimate and animate objects, such as schools of moving fish and even the synchronous flashing of fireflies.

transformer; it receives (absorbs) as well as emits oscillations. If external rhythms are more dominant (i.e., greater than 7.8 Hz), then they force the body to go "out of tune" with itself by entraining to a higher vibration. The most common example of human entrainment is the female menstrual cycle. It has long been recognized, but until recently poorly understood, that in some areas when two or more women live or work together for prolonged periods of time, their menstrual cycles entrain—their menses occur on or about the same day (Weller and Weller 1999). The same phenomenon has been observed in the blinking patterns of fireflies that land on the same bush, as well as the movement patterns of schools of fish and flocks of birds.

The entrainment theory gained support from a series of studies conducted in the early 1970s on the effects of music on the growth of plants, organisms with no known nervous system. Dr. Dorothy Retallack (1973), for example, conducted a study examining leaf growth and water absorption when corn, squash, petunias, zinnias, and marigolds were exposed to music. She found that some types of music induced a "fertilizing effect," promoting plant growth. Interestingly, she discovered that when in the presence of classical music (Bach) and Indian sitar music (Ravi Shankar), plants grew in the direction of the speakers (sometimes even around the speakers), showing a preference for these styles of music. When subjected to loud rock and roll or acid rock, though, they grew away from the speakers. In fact, many of these plants became dehydrated; some even died. Other comparable studies investigating the effects of music on animals have revealed that chickens

Stress with a Human Face

The sound of applause is not usually considered to be a symphony of sorts, but it is music to the ears of singer/songwriter Naomi Judd, who, with her daughter Wynonna, became one of the nation's most renowned country music acts, The Judds. Stricken with a potentially fatal case of hepatitis C, Naomi's singing career was nearly cut short in the summer of 1990. Told she could have only a few years to live, her team of physicians gave a typical forecast for a person in Naomi's condition and then sent her home. A woman of great faith, Naomi decided to listen to the voice in her heart more than the voices of her physicians, and determined that she would not be a passive victim to her condition. Instead, she would become an active participant in her healing journey.

A longtime advocate of the mind-body-spirit connection, Naomi began to apply what she knew in her heart to be true. Setting her focus on healing, she planned a strategy for her recovery. One day, after calling her husband Larry, daughters Wynonna and Ashley, and other family members to her bedside, she informed them of her game plan. In her heart Naomi knew that if she were to disconnect from her profession, her colleagues, and her

music, she would die in record time. She decided to fight back. She announced to those around her that she would go back on tour—a farewell tour. But this would be no ordinary tour. Not only would she give the gift of music, this time she would receive it as well—from the audience. Knowing how powerful the energy of love was, after performing each song, she would soak up the applause, the whistles, the cheers, and direct this energy throughout her body—asking the vibrations to stimulate her immune system to heal the cells of her liver and send the virus into remission. She said, "I would turn each standing ovation, this applause into prayerful support." And it worked! More than two decades later, she is doing well, having tested "negative" 15 years in a row, and sharing the message of faith, hope, and love as essential components of the mind-body-spirit equation.

Music has always held a soft spot in Naomi's heart and that spot continues to grow as she shares her message of the healing journey that we all must take part in to nurture our souls and become whole.

---

lay more eggs and some cows produce more milk when music is piped into their living quarters. Although obviously more complex than either plants or chickens, humans are thought to be influenced in much the same way (Harrelson 2006).

Robert Monroe (1993), former director of the Mutual Broadcasting Network and founder/director of the Monroe Institute, experimented with various frequencies and their effects on brain waves. His findings led him to conclude that specific frequencies (0.5 to 20 Hz), not musical rhythms, were what allowed the brain to entrain to an alpha rhythm, or what he called a frequency-following response. Experimenting further with various frequencies directed toward the right and left ear, he found that he could actually entrain both cerebral hemispheres—which Monroe called "hemi-Sync"—producing a most profound state of relaxation and altered state of consciousness.

Thus, the entrainment theory concludes that relaxing music can have a calming effect because elevated body rhythms entrain with a slower, more natural homeostatic

rhythm produced by a musical composition. Quite literally, relaxation occurs when the body is in harmony with itself and the natural world. Proponents of this theory indicate that many people who listen to upbeat music to relax may in effect throw off their natural body rhythm. This could explain why various parameters measured by biofeedback instruments have not shown a musically induced state of relaxation with all types of music. Currently, musicians such as Steven Halpern and James Owen Matthews are experimenting with incorporating the 7.8 Hz frequency into music, including dolphin "songs" and whale "music" (**FIG. 22.5**).

Metaphysical Theory

The least scientific but perhaps the most intuitively true theory suggests that music has a divine quality. Music is a gift from God, or so Orpheus thought. Greek legend has it that Orpheus was given a lyre by Apollo (the god of music) to offer songs of praise. Although Apollo bequeathed this gift, it was the muses who taught Orpheus to play, hence the word *music*. While

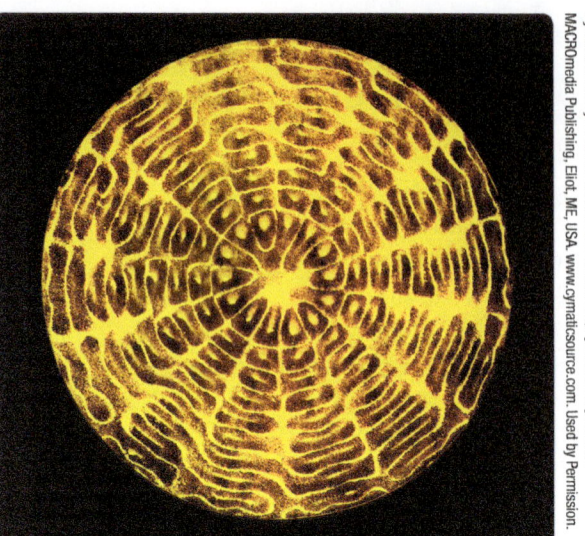

FIGURE 22.5 This mandala-shaped, sonorous figure was created by vibrating a steel plate that was covered with quartz sand, a process referred to as cymatics. The sand collected in the areas of least vibration, along the nodal lines of the steel plate. The plate diameter is 32 cm, the thickness 0.5 mm. This pattern occurred at a frequency of 8,200 Hz.

neurophysiologists like Oliver Sacks have looked for "substance" in the calming effects of music, students of higher consciousness such as Jonathan Goldman have searched for "essence." They theorize that music is a holy (i.e., making whole or healing) gift communicating through the soul or human spirit. Virtually every

> **Metaphysical theory:** A theory that suggests that music is a gift from God.

culture employs music as a vehicle for meditation, from European Gregorian chants, to Native American "sings," to African American gospels. Even classical composers such as Bach, Beethoven, and Mozart were often said to compose through divine inspiration. Bach was once quoted as saying, "The aim and final reason of all music should be nothing else but the glory of God and the refreshment of the spirit." Beethoven once said, "Music is the one incorporeal entrance into the higher world" (Merritt 1990).

Proponents of **metaphysical theory**, including French psychologist and audiologist Alfred Tomatis (1981), hypothesize that music and song have a transcending quality that provides a direct communications link to a higher power. This theory also gives credence to the idea that music is a universal language. Musicologist and composer Dr. Steven Halpern advocates a musical meditation that pairs musical notes with the body's seven metaphysical energy sources, or chakras. In an exercise he titles the spectrum meditation (TABLE 22.2), musical notes are paired with visualization of specific colors, body regions, and meditative thoughts in a particular sequence for a 20-minute period. In research conducted by Halpern (1978) to measure the relaxing effects of musical composition, it was observed that both classical and New Age—specifically Halpern's Spectrum Suite Meditation—produced a significant decrease in the stress response as measured by biofeedback (galvanic skin response).

Music therapist Stephanie Merritt suggests that music has the divine ability to unite or connect the human spirit of all individuals. Citing many examples of the powerful effects of classical music in her book *Mind, Music, and Imagery* (1990), Merritt writes, "Music brings us

TABLE 22.2　Spectrum Meditation

Note	Body Region (Chakra)	Color	Meditative Thought	
B	Crown of head	Violet	I am connected.	
A	Center of forehead	Indigo	I am balanced.	
G	Throat	Blue	My life has a meaningful purpose.	
F	Heart	Green	I choose to love.	
E	Solar plexus	Yellow	I am loved.	
D	Below navel	Orange	I am centered.	
C	Base of spine	Red	I am grounded.	

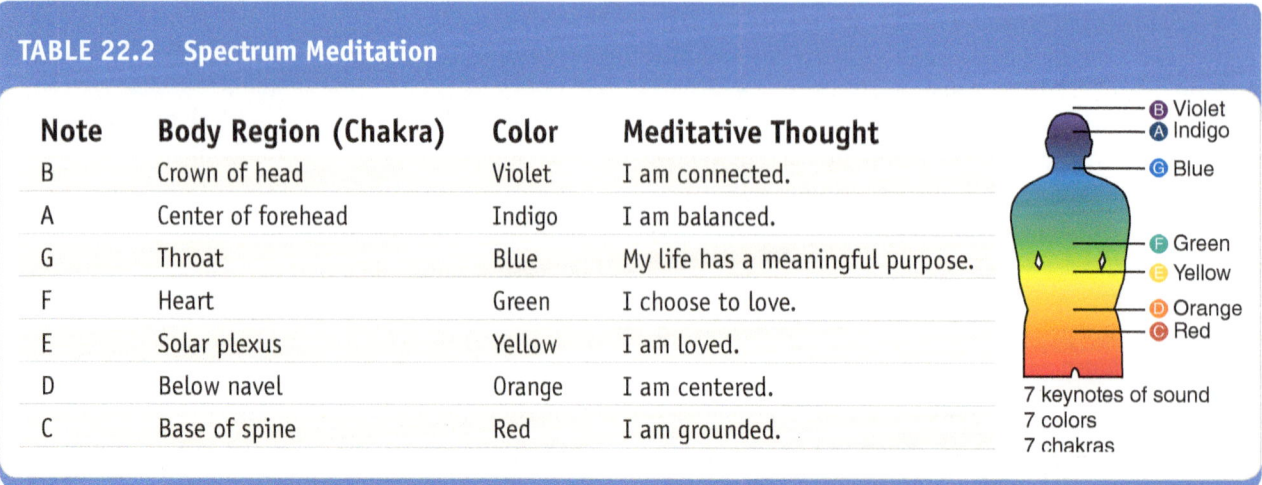

B Violet
A Indigo
G Blue
F Green
E Yellow
D Orange
C Red

7 keynotes of sound
7 colors
7 chakras

back to the consciousness of our oneness and shows us, on a deep level, how much our progress as a human race depends on a mutual love and assistance." Integrating concepts of Jung's theory of individuation and intuition with elements of creativity and right-brain thinking, Merritt hypothesizes that music influences more than just neurons in the body. Although not every type of music can raise one's spirits, the influence of music to provide inspiration of all kinds cannot be argued.

■ Psychological Effects of Music

Perhaps equal to the profound physiological effects produced by music are its apparent effects on attitudes and moods, including fear and depression. Typically, the first thing people say when they hear music they like is how good it makes them feel inside. This was the desired effect when musical recordings were played for several World War II veterans. Exposure to selections of music appeared to decrease symptoms of despondency and in some cases altered mood into modest expressions of joy and pleasure.

The limbic system, particularly the hypothalamus (known as "the seat of the emotions"), is believed to house the neurons that, when stimulated through auditory sensations, can alter mood or emotion. While individuals often recognize at the conscious level the influence music has on mood, auditory stimuli can also penetrate the unconscious mind and promote their own changes in perception and mood. It has long been known in the world of marketing that when slow versions of familiar music, and now even golden oldies, are played in grocery stores, consumers tend to stay longer and make more purchases. This is the intent of the music—to increase sales. Mark Alpert and colleagues validated this marketing ploy in an article published in the *Journal of Business Research* (2005). Slow-tempo music has also been introduced into settings of anxiety such as dentists' and physicians' offices. The premise of this type of music is "stimulus progression," instrumental music that is easily digested by auditory channels. It is the basis for contemporary background music produced by the Muzak Corporation.

Music in all its complexity of arrangement can produce as well as reduce stressful emotions. In the days of silent movies, theaters would hire piano players to compose on-site soundtracks to enhance the emotions of viewers during both dramatic and romantic scenes. With the advent of "talkies," Hollywood incorporated musical soundtracks into its films to highlight emotionally charged scenes and fuel the emotional roller coaster from fear to love, a practice still employed in both movies and television commercials.

Whereas music in elevators and grocery stores may appear normal these days, music in operating rooms may seem a rather novel approach to speeding the healing process. In an experiment to determine the effects of classical music on anxious hospital patients, music therapist Dr. Helen Bonny (Bonny, with Savary 1973) created a series of tapes to be played primarily in the intensive care units at Jefferson General Hospital in Port Townsend, Washington, and St. Agnes Hospital in Baltimore, Maryland. Results revealed significant reductions in both physiological parameters, including blood pressure, heart rate, ventilations, and muscle tension, and increased ability to sleep, as well as reductions in psychological factors including anxiety and depression. Nurses even noticed increased ease in changing intravenous needles.

Music can reach and extend our deepest thoughts and feelings in a way that verbal language cannot. Music has the ability to break down strong emotional defenses and allow for the expression of feelings. Thus, controlled music therapy sessions have been conducted for hundreds of patients as an exercise for the cathartic release of latent or suppressed emotions. Loud, rapid-tempo music has been used by music therapists to assist in the release of latent anger. Uplifting, slow, rhythmic music has been played to both sedate and rejuvenate the body's organ tissues (**FIG. 22.6**).

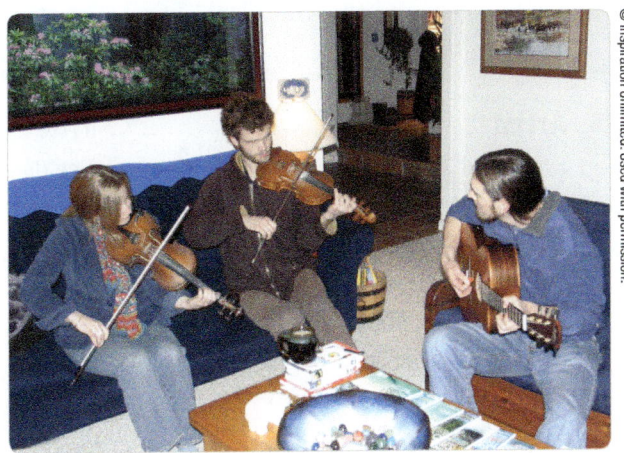

FIGURE 22.6 Listening to calming music can be very relaxing. Music therapy also includes playing music, which can also bring about a sense of tranquility.

Without a doubt music has a profound effect on emotions at both the conscious and unconscious levels. Music heard for the first time often forms associations with the listener's state of mind at that time; hence, emotional attachments are often made to particular pieces of music. Thus, different types of music can be strongly correlated with physical arousal as well as relaxation. In a study to assess the relationship between type of music, musical selection, and enjoyment, and self-reported states of relaxation, Valerie Stratton and Anthony Zalanowski (1984) found no single type of music effective in enhancing relaxation for all subjects. Rather, the critical factor was the degree to which the subject *liked* the music selection. A similar study by McCraty (1998) found similar results. In another investigation, William Davis and Michael Thaut (1989) attempted to determine which types of music people considered relaxing. The music selected by subjects ranging in age from 18 to 43 included U2, Liz Story, Dan Fogelberg, Santana, Mozart, George Thorogood, Wynton Marsalis, Vangelis, William Ackerman, and Beethoven. As might be expected, it was observed that physiological homeostasis (as indicated by heart rate, muscle tension, and finger-skin temperature) was not attained through all musical selections. Subjects indicated, however, that *their* music selection was relaxing to them (TABLE 22.3).

Other musicologists have attempted to study the relationship between performing—singing (the first instrument) or playing an instrument—and well-being.

In his book *The Roar of Silence* (1990), Don Campbell suggests that singing is, in itself, a relaxation technique because it positively alters body rhythms through its changes in ventilation, heart rate, blood pressure, and brain waves. Tone rather than rhythm, however, is believed responsible for these changes. Campbell relates the story of a policy change at a Benedictine monastery in southern France suspending the practice of Gregorian chants. As a result of being denied the opportunity to sing, the Christian monks manifested several symptoms of stress, including repeated bouts of fatigue and illness. When chanting was reinstituted, the health condition of the monks improved significantly. Interestingly, music performed in the form of chants differs markedly from both other lyrical melodies and talking. Halpern notes that singing (specifically Gregorian and Zen chanting) consists of clean vowel sounds, soft in nature, which trail off into a slight hum, creating a tranquil resonance throughout the body. Talking and pop vocals, on the other hand, emphasize consonants, which lend a less tranquil resonance.

Is it true that listening to classical music can make you smarter? Perhaps! According to one study, students who sang or played an instrument scored up to 51 points higher on their SATs than the national average (Rauscher et al. 1993). According to Raymond Bahr, M.D., classical music was proven to be as effective as Valium for some coronary care patients (Bahr 2008). These and other findings have led music therapist

TABLE 22.3   Highly Recommended Playlists of Instrumental Music CDs for Relaxation

Artist	Title	Instrumentation
Eversound Collection	*One Quiet Night*	Various instruments
Jim Wilson	*Northern Seascapes*	Solo piano
Bruce Becvar	*Forever Blue Sky*	Solo guitar
Michael Hoppé	*The Poet*	Solo cello
Michael Hoppé	*The Dreamer*	Solo flute
Secret Garden	*White Stones*	Violin and piano
David Lanz	*Christophori's Dream*	Solo piano
Chris Spheeris	*Eros*	Solo guitar
Yanni	*In My Time*	Solo piano
Deuter	*Sun Spirit*	Synthesizer

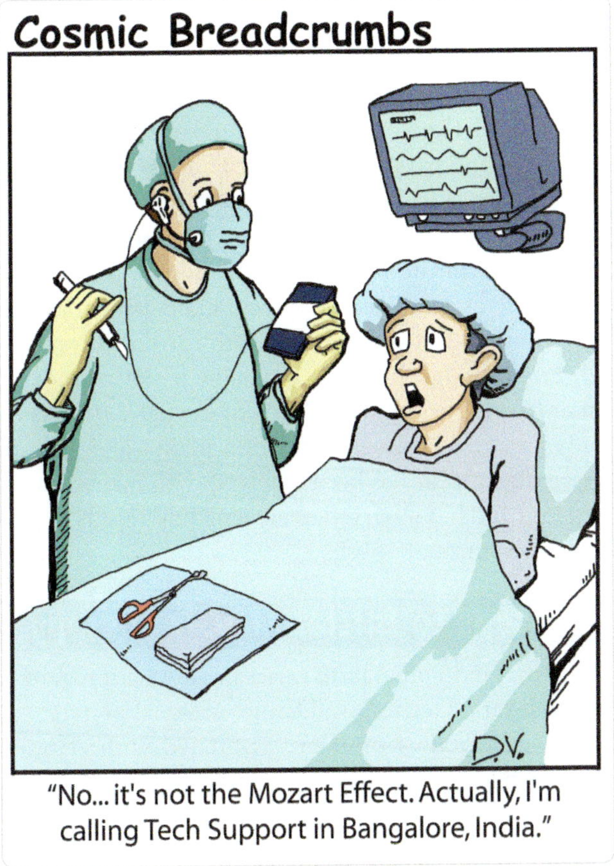

Cosmic Breadcrumbs

"No... it's not the Mozart Effect. Actually, I'm calling Tech Support in Bangalore, India."

FIGURE 22.7 Many hospitals now use music therapy as a form of relaxation for patients, including during some surgical procedures.

Don Campbell to call this the **Mozart effect**. He explains this as music's lifelong effect on health, learning, and behavior. In his book of the same name, Campbell (1997) cites various studies supporting the premise that music not only calms the nerves, but also provides other benefits (**FIG. 22.7**).

Although the concept explaining why music promotes relaxation is not fully understood, this fact hasn't stopped inquiring minds from exploring additional ways to prove the efficacy of music therapy. Music as a means of inducing a deeper sense of homeostasis during grueling gastrointestinal endoscopic procedures was investigated by Rudin (2007). Findings validated the ageless wisdom that, indeed, music therapy is an effective tool for stress relief during these medical procedures. Music also appears to promote quality of sleep for older adults (Lai and Good 2005) and for bone marrow transplants (Sahler et al. 2003). Can music help reduce pain for kids undergoing medical procedures in a pediatric

burn center? That was the research question posed by Whitehead-Pleaux and colleagues (2007). The answer proved to be a resounding yes: "Music therapy reduced pain and anxiety, and that engagement in music therapy enhanced relaxation." A Google search on the topic of current music therapy research provides enough data to boggle even Mozart's mind.

■ Visualization and Auditory Imagery

Music and imagination are wonderful partners. Perhaps the best example of this is the 1940 film *Fantasia*, in which Walt Disney and conductor Leopold Stokowski united cartoon images and several great classical music pieces in a truly inspiring achievement. Another example is the 1936 musical masterpiece by Prokofiev, *Peter and the Wolf*, a musical fable that pairs the sounds of particular musical instruments with animal and human characters (**FIG. 22.8**). Both music and imagination are right-brain capabilities, which may explain the bond between the two. Dr. Sidney Parnes (1988), a creative consultant employed by Disney in the design of Florida's Epcot Center, advocates using music to generate ideas and enhance the imagination and creative processes. In his workshop training sessions, Parnes often plays instrumental pieces to inspire imagination during creative exercises. Music's ability to augment imagination supports the idea that it can be a coping technique as

> **Mozart effect:** A term coined by renowned music therapist Don Campbell to illustrate the lifelong effect of classical music on healing, learning, and behavior.

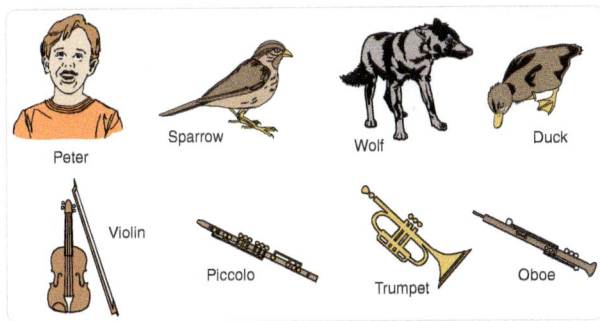

FIGURE 22.8 Russian composer Sergei Prokofiev combined music and imagination in his masterpiece *Peter and the Wolf*, wherein each character is represented by a melody on a different instrument.

well as a relaxation technique; imagination and creativity are essential tools in the resolution of stress. Often during relaxation training sessions, the sounds of natural environments are used to augment participants' imagination, including thunderstorms, ocean waves, mountain streams, and bird sanctuaries.

Merritt also advocates the use of music (classical) to unleash the creative powers of the mind. In workshops conducted for all age groups across the North American continent, she plays a series of classical selections and asks participants to answer the following questions: Did the music calm you? Did it energize you? Did it put you in a dreamlike state? Did it stir up your emotions? Did it focus your mind? Merritt contends that different music styles open up a universe of thoughts and images that leads listeners on a journey of creative expression.

Just as mental imagery can be performed anywhere you have a chance to close your eyes and visualize, the familiar sounds of music can be re-created in your mind. This practice is called **auditory imagery**, or associative recall, and means that a song can be called up and played on the mind's own internal streaming music service. An example might include thinking of the first couple of notes of Beethoven's Fifth Symphony, which then triggers the mind to "play" a portion of the melody or the entire melody. With repeated exposure to and practice of auditory imagery, a desired song that promotes relaxation in an individual can be recalled and played any time, particularly when one feels the need to relax in the midst of stress.

Music Therapy and Chronic Pain

Just as several theories attempt to explain the nature of music's relaxing qualities, so various theories purport to explain music's ability to reduce pain. The most obvious one suggests that music acts as a diversion, by distracting one's thoughts from the origin of pain. This dissociation from pain offers temporary relief. With regard to healing vibrations, the entrainment theory is called upon once again to explain music's ability to decrease pain, with the healing sounds providing a stronger vibration than the energy created by neural pain. Music's healing quality likely combines these two aspects. Current research into approaches utilizing sound vibration, entrainment, and cancer continues to show promise in

Auditory imagery: Imagining or recalling a song or melody in one's head to promote relaxation.

the search for a cancer cure and other immune system illnesses (Lynes 1987; Roberts 2002; Sahler et al. 2003).

In his book *The Healing Power of Sound* (1999), Dr. Mitchell Gaynor discusses the use of music in a variety of healing parameters. Gaynor cites several studies, including research that shows a relationship between music and pain-relieving opiates. He also cites examples where music is used in maternity wards during childbirth as complementary pain management as well as in hospitals at the time of death for the chronically ill. Even though music as medicine is not considered mainstream therapy yet, Deena Spear (2002) thinks it's only a matter of time. As a violin maker and acoustic researcher, Spear has been involved with many healing sessions and has observed many amazing results of pain reduction through music.

Steps to Initiate Music Therapy

Note that individual taste varies greatly with regard to this relaxation technique. Despite personal preferences, however, certain factors are associated with effective music therapy as a relaxation technique (and possible coping strategy). The following suggestions will enhance its effects as a relaxation technique:

1. *Musical selection:* The type of music most conducive to relaxation and return to homeostasis satisfies two criteria.

   a. *The music should be an instrumental or acoustic selection with a slow tempo.* This can include classical, improvisational jazz, New Age, or any music that falls in this domain. There are many types of classical music of varying tempo and rhythm, just as there are many types of jazz, from improvisation to fusion. Not all types of classical or improvisational jazz are slow or relaxing. Typically, classical composers wrote three movements of varying tempos in symphonies and concertos, with the andante and adagio movements being considered by most to be calming in nature. Research conducted by Dr. Charles Schmid (1987) at the Lind Institute found that classical music sequenced in a particular composition of pitch, tempo, and instrumentation proved most conducive to relaxation. The Baroque period was renowned for its calming musical pieces. And now New Age music has begun to integrate synthesized music and sounds of nature, including ocean waves, babbling brooks, dolphins, and songbirds. Particular groups of instruments are credited with contributing to different components of wellness. According to musicologist H. A. Lingerman (1983), brass and percussion instruments parallel the strengths of physical well-being; woodwinds and strings (violins) strengthen emotional well-being; strings (cello and piano) augment mental well-being; and synthesizers and harps nurture the soul.

   b. *The selection should be enjoyable rather than disturbing.* No one piece of music will relax everyone equally. Experimentation with and an open mind to new musical compositions will lead you to a type of music that is right for you. A range of relaxation music can be found online, in special radio programs, and in friends' music libraries. Music that is grating or agitating to listen to will promote stress rather than reduce it. Find something you like and build on this style.

2. *Listening environment:* To fully enjoy the effects of music therapy, all interruptions should be minimized or eliminated so that full attention can be directed toward this special auditory stimulation, and for a sufficient length of time. In his book *Sound Health* (1985), author/composer Steven Halpern states that listening environment is second in importance only to selection of music. He believes that music therapy is best practiced at home in a peaceful environment. Once comfortable with this skill, you can then transfer it to the office or other stress-producing environments.

3. *Postures and cognition:* There are two suggested postures for music therapy. The first and most effective one is similar to a meditative posture, where the individual either sits or reclines in a comfortable position with eyes closed to minimize distractions. In this posture, a right-hemisphere cognitive style is adopted; that is, you accept the music without analysis of composition or instrumentation. Simply surround yourself with the music and let unedited thoughts appear on the mind's screen without subjectivity or emotional attachment. The second posture is an active one where the music serves as background sound to balance other auditory stimulation in your environment, whether you are involved with housework, homework, or office work. This approach also calls for a right-hemisphere cognitive style; that is, you assume an attitude of acceptance and harmony with your environment, seeing yourself as part of the whole, not the whole.

4. *Making your own music:* A more active style of music therapy is making your own music. This can mean singing, humming or whistling a song, or playing an instrument. It can also include programming your smartphone with selections you want to play when you need or want to relax. As was illustrated by the monks who sang Gregorian chants, singing a song you like can be an uplifting experience. Try it sometime when you are down in the dumps. Playing an instrument also can be very rewarding, even if there is no audience but yourself. And at times when you can neither sing nor play an instrument, you can always carry a song in your heart.

■ Best Application of Music Therapy

Thanks to advances in technology (e.g., smartphones), music can be played in a host of environments—while driving a car, sitting in an office, or walking on a sidewalk—to create a more tranquil setting. In these cases, music is often used as background sound, an almost unconscious attempt to promote physiological calmness, while one's attention is directed elsewhere. Although this can certainly be effective, the ideal setting for getting the most out of music therapy is the home environment, with quality time dedicated *solely* to the enjoyment of each note. Perhaps the best application of music therapy today is to create your favorite music playlist to be used at times when you feel the need to unwind from a stressful day or merely end the day on a relaxing note. Audio imagery, like mental imagery, can be done anywhere. Music can affect any mood. Your favorite melody can dissolve anger in milliseconds. And if you have ever heard anyone whistling in the face of fear, remember that this, too, is effective at calming the body.

SUMMARY

- Music therapy is defined as (1) the systematic application of music by the music therapist to bring about helpful changes in the emotional or physical health of the client and (2) the ability to experience an altered state of physical arousal and subsequent mood by processing a progression of musical notes of varying tone, rhythm, and instrumentation for a pleasing effect.

- Music therapy includes both listening to and creating music for a soothing effect.

- Music as therapy has been used for hundreds of generations. Music is also the most popular way to relax for Americans.

- Music is energy made audible through sound waves. These waves are measured in vibrations (oscillations) per second and in terms of decibels (dB). A sound above 120 dB is known to cause damage to neural tissue in the ear. Tinnitus is the clinical name for buzzing and ringing in the ear caused by repeated exposure to high-decibel noises.

- There are three theories for how music promotes the relaxation effect. Biochemical theory states that music is a sensory stimulus that is processed through the sense of hearing. Sound vibrations are chemically changed into nervous impulses that activate either the sympathetic or the parasympathetic nervous system. Entrainment theory suggests that oscillations produced by music are received by the human energy field and various physiological systems entrain with or match the hertz (oscillation) of the music. Metaphysical theory suggests that music is divine in nature.

- Various clinical studies have demonstrated that, under certain conditions, music can alter physiological parameters as well as mood; however, the exact mechanisms underlying these effects are still not completely understood.

- Music therapy can be used as a modality to decrease episodes of chronic pain.

- For music therapy to be fully effective as a relaxation technique, it is best that the music be instrumental (without lyrics). Type of music selected, listening environment, posture, and attitude also affect the quality of the relaxation response.

STUDY GUIDE QUESTIONS

1. What is music therapy?

2. List and explain the three theories of how music is thought to promote relaxation.

3. Listening to music is one form of music therapy. Name two other forms.

REFERENCES AND RESOURCES

Abrams, B. 2001. "Music, Cancer and Immunity." *Clinical Journal of Oncology Nursing* 5(5): 1–3.

Allen, J., and M. Good. 2000. "Music During Crisis: Music Can Be Used to Relieve Symptoms That Interfere with Healing." *American Journal of Nursing* 100(12): 24AA–24FF.

Allen, K. 2001. "Melodies, Mutts Reduce Stress." *Men's Fitness* 52.

Alpert, M., J. I. Alpert, and E. N. Maltzc. 2005. "Purchase Occasion Influence on the Role of Music in Advertising." *Journal of Business Research* 58(3): 369–376.

Alvin, J. 1975. *Music Therapy.* New York: Basic Books.

American Music Therapy Association. 8455 Colesville Road, Suite 100, Silver Spring, MD 20910. www.musictherapy .org.

Andrade, P. E., and J. Bhattacharya. 2003. "Brain Tuned to Music." *Journal of the Royal Society of Medicine* 96: 284–287.

Assagioli, R. 1991. "Music: Cause of Disease and Healing Agent." In *Music Physician for Times to Come*, edited by D. Campbell. Wheaton, IL: Quest Book, 97–110.

Bahr, R. 2008. Personal communication (Effects of Classical Music on Critical Care Patients: Discussion with Helen Bonny), April 9. St. Agnes Hospital, Baltimore, MD.

Barr, F. 1983. "Melanin." *Medical Hypothesis* 11: 1–140.

Becker, R. 1990. *Cross Currents.* Los Angeles: Tarcher Press.

Bentov, I. 1988. *Stalking the Wild Pendulum: On the Mechanics of Consciousness.* Rochester, VT: Destiny Books.

Bhattacharya, J., and H. Petsce. 2005. "Phase Synchrony Analysis of EEG During Music Perception Reveals

Changes in Functional Connectivity Due to Musical Expertise." *Signal Processing* 85(11): 2161–2177.

Bonny, H. L. 1997. "The State of the Art of Music Therapy." *The Arts in Psychotherapy* 24(1): 65–73.

Bonny, H., and L. Savary. 1973. *Music and Your Mind: Listening with a New Consciousness.* New York: Harper & Row.

Borling, J., and J. Scartelli. 1986. "The Effects of Sequenced Versus Simultaneous EMG Biofeedback and Sedative Music on Frontalis Relaxation Training." *Journal of Music Therapy* 23: 157–165.

Bradt, J. 2010. "The Effects of Music Entrainment on Postoperative Pain Perception in Pediatric Patients." *Music and Medicine* 2(3): 150–157.

Bryant, D. R. 1987. "A Cognitive Approach to Therapy Through Music." *Journal of Music Therapy* 24: 27–34.

Burns, D. 2001. "The Effect of the Bonny Method of Guided Imagery and Music on the Mood and Life Quality of Cancer Patients." *Journal of Music Therapy* 1: 51–65.

Campbell, D. 1984. *Introduction to the Musical Brain.* St. Louis, MO: Magnamusic-Baton.

Campbell, D. 1990. *The Roar of Silence.* Wheaton, IL: Theosophical Society.

Campbell, D. 1991. *Music: Physician for Times to Come.* Wheaton, IL: Quest Books.

Campbell, D. 1997. *The Mozart Effect.* New York: Avon Books.

Campbell, D. 2001. "Do You Hear What I Hear?" *Alternative Therapies* 7(1): 34–37.

Campbell, D. 2010. Personal communication, June. Boulder, CO.

Chance, P. 1984. "Music Hath Charms to Soothe a Throbbing Head." *Psychology Today* 21(2): 14.

Chou, M. H., and M. F. Lin. 2006. "Exploring the Listening Experiences During Guided Imagery and Music Therapy of Outpatients with Depression." *Journal of Nursing Research* 14(2): 93–102.

Clynes, M. (Ed.). 1982. *Music, Mind, and Brain: The Neuropsychology of Music.* New York: Plenum Press.

Cousins, N. 1979. *Anatomy of an Illness as Perceived by the Patient.* New York: Bantam Books.

Crussi-Gonzalez, F. 1989. "Hearing Pleasures." *Health* 21(3): 65–71.

Darnley-Smith, R., and H. Patey. 2003. *Music Therapy.* London: Sage Publications.

Davis, W., K. E. Gfeller, and M. H. Thaut. 1999. *An Introduction to Music Therapy: Theory and Practice.* Boston, MA: McGraw-Hill.

Davis, W., and M. Thaut. 1989. "The Influence of Preferred Relaxing Music on Measures of State Anxiety, Relaxation, and Physiological Responses." *Journal of Music Therapy* 26: 168–187.

Diamond, J. 1983. *The Life Energy in Music,* vol. I & II. New York: Archaeus Press.

Elligan, D. 2004. *Rap Therapy.* New York: Dafina Publishing.

Espring, A. 2000. *Sympathetic Vibrations: A Guide for Private Music Teachers.* Springfield, IL: Charles C. Thomas.

Evans, D. 2002. "Review: Music as a Single Session Intervention Reduces Anxiety and Respiratory Rate in Patients Admitted to Hospital." *Evidence-Based Nursing* 5(3): 86.

Floyd, J., J. Kirkpatrick, and M. Rider. 1985. "The Effect of Music, Imagery, and Relaxation on Adrenal Corticosteroids and the Re-entrainment of Circadian Rhythms." *Journal of Music Therapy* 22: 46–58.

Gardner, K. 1990. *Sounding the Inner Landscape: Music as Medicine.* Stonington, ME: Caduceus Publications.

Gaynor, M. 1999. *The Healing Power of Sound.* Boston, MA: Shambhala Books.

Goldman, J. 1991. "Sonic Entrainment." In *Music Physician for Times to Come,* edited by D. Campbell. Wheaton, IL: Quest Book, 217–233.

Goldman, J. 1998. "Sound as Subtle Energy." Sound Colloquium, Loveland, CO, August.

Golin, M. 1988. "New Age Prescription for Sound Health." *Prevention* 40: 66.

Gutheil, E. 1952. *Music and Your Emotions.* New York: Liveright.

Halpern, S. 1978. *Tuning the Human Instrument.* Belmont, CA: Spectrum Research Institute.

Halpern, S., with L. Savary. 1985. *Sound Health: The Music and Sounds That Make Us Whole.* San Francisco: Harper & Row.

Hanser, S. 1985. "Music Therapy and Stress-Reduction Research." *Journal of Music Therapy* 22: 193–206.

Hanser, S. B. 2000. *The New Music Therapist's Handbook.* Milwaukee, WI: Berklee Press.

Hanser, S. B., S. C. Larson, and A. O'Connell. 1983. "The Effects of Music on Relaxation of Expectant Mothers During Labor." *Journal of Music Therapy* 20: 50–58.

Harrelson, J. 2006. "Making an Eggs-cellent Discovery." *Palo Alto News,* October 8.

Haun, M., R. O. Mainous, and S. W. Looney. 2001. "Effect of Music on Anxiety of Women Awaiting Breast Biopsy." *Behavioral Medicine* 27: 127–132.

Heline, C. 1969. *Healing and Regeneration Through Music.* Santa Barbara, CA: New Age Press.

Hodges, D. 1980. *Handbook of Music Psychology.* Lawrence, KS: National Association of Music Therapy.

Hoffman, N. 1974. *Hear the Music! A New Approach to Mental Health.* Boynton Beach, FL: Star.

International Medical News Group. 2000. "Music Therapy for Parkinson's." *Family Practice News* 30(6): 18.

Jenny, H. 2001. *Cymatics: A Study of Wave Phenomena.* Newmarket, NH: MACRO Media Publishing.

Kenny, C. B. 1985. "Music, a Whole Systems Approach." *Music Therapy* 5: 3–11.

Kim, D. 2004. "A Spiking Neuron Model for Synchronous Flashing of Fireflies." *Biosystems* 76(1–3): 7–20.

Knight, W. 2001. "Relaxing Music Prevents Stress-Induced Increases in Subjective Anxiety, Systolic Blood Pressure, and Heart Rate in Healthy Males and Females." *Journal of Music Therapy* 38(4): 254–272.

Kumar, A., F. Tims, D. Cruess, et al. 1999. "Music Therapy Increases Serum Melatonin Levels in Patients with Alzheimer's Disease." *Alternative Therapies in Health and Medicine* 5(6): 49–57.

Kwekkeboom, K. 2003. "Music Versus Distraction for Procedural Pain and Anxiety in Patients with Cancer." *Oncology Nursing Forum Online* 30(3): 433–440.

Lai, H. L., and M. Good. 2005. "Music Improves Sleep Quality in Older Adults." *Journal of Advanced Nursing* 49(3): 234–244.

Lai, Y. 1999. "Effects of Music Listening on Depressed Women in Taiwan." *Mental Health Nursing* 20: 229–246.

Larkin, M. 1985. "Musical Healing." *Health* 17: 12.

Lauterwasser, A. 2006. *Water Sound Images*. Newmarket, NH: MACRO Media Publishing.

Leblanc, A. 1982. "An Interactive Therapy of Music Preference." *Journal of Music Therapy* 19: 28–42.

Lehmann, A. C. 1997. "Affective Responses to Everyday Life Events and Music Listening." *Psychology of Music* 25: 84–90.

Leonard, G. 1981. *The Silent Pulse*. New York: Bantam New Age Books.

Levitin, D. 2007. *This Is Your Brain on Music*. New York: Plume Books.

Licht, S. 1946. *Music in Medicine*. Boston: New England Conservatory of Music.

Lingerman, H. 1983. *The Healing Energies of Music*. Wheaton, IL: Theophysical Society.

Llaurado, J. G., and A. Sances. 1974. *Biological and Clinical Effects of Low-Frequency Magnetic and Radiational Fields*. Springfield, IL: Charles Thomas.

Logan, T., and A. Roberts. 1984. "The Effects of Different Types of Relaxation Music on Tension Levels." *Journal of Music Therapy* 21: 177–183.

Lynes, B. 1987. *The Cancer Cure That Worked*. Queensville, Canada: Marcus Books.

Marwick, C. 2000. "Music Therapists Chime in with Data on Medical Results." *JAMA* 283: 731–734.

McClellan, R. 1988. *The Healing Forces of Music*. Amity, NY: New House Publications.

McCraty, R. 1998. "The Effects of Different Types of Music on Mood, Tension and Mental Clarity." *Alternative Therapies in Health and Medicine* 4(1): 75–84.

McKinney, C. H., M. H. Antoni, M. Kumar, F. C. Tims, and P. M. McCabe. 1997. "Effects of Guided Imagery and Music (GIM) Therapy on Mood and Cortisol in Healthy Adults." *Health Psychology* 16(4): 390–400.

Merritt, S. 1990. *Mind, Music, and Imagery*. New York: Plume Books.

Michael, D. E. 1985. *Music Therapy*. New York: Thomas Books.

Mitchum Report on Stress. 1990. New York: Research & Forecast.

Monroe, R. 1993. *Journeys Out of the Body*. New York: Bantam Books.

Nelson, N., and R. Weatherbs. 1998. "Necessary Angels: Music and Healing in Psychotherapy." *Journal of Humanistic Psychology* 38: 101–108.

O'Kelly, J. 2002. "Music Therapy in Palliative Care: Current Perspectives." *International Journal of Palliative Nursing* 8(3): 130–136.

Overy, K. 2000. "The Potential of Music as an Early Learning Aid for Dyslexic Children." *Psychology of Music* 28(2): 218–229.

Parnes, S. J. 1988. *Visionizing*. East Aurora, NY: D. O. K. Publishers.

President and Fellows of Harvard College. 2003. "Music as Medicine." *Harvard Men's Health Watch* 7(8): 5–6.

Priestly, M. 1975. *Music Therapy in Action*. New York: St. Martin's.

Rauscher, F. H., G. L. Shaw, and K. N. Ky. 1993. "Music and Spatial Task Performance." *Nature* 365: 611.

Retallack, D. 1973. *The Sound of Music and Plants*. Santa Monica, CA: DeVorss.

Rider, M. S., J. W. Floyd, and J. Kirkpatrick. 1985. "The Effect of Music, Imagery, and Relaxation on Adrenal Corticosteroids and the Re-entrainment of Circadian Rhythms." *Journal of Music Therapy* 22(1): 46–58.

Robb, S. 2000. "Music Assisted Progressive Muscle Relaxation, Progressive Muscle Relaxation, Music Listening, and Silence: A Comparison of Relaxation Techniques." *Journal of Music Therapy* 37(1): 2–21.

Roberts, S. 2002. "Music Therapy; Pain—Treatment." *Music Therapy for Chronic Pain* 55(9): 26–28.

Rosenfeld, A. 1985. "Music: The Beautiful Disturber." *Psychology Today* 19: 48–57.

Rudin, D. 2007. "Frequently Overlooked and Rarely Listened To: Music Therapy in Gastrointestinal Endoscopic Procedures." *World Journal of Gastroenterology* 13(33): 4533.

Sacks, O. 2007. *Musicophilia: Tales of Music and the Brain*. New York: Knopf Books.

Sahler, O. J., B. C. Hunter, and J. L. Liesveld. 2003. "The Effect of Using Music Therapy with Relaxation Imagery in the Management of Patients Undergoing Bone Marrow Transplantation: A Pilot Feasibility Study." *Alternative Therapies in Health and Medicine* 9(6): 70–74.

Scarletti, J. 1982. "The Effect of Sedative Music on Electromyographic Biofeedback-Assisted Relaxation

Training of Spastic Cerebral Palsied Adults." *Journal of Music Therapy* 14: 210–218.

Scarletti, J. 1984. "The Effect of EMG Feedback and Sedative Music, EMG Biofeedback Only, and Sedative Music Only on Frontalis Muscle Relation Ability." *Journal of Music Therapy* 21: 67–78.

Schmid, C. 1987. *Relax with the Classics.* San Francisco, CA: Lind Institute.

Schrader, C. 1988. "Modern Alchemy: Holistic High Tech." *Harper's Bazaar* 3316 (April): 161.

Scofield, M., and M. Teich. 1987. "Mind-Bending Music." *Health* 19: 69–76.

Shaw, G. 2000. *Keeping Mozart in Mind, Listening to Mozart Sonata (k.488) Enhances Spatial-Temporal Reasoning: The "Mozart Effect."* San Diego, CA: Academic Press.

Simkin, B. 2001. "Mozart (Medical and Musical Byways of Mozartiana)." *Journal of the American Medical Association* 286(12): 1514.

Solomon, A., and G. Heller. 1982. "Historical Research in Music Therapy." *Journal of Music Therapy* 19: 161–177.

"Sound, Mind and Body; Music's Healing; Mozart's Healing Powers." 2001. *The Economist (US)*, January 13, p. 8.

Spear, D. Z. 2002. *Ears of the Angels.* Carlsbad, CA: Hay House.

Staum, M. 2000. "The Effect of Music Amplitude on the Relaxation Response." *Journal of Music Therapy* 37(1): 22–39.

Stratton, V., and A. Zalanowski. 1984. "The Relationship Between Music, Degree of Liking, and Self-Reported Relaxation." *Journal of Music Therapy* 21: 184–192.

Summer, L. 1985. "Imagery and Music." *Journal of Mental Imagery* 9: 83–90.

Thayer, G. 1968. *Music in Therapy.* New York: Macmillan.

Tomatis, A. 1981. *La Nuit Uterine.* Paris: Editions Stock.

Trapp, M. A. 1949. *The Trapp Family Singers.* New York: Doubleday.

Treurnicht Naylor, K., S. Kingsnorth, A. Lamont, P. McKeever, and C. Macarthur. 2011. "The Effectiveness of Music in Pediatric Healthcare." *Evidence Based Complement Alternative Medicine* 2011: 464759.

Waldon, E. 2001. "The Effects of Group Music Therapy on Mood States and Cohesiveness in Adult Oncology Patients." *Journal of Music Therapy* 38(3): 212–238.

Waldrop, M. 1985. "Why Do We Like Music?" *Science* 227: 36.

Watson, A., and N. Drury. 1987. *Healing Music: The Harmonic Path to Wholeness.* Dorset, England: Prism Press.

Weller, L., and A. Weller. 1999. "Menstrual Term Synchrony in a Sample of Working Women." *Psychoneuroendocrinology* 24(4): 449–459.

Westle, M. 1998. "Music Is Good Medicine." *Newsweek,* September 21, p. 103.

Wheeler, B. (Ed). 2016. *Music Therapy Handbook.* New York: Guilford Press.

Whitaker, M. H. 2010. "Sounds Soothing: Music Therapy for Postoperative." *Nursing* 40(12): 53–54.

Whitehead-Pleaux, A. M., N. Zebrowski, M. J. Baryza, and R. L. Sheridan. 2007. "Exploring the Effects of Music Therapy on Pediatric Pain: Phase 1." *Journal of Music Therapy* 44(3): 217–241.

Winkelman, M. 2003. "Complementary Therapy for Addiction: 'Drumming out Drugs.'" *American Journal of Public Health* 93(4): 647–652.

Zare, M., A. A. Ebrahimi, and B. Birashk. 2010. "The Effects of Music Therapy on Reducing Agitation in Patients with Alzheimer's Disease: A Pre-Post Study." *International Journal of Geriatric Psychiatry* 25(12): 1309–1310.

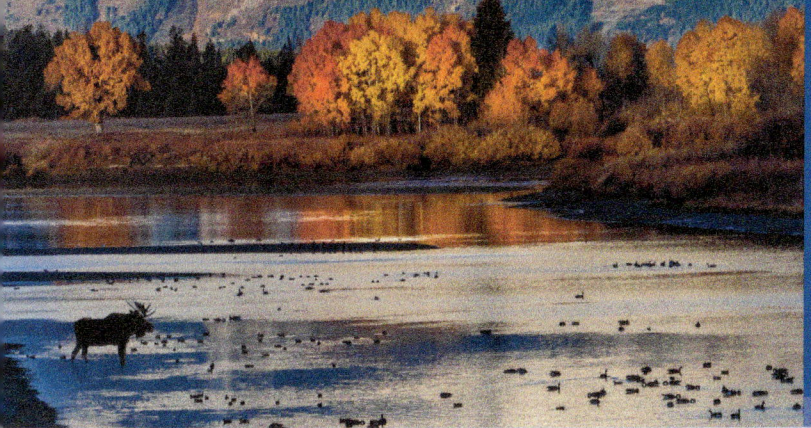
© Inspiration Unlimited. Used with permission.

CHAPTER 23

Massage Therapy

Oh, that the water softens the rocks with time, may thy hands craft my body soft like the weathered rocks.

—Anonymous

Of all the relaxation techniques available for reducing symptoms of stress, one requires special assistance: the muscle massage. Although you can certainly rub and knead your own muscles to relieve soreness in some reachable body regions, an extra set of hands is a virtual necessity to get the full relaxation effect. Muscle tension is the premier symptom of the stress response, and massage therapy (also known as bodywork) is the best technique to diminish it. Professional muscle massage is defined as the manipulation of skin, muscles, ligaments, and connective tissue for the purposes of decreasing muscle tension and increasing physical comfort of musculature and its surrounding joints. But massage therapy has a more profound effect than manipulation of tissue. In a very "touch-conscious" society, professional physical contact can nurture a sense of connectedness otherwise missing in our lives. In its own way, muscle massage creates harmony among the body, mind, and spirit.

In the past decades, as the world has grown smaller through increased accessibility of information and travel, a greater appreciation of muscle massage has spread throughout the global village, particularly the United States. According to articles in *U.S. News and World Report, Time*, and *Newsweek*, **massage therapy** has now hit the mainstream as an acceptable healing modality. This technique gained acceptance in Western cultures as a result of the health and fitness boom of the 1980s, especially in health clubs and corporate settings in addition to the routine practices in professional- and amateur-sport locker rooms (**FIG. 23.1**).

Massage therapy is now a bona fide practice. Massage therapists can receive certification from accredited schools across the United States. Certification requirements vary from state to state, but most massage therapy schools require about 500 hours of classroom instruction combined with practicum experience. Since the inception of the **American Massage Therapy Association (AMTA)** in 1943, the popularity of massage as a therapeutic

Massage therapy: A relaxation technique; the manipulation of skin, muscles, ligaments, and connective tissue for the purpose of releasing muscle tension and increasing physical comfort of musculature and surrounding joints.

American Massage Therapy Association (AMTA): The governing body that accredits massage therapy schools and certifies graduates in massage therapy.

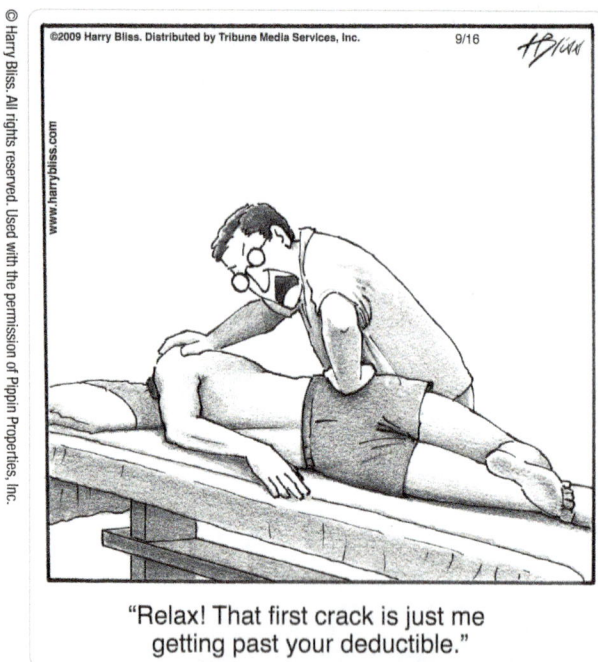

"Relax! That first crack is just me
getting past your deductible."

FIGURE 23.1   Ignore the cracks, enjoy the experience.

modality has grown exponentially over the decades, with hundreds of approved massage therapy schools and hundreds of thousands of licensed massage therapists. Massage therapy was even offered to athletes at the most recent Olympic Games.

To be sure, an extra set of hands does not come cheap. Rates range from $50 to $120 per massage, depending on length of time and location involved. (Home visits are usually more.) In some cases, corporations and insurance companies now cover the cost as a medical benefit for employees. Despite the expense, anyone who has had a professional muscle massage will testify that the benefits are well worth it. For decades, if not centuries, muscle massage was considered a luxury affordable only by the elite. With the current prolific use of desktop and laptop computers, bodywork has become a necessity for nearly everyone in the effort to maintain personal health and well-being. The recent focus of massage therapy has been on the use of warm stones (stone therapy) to heat muscle tissue to relieve soreness, stiffness, and pain. Regardless of the approach, the use of touch relieves stress.

Historical Perspective

Massage therapy has been in use for more than 3,000 years; the earliest references to it are in Chinese treatises on medicine. It was believed that touch not only relieved muscle soreness, but also contributed a profound healing quality to one's life force or spiritual energy. Greek philosopher and physician Hippocrates, the "father of modern medicine," advocated a mind-body approach to physicians' care. In one of his writings he stated, "The physician must be experienced in many things, but most assuredly in rubbing." Muscle massage was apparently practiced in several other ancient cultures as well; records of the Persians, Hindus, and Egyptians all refer to it. The practice of healing touch is not even specific to the human species: Many other members of the animal kingdom are known to use elements of therapeutic touch as well (Downing 1972).

Although there are several types of massage therapies, they all seem to fall into two categories: those originating in the East, particularly China and India, and those deriving from Scandinavian forms. Through the influences of these cultures, massage has long flourished as a viable relaxation technique in Asia and Northern Europe. By contrast, Victorian cultural influences on the United States of a century ago made this therapeutic method less than socially acceptable. Even today, physical contact (of any kind) is not a dominant behavior in America. Nevertheless, human beings in every culture need some regular form of healthy touch for their well-being.

The Need for Human Touch

In 1999, John Naisbitt, author of *Megatrends 2000*, said, "The more high technology around us, the greater the need for human touch." As he mentions in his book, high technology has been repeatedly cited as a reason for increased stress. Naisbitt's prophetic comments have proved themselves true. They also reveal the insight that as we move closer and closer to a full technology society, we distance ourselves further and further from the basic elements that used to provide physical, emotional, and spiritual sustenance. Even before the high-tech age, though, American culture was known for its habits and customs minimizing physical contact. In Naisbitt's opinion, technological advancement has only exaggerated this cultural idiosyncrasy. Naisbitt is not alone in his thinking. Several health practitioners recognize what they call a "famine of touch," or touch deprivation, in the United States. But human touch is as much a necessity as air, food, and water. Reports from orphanages assert that babies deprived of touch can actually die (Field 2008). Tongue in cheek, but very serious about their message, health practitioners Bob Czimbal and Maggie Zadikov explain that people need vitamin T (touch) for their well-being (TABLE 23.1) just like the other vitamins. So, as the mind-body-spirit relationship continues to be acknowledged in the United States, active interest in the effects of massage therapy has developed, leading to several research studies on this topic.

Almost 30 years ago, when futurist John Nesbitt suggested that massage and bodywork would become a popular part of the social fabric, even he didn't foresee the problems with spinal deformity via the use of handheld screen devices like smartphones and tablets. But such is becoming the norm today, so much so that specialists now call it "text neck." This syndrome, common among millennials, results from the 60-degree head tilt used when looking at a smartphone. This tilt puts 60 pounds of pressure on the upper vertebrae, causing curvature of the spine and contorted musculature of the head, neck, and shoulders (Bever 2014).

■ Massage Therapy Research

Research in the area of massage therapy has involved several demographic populations, including premature babies, cocaine-addicted babies, college students, recovering alcoholics, and the elderly, to name just a few. Overall, the findings of these studies indicate that massage (primarily Swedish massage, described later in this chapter) is a very viable technique to promote physical relaxation as well as other health-related benefits. Dr. Tiffany Field, who heads the Touch Research Institute at the University of Miami School of Medicine, has conducted several studies on the effect of massage on infant health. In a reliability study with Scafidi and associates (1990) (designed to validate previous findings), it was revealed that three 15-minute periods of massage therapy for three consecutive hours over a 10-day period stimulated growth in premature babies. In 20 babies who received "tactile kinesthetic stimulation," a 21 percent average increase in weight gain per day was observed. Perhaps more impressive, these babies left the hospital an average of 5 days earlier than control subjects did. Thus, Field is of the opinion

TABLE 23.1 Vitamin T (Touch)

Type	Level	Examples
Public touch	T7	Introductions with handshakes
Professional touch	T6	Touch dispensed by professionals
Social touch	T5	Greetings, talk touch, social dance
Friendly touch	T4	Hugging, playful touch, comforting
Family touch	T3	Cuddling, hugging, kissing
Special touch	T2	Holding, sleeping, hugging, dancing
Personal touch	T1	Massage, bathing, time in nature
Sexual touch	TS	Passionate pleasure involving consenting adults

Vitamin T Terminology

Leveling: Achieving harmony between two people with differing comfort levels regarding touch, usually by expressing the less intimate level (e.g., T7 or T6).

Intimacy: Level of friendship, familiarity, or closeness with another person, reflected by the frequency, intensity, and duration of contact.

Primary deficiency: An inadequate supply of vitamin T.

Space invaders: People who invade your personal space, physically or verbally.

Ouch: A painful touch experience (Touch minus T = Ouch).

Stop: Refusal skills for dealing with space invaders or ouches.

Reproduced from B. Czimbal and M. Zadikov. 1991. *Vitamin T: A Guide to Healthy Touch.* Portland, OR: Open Book. Used with permission from Bob Czimbal.

that touch therapy is crucial in the development of the infant into childhood. Her theory is that those infants who are "touch deprived" (receive less than adequate physical nurturing) manifest several mind-body problems throughout life.

Massage was also studied by McKechnie and colleagues (1983). They found that connective tissue massage aided in reducing resting heart rate, skin resistance, and muscle tension (as recorded by EEG), thus indicating that this mode of relaxation was beneficial in reducing the symptoms associated with anxiety. The combined effects of exercise and muscle massage on mood in college students were examined by Weinberg et al. (1988), who discovered that, when combined, these two variables produced mood enhancement exceeding that by exercise alone. Subjects maintained high levels of "vigor," while at the same time they reported noticeably decreased levels of muscle tension, fatigue, anxiety, depression, and anger. In a similar study, Channon (1986) compared massage therapy with progressive muscular relaxation. She found that, as a relaxation technique, massage was far more effective in reducing muscle tension than Jacobson's relaxation technique. Using biofeedback technology, Naliboff and Tachiki (1991) looked at the effect of muscle massage on skin conductance, skin temperature, and electromyographical activity in subjects receiving a 30-minute dermapoint massage to forearm and trapezius muscles. This treatment resulted in a significant decrease in muscle activity and an increase in skin temperature of the forearm.

In the then–Soviet Union, Kolpakov and Rumyantseva (1987) conducted a study to determine what effect regular eye massage would have on vision and eye fatigue in factory employees. They found that this treatment was effective in decreasing visual strain and recommended massage as a viable form of medical treatment. In Japanese subjects, a daily 20-minute facial massage, as reported by Jodo and colleagues (1988), seemed to produce greater physiological homeostasis, including a greater sense of perceived relaxation, compared to controls. There have been many claims that massage influences biochemical reactions (hormones and enzymes) within the body as well as changes to peripheral body tissues. In an attempt to investigate these claims, one study by Green and Green (1987) measured the effect of massage therapy on biochemical constituents in saliva (SIgA) and cortisol. They found that a 20-minute massage significantly increased salivary immunoglobulin, suggesting that massage may actually enhance immune function. Likewise, Day and associates (1987) found that massage therapy had a significant effect on serum levels of beta-endorphins and B-lipoproteins.

With regard to chemical dependency, a study conducted by Adcock (1987) noted that when patients combined drug or alcohol treatment with massage therapy, the detoxification period was shorter, and subjects reported a greater sense of physical relaxation and self-acceptance and self-esteem. Gauthier (1990) studied the use of massage therapy in children diagnosed as emotionally deprived as an effective part of a multimodal-therapy approach. Massage continues to be a topic of academic interest well into the 21st century with a focus on specific populations, many with positive outcomes. The following is a sample of findings with positive outcomes: massage for cancer patients (Liu 2008; Stringer et al. 2008), massage for patients with carpal tunnel syndrome (Moraska et al. 2008), and massage for patients who have chronic lower-back pain (Imamura et al. 2008). One study went back to examine health claims suggested decades ago: Kaye and colleagues (2008) investigated the effect of deep-tissue massage on the vital signs of heart rate and blood pressure, revealing a significant reduction of both systolic and diastolic values as well as a decrease of one's resting heart rate by 10 beats per minute. Tiffany Field's research on touch (2010) involved massage for pregnant women. Subjects who received massage therapy reported not only decreased leg and back pain (common with pregnancy), but also noticeable decreases in depression and anxiety. Moreover, levels of the stress hormone cortisol decreased. Not only was labor pain reduced with massage, but also labor periods were noticeably shorter (by 3 hours) and there was less need for medication. From these and other studies, it can be concluded unequivocally that massage therapy is a viable technique to promote relaxation and several other health-related benefits.

■ Types of Massage

Massage can take many forms. Typically, licensed massage therapists are trained in most, if not all, of these techniques and then go on to specialize in one particular style. Some integrate various types in a synthesis all their own. This chapter focuses on five major types of massage—shiatsu, Swedish, Rolfing, myofascial release, and sports massage—each with its own nuances. Additional methods worth mentioning, all classified as bodywork, include Trager, zero balancing, postural integration, cranial-sacral therapy, reiki, Feldenkrais, reflexology, and trigger-point therapy.

Stress with a Human Face

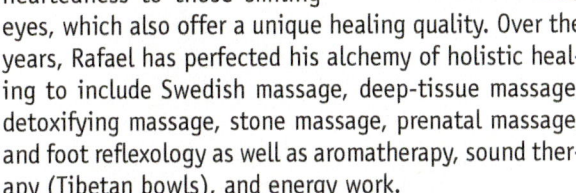

Courtesy of Rafael O'Neil.

If you ever happen to be traveling to, or living in, Houston and need a massage, the first person to call for an appointment is Rafael O'Neil. Why? Because he was voted the Best Massage Therapist in Houston, that's why. His clients, including several professional athletes and celebrities, say it's not only his hands that work magic, but also that the whole ambiance of his office radiates healing. Rafael has been a licensed massage therapist since 1992. His training has taken him all over the world, including Spain, Switzerland, France, and Mexico. Wherever he goes, success follows, including an enviable list of day spas often cited in the "Best of" section of the *Houston Business Journal*.

To look at Rafael you might not guess he is half Irish, yet it's his Mexican roots, passed down from his mother and grandmother, that inspired a career in healing. It's

the Irish side, however, that adds an element of light-heartedness to those smiling eyes, which also offer a unique healing quality. Over the years, Rafael has perfected his alchemy of holistic healing to include Swedish massage, deep-tissue massage, detoxifying massage, stone massage, prenatal massage, and foot reflexology as well as aromatherapy, sound therapy (Tibetan bowls), and energy work.

"Every person I work on today has stress, and lots of it. Stress begins in the mind, but quickly becomes physical tension. Years ago people thought of a massage as a luxury. Today it's a necessity in this frenetic society," he explains. What does Rafael do to relax? At the top of his list is spending quality time with his son, Rafael Jr. "That, to me," he said, "is healing!"

Although the primary benefit of massage is muscle relaxation, several therapists claim additional health effects, including increased blood and lymph flow (making one less susceptible to illnesses), and a general sense of well-being. Many people add emotional well-being, which also contributes to the overall health of the individual. Knowing that emotional well-being is so closely tied to physical health, these claims are not unfounded. The healing power of touch has long been accepted in many cultures, and is now gaining recognition in the United States, as made evident by the proliferation of massage therapy certification programs and the boom in the profession of massage therapists nationwide. Whereas the techniques of massage are clearly directed toward physical constituents, primarily muscle, connective tissue, and bone and nerve endings, the neural, hormonal, and immune systems may unite for a healing effect yet to be clinically understood. Above all else, it is important to remember that the mind and body are one, not two separate entities, and relaxing the body through massage may certainly have a cross-over effect on other aspects of well-being. For this reason, massage therapy is now being fully integrated into medical practices, as well as into nursing, physical therapy, and other aspects of clinical medicine. The seven styles presented here are among the most popular styles of muscle-massage therapies.

Shiatsu

Shiatsu, also known as acupressure, is based on the concept of freeing blocked energy currents within the body. The term *shiatsu* translates as "finger pressure" (*shi* = "finger," *atsu* = "pressure"). It is a distant cousin of acupuncture, and applies force through finger pressure as well as forearm, elbow, knee, and palm pressure instead of needles to unblock energy congestion (**FIG. 23.2**). In this ancient Japanese practice, based on the concept of *chi* or life force, pressure is applied to specific body locations that house the crossroads or meridians of energy. These energy paths in the body seem to parallel, yet are unrelated to, the nervous system. The manual application of gentle pressure relieves blockage, thus allowing free-flowing energy essential to health and longevity. On the surface, shiatsu appears only to relax muscle tension. Upon closer examination, it is believed to have a healing quality through the subtle anatomy as well. The philosophy of shiatsu, derived from the concepts of yin and yang, is that interruptions in the flow of energy

> **Shiatsu:** A type of massage, also known as acupressure, in which pressure is placed on various points (*tsubos*) to release blocked energy and thus promote relaxation.

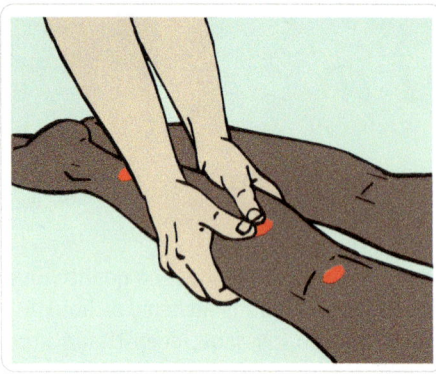

FIGURE 23.2   The practice of shiatsu is based on the premise that pressure applied to specific points on the body can release energy congested in the meridians of the body's subtle anatomy. Not all pressure points directly correspond to the area of the body that is sore or distressed.

create an imbalance in the life force that may become manifest in a host of physical ailments. Restoration of energy through energy channels is thought to relieve ailments specific to the site of blockage, which in many cases is distant from the region of discomfort.

The body has 14 segments, or major meridians. Points along these meridians, where pressure is applied, are called *tsubos*. The application and release of pressure to *tsubos* is thought to remove an energy block caused by muscle tension or toxins in the muscle tissue that can cause cramps. Once a specific *tsubo* is located, about 20 pounds of pressure is applied in a brisk, circular motion

---

Tsubos: The specific points on the meridian that are used in acupressure to release tension.

Swedish massage: The most common and well-known type of massage in Western culture; uses a variety of hand motions (e.g., kneading, stroking, and karate-type chops) to relieve the tension for muscle tissue, often expressed as knots.

Effleurage: The first of five progressive steps/hand maneuvers in Swedish massage that consists of long strokes along the length of the muscle tissue.

Petrissage: The second of five progressive steps/hand maneuvers in Swedish massage; it consists of a series of rolls, rings, and squeezes made by the fingertips or palm of the hand.

Friction: The third of five progressive steps/hand maneuvers in Swedish massage, also known as kneading the muscle tissue.

---

for 15 to 20 seconds. This is then repeated on the equivalent pressure point on the opposite side of the body. Shiatsu uses primarily the thumbs to single out pressure points on the body with both a soft approach (the first interphalangeal joint) or a hard approach (the tip of the distal phalanx).

Although shiatsu is used specifically to reduce muscle tension, it has also been practiced to relieve sinus aches and tension headaches. Research investigating *tsubos* has found they are indeed in close proximity to neural plexuses and stretch receptors, validating the premise of this pressure-relief technique (Lundberg 2003). Although the effects of acupressure can be felt immediately, practitioners agree that daily applications for 7 to 10 days bring full restoration and energy balance. Shiatsu is often preferred over other types of massage for its simplicity; individuals can remain fully clothed while being treated. This type of massage is often used by individuals in the performing arts such as ballet. Other advantages of shiatsu include that (1) it has no adverse side effects, (2) it can be practiced on individuals of any age, and (3) it allows for relaxation of the entire body.

Swedish Massage

Known to Americans as the total body massage, the Swedish or Western massage, created by Swedish fencing master and gymnast Peter Heinrik Ling, emphasizes decreased muscle tension and increased circulation. It is currently the most commonly practiced massage style in the United States and Europe, as noted by the AMTA. In **Swedish massage**, the individual disrobes and lies face down on the table with a sheet over the buttocks. Massage oils or lotions are used on the regions of application to nourish the skin and avoid irritating friction by the massage therapist's hands. Relaxing music is often played in the background (**FIG. 23.3**).

Swedish massage involves five steps. The first step, **effleurage** (**FIG. 23.4**), is a smooth, gliding stroke along the length of the muscle fibers. Both hands are used to relax soft tissue, generally in the direction of the heart. A motion to begin to limber muscles and prepare the body for the next phase, it may also include light strokes along the spine up to the base of the head. The second step, **petrissage** (**FIG. 23.5**), is a series of rolls, rings, and squeezes made with either the fingertips or the palm of the hand. Petrissage motions include a little more pressure than is involved in the first stage. The third step of Swedish massage is referred to as **friction**

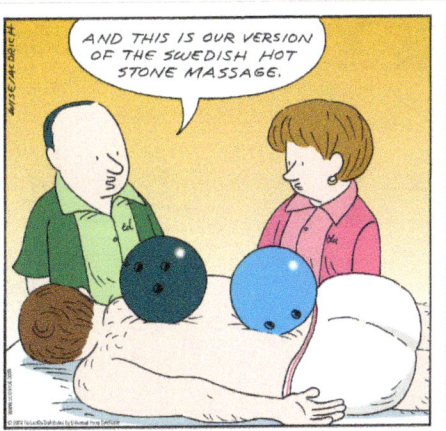
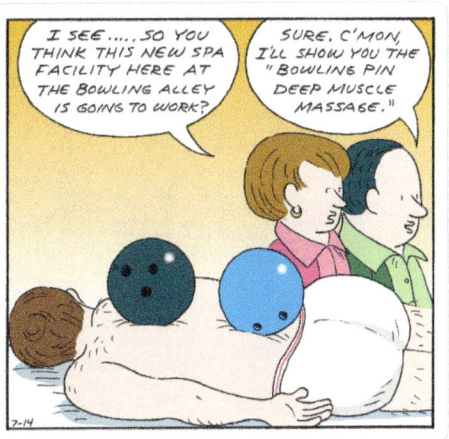

FIGURE 23.3   If you have never had a stone massage, give it a try (note: the stones are NOT this big).

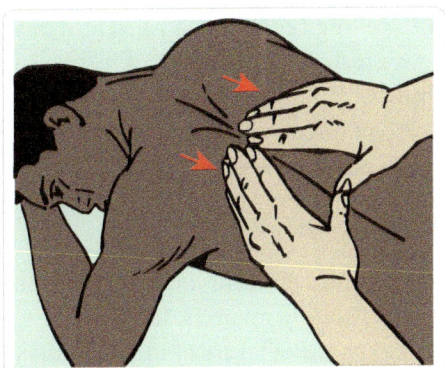

FIGURE 23.4   Effleurage.

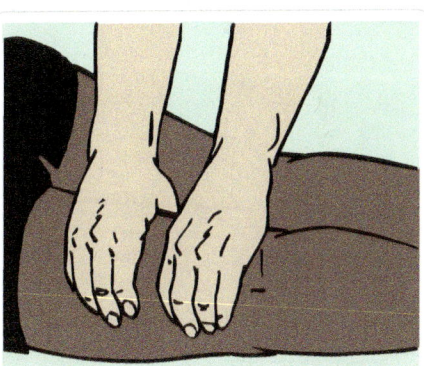

FIGURE 23.6   Friction (kneading).

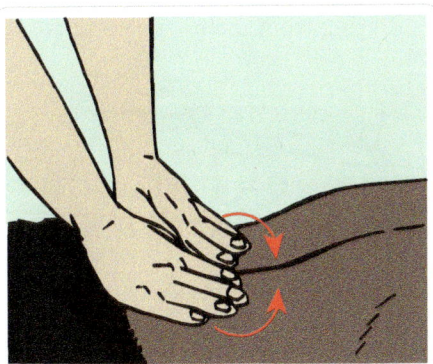

FIGURE 23.5   Petrissage.

tapotement (**FIG. 23.7**), similar in appearance to the percussive strokes of karate chops, is performed in specific regions to activate or revive nerve cells within extremely hard muscle tissue. The last step, **vibration** (**FIG. 23.8**), is described as a "trembling shaking gesture" to increase circulation throughout a desired body region.

The area targeted by Swedish massage is the posterior side of the body—calves, hamstrings, lower back, neck,

(**FIG. 23.6**) and involves a deep **kneading** action of muscle tissue between the fingers and thumbs. Friction can also include deep, small circular motions with the thumb, knuckles, or finger points to extend the penetration of friction beyond the surface of the skin. The fourth step,

Kneading: Also known as friction in Swedish massage, when the hands knead the muscle tissue to promote relaxation.

Tapotement: The fourth of five progressive steps/hand maneuvers in Swedish massage that looks like karate chops on the belly of the muscle.

Vibration: The fifth of five progressive steps/hand maneuvers in Swedish massage that resembles a type of shaking gesture to promote increased circulation.

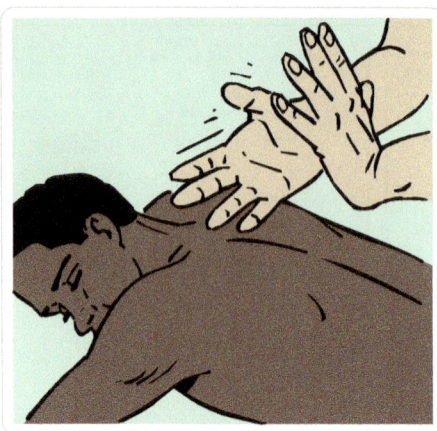

FIGURE 23.7 Tapotement.

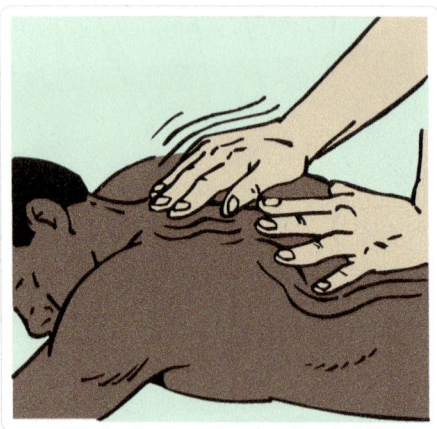

FIGURE 23.8 Vibration.

and shoulders. These muscle groups are most prone to tension from sleeping, walking, standing, and sitting postures because in these positions muscles are shortened (contracted) for an extended period of time. Sleeping in a fetal position, for example, leaves the hamstrings and calf muscles contracted for 6 to 8 hours. These lifestyle postures can create imbalance and malalignment in both anterior and posterior muscles.

Rolfing

If styles of massages were classified, as are the martial arts, from softest to hardest, **Rolfing** would be designated as the hardest of all the massage techniques. In fact,

> **Rolfing:** Deep-tissue massage created by Ida Rolf to promote better posture by working with the soft connective tissue around and between muscles.

there are those who would describe Rolfing as physical torture because of the deep-tissue work. Rolf therapists deny that Rolfing is a type of massage at all, although like massage, they define it as a manipulation of muscle and soft connective tissue (**FIG. 23.9**). The technique of Rolfing was developed by Ida Rolf over a 50-year period starting in 1925. Rolf, a researcher for the Rockefeller Foundation specializing in the study of collagen and connective tissue, hypothesized that human musculature begins to lose alignment from repeated movement established in childhood and carried through to adulthood. These imbalances result from a shortening and thickening of the myofascia surrounding muscle fibers. Rolf's theory suggests that because the human skeletal structure is held in place by soft tissue (muscles, tendons, and ligaments), a muscle contracted for prolonged periods of time will pull the skeletal frame out of its natural alignment. Rolfing borrows the concept that the physical whole is greater than the sum of its muscular parts. The premise of Rolfing is that deep muscular penetration can correct imbalances through slight but repeated alterations of body structure. If body segments become realigned, then the body as a whole can function more efficiently (Jones 2004).

Whereas other massage techniques apply gentle to moderate pressure, Rolfing involves deep "digging" into soft tissue, often separating layers of muscles and stretching and lengthening them with the hands, elbows, and sometimes the entire body weight of the massage therapist. This technique is not advocated for everyone. Rather, it is suggested for highly muscular individuals or those suffering from intense stress-related problems

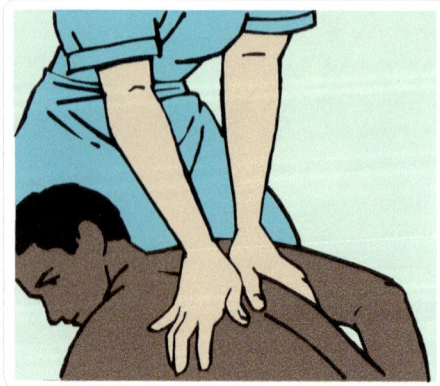

FIGURE 23.9 Rolfing is a very deep, penetrating massage used to realign muscles that have become shortened because of poor posture or maladaptive body positions such as sitting at computers or desks.

that manifest in extreme muscular tightness such as low back pain resulting from poor hip alignment and neck and shoulder pain. Rolfing therapists assert that changes in "pressure stretches" and muscle fascia alignment over 10 sessions can be maintained for improved health. Although the initial manipulation is considered painful, individuals who experience this technique indicate that overall the effects are quite satisfying.

Myofascial Release

Not all forms of physical therapy are created equal, especially when one considers the holistic focus of **myofascial release**. Frustrated with the mechanistic approach to health care, specifically as it applied to physical manipulation, John Barnes, a physical therapist, searched for a greater understanding of the mind-body connection as it applied to the more clinical applications of bodywork. What led Barnes on this search early in his career was the frustration he felt when, after restoring a sense of alignment and pain-free comfort in his patients, he would notice that their symptoms would reappear soon after they left his office. His search led him to all corners of the globe, to courses in acupuncture, joint mobilization, muscle energy, and bioenergy techniques. The synthesis of his experiences, well grounded in the fundamentals of physical therapy, soon became known as myofascial release. In the words of Barnes (1995), "Myofascial release is the three-dimensional application of sustained pressure and movement into the fascial system in order to eliminate fascial restrictions and facilitate the emergence of emotional patterns and belief systems that are no longer relevant or are impeding progress."

Rather than placing the emphasis on muscular manipulation, as so many bodyworkers do, Barnes focuses on the fascial (connective) tissue itself, which in truth holds the muscles in place. When fascial strains occur throughout the body, as they will from vigorous movements, trauma, surgery, or the subtleties of the aging process, tightness occurs, resulting in a loss of flexibility and spontaneity of movement. Eventually, fascial tension can distort one's posture through the three-dimensional alignment of the vertebral column. Barnes notes that current estimates suggest that more than 90 percent of patients treated in physical therapy have some level of myofascial dysfunction. Unlike various forms of bodywork that are often symptom specific (massaging the lower back for low back pain), the technique of myofascial release is holistic in that connections among muscles through the fascia may require distant musculature to be worked to release the tension formed through the strands of connective tissue.

How does myofascial release differ from a Swedish or sports massage? First, an assessment is made by visually analyzing the human frame, searching for symptoms of distortion and imbalance. Next, by palpating the tissue texture of the various fascial layers, the therapist evaluates symmetry, rate, quality, and intensity of craniosacral rhythm, and possible energy disturbances in the gross or subtle anatomy. Upon locating an area of fascial tension, gentle pressure is applied in the direction of the restriction. With a gentle, sustained pressure, rather than a forced manipulation, the restriction is released. As the collagenous barrier is released, the tissue length is increased. And that's not all. Barnes notes that, because of the dynamic connection between mind and body, a release of fascial tension is often accompanied by an emotional release as well. In Barnes's words, "The tissue seems to hold a consciousness all its own. As releases occurred, patients reported memories or emotions emerging that were connected to past events or traumas. As their fascial systems changed, and the memories or emotions surfaced, patients improved, even though they previously were unresponsive to all forms of traditional care" (1995). The goal of myofascial release is to eliminate fascial tension, reduce pain and headaches, restore motion, and restore the body's equilibrium. When the body reaches a state of balance or equilibrium, full health is restored, and this, says Barnes, is what life is all about: finding balance.

Sports Massage

In the pursuit of athletic excellence, individuals now train three times as long per day as their colleagues did less than a decade ago. Since the creation of ultra-endurance sports, including the triathlon (swimming, cycling, and running), Ride Across America (RAAM), and ultramarathons (50+ miles), athletes have been pushing their bodies beyond where they have ever been before (Johnson 1995). The last thing any competitive athlete wants to encounter is damage to muscle tissue, which may result in prolonged injury. In the world of competitive athletics, any method or device to gain a competitive edge over one's opponent has merit. This

> **Myofascial release:** Deep-tissue massage created by John Barnes to release tension by working with the myofascial (soft connective) tissue.

edge is often found in **sports massage**, which has quickly gained acceptance throughout the athletic community. Since the 1984 Los Angeles Olympics, where sports massage was made available to all athletes at no cost, the demand for such therapists has increased dramatically for all athletic purposes, from high school and college competitions to all levels of amateur and professional sports. It is now considered one of the responsibilities of professional physical trainers.

Sports massage appears to be a hybrid of shiatsu, Swedish massage, and deep-tissue massage in its emphasis on both compressive and rhythmic pumping movements to remove the buildup of lactic acid in the muscles because of repeated contractions. Metabolic by-products of physical exercise, of which the most common is lactic acid, have fatiguing effects on muscle tissue. It is the repeated pumping motion to circulate metabolites for removal that has made sports massage so popular. In addition, however, repetitive movement often promotes microtears, most commonly at sites where connective tissue attaches to bone. So, another purpose of sports massage is the restoration of cell tissue by increasing circulation to stimulate new cell growth. One method often used in sports massage is **trigger point therapy**, in which pressure is placed on "hyperirritable" points of the muscle that are causing a radiating pain in a region. Manipulation (deep-tissue work) of specific trigger points releases tension throughout the entire muscle tissue and associated areas.

Spectators at athletic events can watch sports massages being given to athletes during pre-event warm-ups, as a means to prepare muscles for activity; for postevent restoration; and occasionally during competition, between stages of coupled events. Most commonly, though, they are performed during training seasons to improve the rate of tissue regeneration after each workout. Although to date there is no scientific evidence that lactic acid is removed in this manner (Hemmings et al. 2000; Moraska 2005)—lactic acid clears the muscles within 2 hours (Fox, Bowers, and Foss 1989)—sports

> **Sports massage:** A combination of Swedish massage, shiatsu, and some type of deep-tissue bodywork now popular among professional and amateur athletes.
>
> **Trigger point therapy:** Applied pressure to and manipulation of hyperirritable points of muscle that are causing radiating pain in a region; used in sports massage.

massage enjoys the greatest degree of medical acceptance for healing muscle tissue.

Thai Massage

Thai massage is believed to date back to the dynasty of Thai King Rama III one thousand years ago. To ensure the legacy of this type of bodywork, he had his healers etch epigraphs of the human body with energy lines in stone as texts for future healers. Thai massage is perhaps best described as a complex sequence of soft tissue pressure (massage) combined with stretching, twisting, and joint manipulations. Pressure is used to achieve stretching and twisting, which requires several different positions to achieve the desired result of alignment, flexibility, and relaxation. Proper leverage is essential for this style of bodywork, and typically a small effort by the practitioner results in a large effect for the client. It is not uncommon for the body worker to twist, pull, push, and rotate segments of body parts and joints for the optimal effect. The session is typically divided into zones (e.g., feet and legs, legs and back, chest and abdomen, arms and hands, neck and face), and the client will either lay down or sit during different parts of the session. It is also not uncommon for the body worker to use their hands, elbows, feet, and knees for the specific leverage desired. Like acupressure, Thai massage works with the body's energy patterns to establish a correct alignment for optimal energy flow. Each technique in Thai massage is designed to stimulate and access the flow of intrinsic energies by allowing the release of blocked energies that inhibit a sense of balance for mind, body, and spirit. Although it may look and feel painful, the peaceful nature of Thai massage is based on the principles of Buddhist compassion, and like a good yoga session it feels quite refreshing.

Chinese Massage

If you live in or near a moderate-sized city, you may have noticed that massage therapy centers not only include Swedish and Thai approaches, but also a Chinese influence. Unlike traditional massage centers where customers have their own private room, the Chinese American style of massage offers an open room format with limited privacy (three walls), yet the client remains fully clothed (men can remove their shirts if desired). Before the massage begins, the client states his or her preference (on a scale of 1 to 7, with 1 being light and 7 being hard). Oil or lotion and sometimes hot stones are used. Once situated on a massage table lying face down, the client is covered with a clean sheet, and the massage begins. Like other styles of massage, Chinese massage includes kneading of muscles, and in some cases positioning limbs for an added stretch. By and large, this style might be best described as a cookie-cutter approach (i.e., same massage for all people). Yet for those who are new to massage, this serves as a nice, comfortable experience for a very reasonable price.

Other Touch Therapies

Other techniques are closely associated with the concepts and practice of muscle massage, so they have been placed in this chapter (**BOX 23.1**). These types of touch, although not new, have not been studied extensively, and therefore their dynamics for apparently causing relaxation effects are not completely understood. Be that as it may, they make for interesting additions to the category of therapeutic touch.

Aromatherapy. **Aromatherapy** is a technique where perfumed scents are used to promote feelings of calmness. The practice of rubbing natural essences on the body to create tranquility dates back to the age of

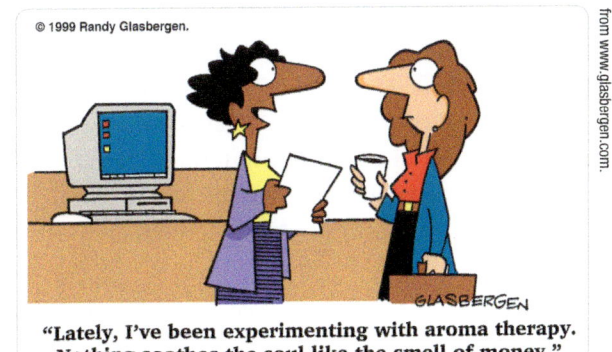

"Lately, I've been experimenting with aroma therapy. Nothing soothes the soul like the smell of money."

FIGURE 23.10 For some people aromatherapy is very relaxing.

Egyptian pharaohs, when it was commonly believed that the fragrance of flowers and herbs forged a unique bond between body and soul. The technique was revived in the New World in the late 1920s by Dr. Edward Bach, a homeopathic physician, and again in 1990 in Japan, where various fragrances (e.g., peppermint) were introduced into the workplace as a means to stimulate productivity. There appear to be two theories to explain the effectiveness of aromatherapy. The first is that it replaces threatening sensations with pleasurable ones. More specifically, aromatherapy works to desensitize conscious thought, or sensory overload of all five senses, through fragrances perceived to be appealing to the olfactory sense. Many fragrances also elicit powerful thoughts and memories (**FIG. 23.10**).

Many research studies have been conducted on the efficacy of aromatherapy, mostly in Europe and Asia. The National Association for Holistic Aromatherapy now publishes the *Aromatherapy Journal* with the mission to revive the knowledge of medicinal use of aromatic plants and essential oils to its fullest extent. Essential oils have been used in the healing process of cancer patients. One study revealed that cancer patients became more relaxed with Roman chamomile essential oils (Wilkinson et al. 1999). And it is well known that the Sloan Kettering Cancer Hospital uses vanilla extract as a means to relax patients who appear anxious to enter the CAT scan apparatus, just as many maternity wards use lavender to relax women ready to give birth.

BOX 23.1   What are the Havening Techniques?

At first glance, the Havening Techniques (based on the concept of a "safe haven") might seem like a quick self-massage, but that would be too simple an explanation. Created by Dr. Ronald Ruden, Havening is known in counseling circles as a tactile technique, among many, in a group of psychosensory therapies that are used to add comforting sensory input to alter one's thought, mood, or behavior by promoting Delta brain waves for relaxation. The Havening Techniques, known to rapidly reduce anxiety, can best be described as a gentle stroking action along the muscles of the arms, hands, and legs.

The protocol:

1. Wash hands.
2. Apply Havening touch on the upper arms (shoulders to elbows).
3. Close your eyes and take several slow, deep breaths.
4. Recall the more challenging memories and moments of your day.
5. Repeat the words "safe," "peaceful," "hopeful," "calm" (four times).
6. Repeat on arms, hands, or legs as desired.

Aromatherapy: The use of essential oils to promote relaxation through the sense of smell; often used in many types of bodywork as a complementary relaxation method.

The part of the brain that processes olfactory sensations is in close proximity to the hypothalamus, which may explain why specific fragrances can elicit memories and their related emotions quite quickly. Furthermore, emotions are part of the right-brain domain, and it is accepted that when one part of the cerebral hemisphere is activated, in this case by positive emotions, then other hemispheric functions are enhanced.

The second theoretical approach to aromatherapy involves the application of fragrance-laced oils to the skin during massage. The pores of the skin are believed to soak up the oils and circulate these essences through the body via the circulatory and lymphatic systems, cleansing the body internally and instilling a sense of physiological calmness.

The topic of aromatherapy has gained much interest in the past 20 years, in both aesthetic and clinical practices. Clinical aromatherapy, as defined by Peter Holmes (1995), is a unique healing process achieved through aroma or scent by three means—physiologically, topically, and psychologically. According to Holmes, the main function of clinical aromatherapy is to affect "the specific actions for the purpose of altering human physiology (decreased stress hormone secretion), nurture the skin (through essential oils), and affect the psyche by promoting a sense of mental and emotional relaxation." Most frequently combined with massage therapy, acupuncture, and some nursing practices, clinical aromatherapy is thought to provide a unique dynamic to the integrity of the mind-body-spirit connection in terms of relaxation.

Lavender, widely accepted for its calming effects, has been the topic of scientific interest over the past several years, perhaps more than any other aromatherapy essential oil. The results are mixed. Kiecolt-Glaser and colleagues (2008) investigated the effects of lavender and lemon on mood and endocrine and immune function. Results revealed that fragrances had no reliable effect on salivatory cortisol levels, heart rate, blood pressure, or immune function, though subjects found the scent of lemon boosted one's mood. Conversely, Shiina and colleagues (2007) found that the scent of lavender significantly reduced serum cortisol levels and improved coronary flow in healthy men, yet blood pressure and heart rate appeared not to be affected.

The following are some popular aromatherapy essences and their biomedical applications for stress reduction:

- *Lavender*: Lavender is known primarily as a neurocardiac sedative, triggering the nervous system to decrease neural firing, thus allowing a decrease in resting heart rate and blood pressure. Used in a state of tension, this fragrance is said to calm, uplift, and relax the mind and body.

- *Juniper*: Best known for its muscle-relaxant qualities, juniper is recommended for muscle spasms, fibromyalgia, intestinal and uterine cramps, and peptic ulcers.

- *Chamomile/Moroccan blue*: A fragrance that calms, nurtures, and regenerates, chamomile is also known as a nervous sedative/relaxant with the ability to help promote decreased blood pressure, act as a bronchodilator, and be an anti-allergenic. It is used primarily for situations resulting in suppressed anger, irritability, and resentment.

- *Vetiver*: Vetiver is known as an immunoregulator in that it is said to help boost the integrity of the immune system. It is used for immunodeficiency and autoimmune disorders. This fragrance is noted for its ability to make a person feel more grounded and centered.

- *Palmarosa*: The palmarosa essence is used as an anti-infective agent for cases involving bacteria, viruses, or fungi, as well as sinus infections, candidiasis, and chlamydia. The healing vibration of palmarosa is thought to help boost the constituents of the immune system and bring the body back to a state of homeostasis.

Hydrotherapy. Baths, hot tubs, and **flotation tanks**, which collectively make up the category of **hydrotherapy**, are distant relatives to muscle massage. The use of hot baths can be traced back to several ancient cultures, from the Romans and Japanese to the Maori of New Zealand. When the body is immersed in hot water, peripheral blood vessels (those nearest the skin and muscles) dilate. Blood is then shunted from the body's core to the periphery to dissipate heat. This influx of blood to the muscles reduces tension by decreasing neural firing at the site of the motor end plate, and the muscles

---

Flotation tanks: A moderate sensory deprivation tank in which a person floats on his or her back in warm water to calm the nervous system through decreased stimulation.

Hydrotherapy: The use of baths, hot tubs, Jacuzzis, and flotation tanks to augment the sense of touch to promote relaxation.

soon become pliable and incredibly relaxed. The addition of water jets to the hot bath by Candido Jacuzzi in the early 1950s increased the effects of hot tubs, and this relaxation technique remains quite popular today.

In 1980, the cult movie *Altered States* introduced flotation tanks to the American public. Whereas the movie was science fiction, flotation tanks are very real. The first such tank was created by Dr. John C. Lilly in 1954 at the National Institutes of Health. It was designed to eliminate all external stimuli, including gravity. The subject disrobed and was suspended vertically in water. All senses were basically "turned off." Early changes in tank design included the addition of Epsom salts, which allowed the body to float horizontally, and controlled water temperature. Today, commercial flotation tanks are similar in concept, but with the use of computer technology they feature lighting, ultraviolet water purification, underwater stereos, and even optional video screens to cater to the preference of clients who can afford the $50 to $100 per flotation hour. Without a doubt, the cessation of sensations has a profound effect on both mind and body, sometimes lasting 4 to 5 days after immersion. Research conducted at the National Institutes of Health revealed that flotation-tank therapy decreases the following: depression, insomnia, muscle tension, plasma stress hormones (cortisol and ACTH), resting heart rate, resting blood pressure, anxiety, and physical (musculoskeletal) pain (Hutchinson 1984). As a result, overall well-being is dramatically increased. Flotation tanks, in fact, are said to provide the ultimate relaxation experience (Harby 1988). As people around the world become more stressed with sensory bombardment, interest in flotation tanks has resurfaced for purposes of relaxation, obstetrics, and rehabilitation therapy (Kjellgren 2003; Kotz 2008; Stark et al. 2008).

Pet Therapy. With the recent discovery of a special neuropeptide called beta-endorphin, a natural substance similar to morphine secreted by the brain, lymphocytes, and perhaps other cells, new theories quickly developed about its relationship to positive mood change as well as factors that may release it in the body. About the same time, a therapeutic practice was started in several nursing homes, clinical care settings, prisons, and some schools: **pet therapy** (**FIG. 23.11**). It was noticed that physical and psychological responses were altered favorably when people came in contact with pet animals, suggesting a link between the two discoveries. Pet therapy involves the integration of animals into clinically directed therapeutic activities, particularly through

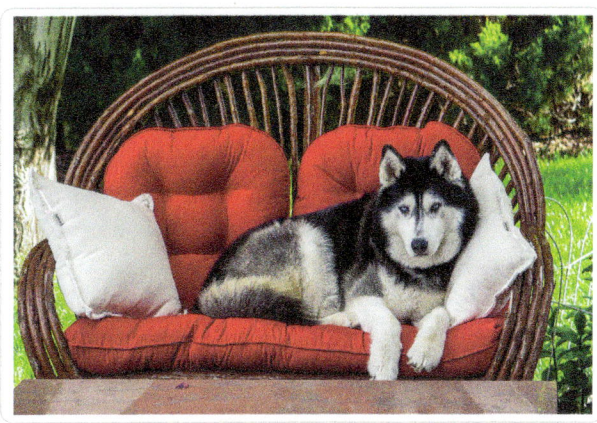

FIGURE 23.11   By and large, people who own or care for pets are less stressed and more healthy than people who do not have pets. Many pet therapy programs exist around the country, serving a spectrum of stressed people, from hospital patients and quadriplegics to members of various cancer support groups.

holding and petting small domestic animals, such as cats and dogs, and in some rare cases, swimming with dolphins. In the past few years, pet therapy has moved from cats and dogs making the rounds in nursing homes to riding horses in Virginia and swimming with dolphins in Florida and Hawaii. The new name given to pet therapy is pet-assisted therapy. Several years ago, a "pet partners" program was developed for burn victims through the Hope Therapy Program of the University of Texas in Houston, in conjunction with the Moody Gardens in Galveston, Texas. Pet Partners, a national pet therapy program, is now located in 45 states and four countries.

The results of pet therapy are quite remarkable: The tactile contact, combined with new companionship, seems to have a special healing quality. Although changes in muscle tension have not been investigated, significant changes in resting heart rate, blood pressure, and mood have been observed with interest (Burke 1992; Cusack and Smith 1984; Holden 1984). In the company of pets, resting heart rate and blood pressure showed significant decreases while perceived mood improved. In addition, pet owners felt physically better when they touched and petted their animals. Professor

Pet therapy: The use of hand contact with pets to promote relaxation among hospital patients, nursing home patients, and now everyday pet owners who claim better health through decreased resting heart rate and blood pressure.

Erika Friedman notes that survival rates for coronary patients are higher among pet owners than those who do not own pets, and that elderly people who own pets make fewer visits to their physicians (Burke 1992). The conclusion from these and other findings suggests that physical contact with friendly animals promotes relaxation similar to that associated with meditation and biofeedback. Although the specific physiological factors associated with improved mood remain a mystery in the field of psychoneuroimmunology, current conventional wisdom suggests a strong link between the release of beta-endorphins and other neuropeptides and touch, which can indeed have a healing or restorative effect on the body. Researchers may one day find that the relaxing effect is related to entrainment of the animals' energy field with that of humans.

Therapeutic Touch. Clinical medicine, which for centuries shunned the metaphysical aspects of healing through touch, is slowly beginning to acknowledge the possibility that this type of healing can augment standard medical treatment. **Therapeutic touch (TT)** was made popular by Dolores Krieger, RN, and has been taught to thousands of nurses worldwide. In her book *Hands of Light* (1987), healer Barbara Ann Brennen discusses her collaborative efforts with prominent physicians, particularly in the field of oncology. Like shiatsu, therapeutic touch and bioenergy healing involve the manipulation of blocked energy centers, thus clearing the pathways (chakras) of the human energy field. Rather than applying pressure with the thumbs or palms, however, healing occurs through the laying on of the hands, which "conducts" positive or healing energy through the body's energy field. Similarly, the ancient Japanese Reiki method integrates physical manipulation of muscle and connective tissue with universal energy (*ki*). As the disciplines of physics and clinical medicine expand and the gap of understanding narrows regarding the dynamics of human matter, a greater collaboration of all aspects of healing may unfold.

■ Physiological and Psychological Benefits

Perhaps the most notable effect of massage therapy is the state of complete physical relaxation one experiences during and immediately after the experience. The appli-

Therapeutic touch: An energy-based healing modality using the science of subtle energy to restore homeostasis (also similar to Reiki and healing touch).

cation of touch at the site of tense muscles first increases neural reflex receptor activity, causing a dilation of blood vessels and increased circulation. This increase in blood supply apparently decreases neural drive through the afferent neural mechanism. In effect, this desensitizes the nerve endings receiving messages from the brain, thus decreasing muscle tension. Repeated claims have been made that massage cleans the muscles of metabolic waste products through gentle pumping of the circulatory and lymphatic systems; however, no scientific evidence supports this theory. A more likely theory, yet to be proven, is that touch triggers the release of neuropeptides, including beta-endorphins, which may neutralize or diminish the effects of metabolic by-products. Despite the fact that many claims are yet unproven scientifically, it is commonly accepted that the effects of massage therapy on the musculoskeletal and neuromuscular systems, including increased flexibility and decreased muscle tension, are unrefuted (Harrison 1986; Moraska 2005). In fact, physicians are increasingly referring their patients with low back pain, bone fractures, multiple sclerosis, structural bone disease, and arthritis to massage therapists for treatment complementary to their own prescribed medical therapy for these ailments (Bailey-Lloyd 2007).

The physical effects of massage are only superseded by the emotional experience of relaxation. It appears the mind also benefits from the powers of touch, as described earlier. When the mind is cleared of thought, stress is minimized. The nursing community reports that massages also provide a sense of serenity and security to patients. In a study reported by Cohen (1987), where massage therapy was administered to cancer patients, questionnaires measuring mood and symptoms of distress revealed that massage promoted a greater sense of tranquility and vitality with less lethargy, compared to just relaxing in a prone position.

The reduction of tension headaches and other stress-related ailments suggests that there is a significant relationship between mind and body, and that both benefit from this relaxation technique. Massage therapists often comment on the ease with which their clients express themselves verbally while being massaged, suggesting the loosening of mental and emotional blocks as well as muscular knots. Note that there are times when massage is not recommended—for example, when people have skin rashes, severe bruises, and muscle strains—contraindications with which massage therapists are well acquainted.

Massage therapy can be a wonderful supplement to your collection of relaxation techniques. It is suggested, however, that you check the qualifications of the massage therapist because there are many practitioners who have no certified training. In addition to certification, many states now require that massage therapists become licensed. (The state of New York, for example, requires competence in anatomy, physiology, kinesiology, neurology, pathology, hygiene, and first aid and CPR, in addition to massage techniques.) For more information on massage therapy and certification and/or licensing, visit the AMTA website at https://www.amtamassage.org.

Massage Therapy and Chronic Pain

With muscle tension being the number one symptom of pain, massage therapy is often recommended as the first healing modality for acute and chronic pain, particularly muscular pain involving the neck and shoulder region, lower back, and legs. Bodywork is available in the forms of sports massage, Rolfing, myofascial release, and others, all of which offer their own unique style of physical manipulation to relieve pain (**FIG. 23.12**). The literature is loaded with books and articles supporting the premise and efficacy of pain relief through a host of bodywork modalities (Imamura et al. 2008; Schatz 2001). Research also supports the use of aromatherapy for pain reduction (Buckle 1999).

Best Application of Massage Therapy

Muscle tension is cited as the number one symptom of stress. Bodywork, in all its forms, can be used to help decrease muscle tension, lessen muscle stiffness, and help restore a sense of physical (and mental) homeostasis. People in service professions (from food servers and

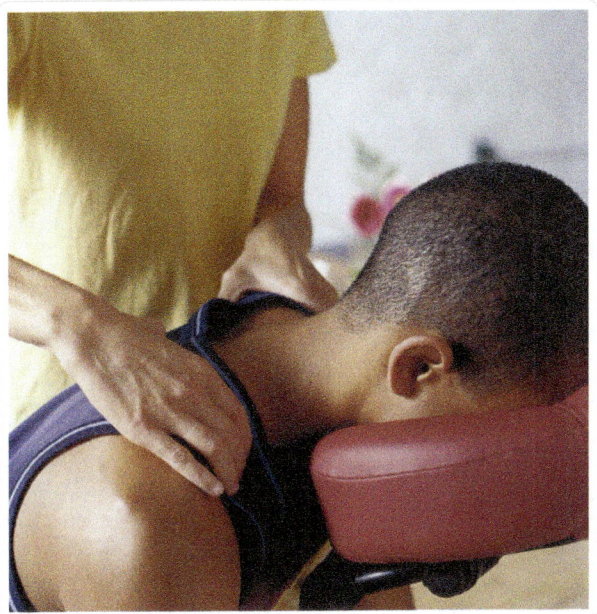

FIGURE 23.12 Muscle tension is considered to be the number one symptom of stress. Muscle massage in the form of Swedish massage is the most common type of massage. Also popular are shiatsu, sports massage, and myofascial release. Some types of bodywork include aspects of all of these.

nurses to store clerks and shelf stockers) who stand and walk in their jobs would benefit greatly from massage therapy as a means to reduce muscle tension. As people spend less time being active and more sedentary time in front of their computer screens, muscles of the neck, shoulders, and upper back receive undue stress from a specific posture associated with screen viewing. As a result, bodywork offers a powerful means to intercept the stress response and promote relaxation in overworked, stiff, or tired muscles.

SUMMARY

- Muscle massage is the manipulation of skin, muscles, ligaments, and connective tissue for the purpose of decreasing muscle tension and increasing physical comfort in musculature and surrounding joints. This is the one relaxation technique that requires the assistance of someone else to achieve the full effect.

- Massage therapy is now a bona fide practice, with more than 56,000 practitioners certified through the American Massage Therapy Association. Massage therapists must go through formal education (500 hours of classroom instruction) as well as 3 years of practice before becoming certified.

- Massage therapy not only aids in the reduction of muscle tension, but also provides an essential human need: touch. Research indicates that human touch is vital for well-being, and that as people become more involved with technology there is less human contact, resulting in what some call touch deprivation.

- Landmark studies by Field showed that infants require human touch to thrive; speculation is that people of all ages need it as well. Other research shows that massage therapy is as effective in promoting the relaxation response as are other forms of relaxation.

- There are several different types of massage, or bodywork. Swedish massage is the most widely recognized style in the West, but shiatsu, Rolfing, myofascial release, and sports massage, well known in other parts of the world, are gaining popularity.

- Aromatherapy, hydrotherapy, pet therapy, and therapeutic touch are other related touch therapies.

- Studies involving various massage therapies indicate that there is not only a physical relaxation effect, but in many cases an emotional benefit as well.

- Since the advent of the fitness boom in the late 1970s and early 1980s, massage has become a significant aspect of health maintenance. Today, several corporations offer muscle massage as part of wellness programs for employees who spend their workdays in front of a computer terminal.

- Massage therapy is used as a modality to decrease episodes of acute and chronic pain.

STUDY GUIDE QUESTIONS

1. What is massage therapy, and why is it thought to be an effective means to relax?

2. List and describe five styles of massages (bodywork).

3. What is aromatherapy, and why is this technique thought to be relaxing?

4. What is hydrotherapy, and why is this technique thought to be relaxing?

5. What is pet therapy, and why is this technique thought to be relaxing?

REFERENCES AND RESOURCES

Adcock, C. L. 1987. "Massage Therapy in Alcohol/Drug Treatment." *Alcoholism Treatment Quarterly* 4(3): 87–101.

Allen, K. 2001. "Melodies, Mutts Reduce Stress." *Men's Fitness* 17: 52–54.

American Massage Therapy Association, 500 Davis Street, Evanston, IL 60201. 1-877-905-0577. www.amtamassage.org.

American Massage Therapy Association. 1986. *Sports Massage*. Chicago, IL: Author.

American Massage Therapy Association. 1989. *A Guide to Massage Therapy in America*. Chicago, IL: Author.

Ashton, J. 1984. "Holistic Health Six: In Your Hands." *Nursing Times* 80(19): 54.

Auckett, A. 1981. *Baby Massage: Parent–Child Bonding Through Touching*. New York: Newmarket Press.

Bach, E. A. 1921. "Clinical Comparison Between the Action of Vaccines and Homeopathic Remedies." *British Homeopathic Journal* 9: 21–24.

Bailey-Lloyd. C. 2007. What's all the buzz about Massage Therapy. http://ezinearticles.com/?Whats-All-the-Buzz-about-Massage-Therapy?&id=879643

Barber, B. 1978. *Sensual Water, A Celebration of Bathing*. Chicago: Contemporary Books.

Barker, S. B., and K. S. Dawson. 1998. "The Effects of Animal-Assisted Therapy on Anxiety Ratings of

Hospitalized Psychiatric Patients." *Psychiatric Services* 49(6): 797–801.

Barnes, J. 1990. *Myofascial Release: The Search for Excellence.* Paoli, PA: RSI-T-A, Myofascial Treatment Centers.

Barnes, J. 1995. Personal communication, August 5. Sedona, AZ.

Bentley, E. 2000. *Head, Neck, and Shoulders Massage: A Step-by-Step Guide.* New York: St. Martins Griffin.

Bever, L. 2014. "'Text Neck' Is Becoming an Epidemic and Could Wreak Your Spine." *Washington Post,* November 14.

Box, D. 1985. "Putting on the Pressure." *Nursing Mirror* 160: 22.

Brennen, B. A. 1987. *Hands of Light.* New York: Bantam Books.

Buckle, J. 1999. "Use of Aromatherapy as a Complementary Treatment for Chronic Pain." *Alternative Therapies* 5(5): 42–50.

Buckle, J. 2000. "The Smell of Relief." *Psychology Today* 33(1): 24.

Burke, S. 1992. "In the Presence of Animals." *U.S. News and World Report,* February 24, pp. 64–65.

Caddy, S. H., and G. Jones. 1997. "Massage Therapy as a Workplace Intervention for Reduction of Stress." *Perceptual & Motor Skills* 84(1): 157–158.

Cassar, M. 1999. *Handbook of Massage Therapy.* Woburn, MA: Butterworth-Heinemann.

Channon, L. D. 1986. "Relaxation Techniques: Alternatives to Progressive Relaxation." *Australian Journal of Clinical and Experimental Hypnosis* 14(2): 133–137.

Ching, M. 1999. "Contemporary Therapy: Aromatherapy in the Management of Acute Pain?" *Contemporary Nurse* 8(4): 146–150.

Cohen, N. 1987. "Massage Is the Message." *Nursing Times* 83(19): 19–20.

Cunningham, S. 2000. *Magical Aromatherapy: The Power of Scent.* St. Paul, MN: Llewellyn Publications.

Cusack, O., and E. Smith. 1984. "Pets and the Elderly: The Therapeutic Bond." *Activities, Adaptations, and Aging* 4(2–3): 33–49.

Cuva, L. 2000. "Is Your Company at Risk?" *Corporate Health Solutions* 1(1).

Czimbal, B., and M. Zadikov. 1991. *Vitamin T: A Guide to Healthy Touch.* Portland, OR: Open Book.

Day, J. A., R. R. Mason, and S. E. Chesrown. 1987. "Effect of Massage on Serum Level of β-Endorphin and β-Lipoprotein in Healthy Adults." *Physical Therapy* 67: 926–930.

Dion, K. 2001. "Massage Therapy—What Is It?" *Healthcare Review* 14(3): 5.

Downing, G. 1972. *The Massage Book.* New York: Random House.

D'urso, M. A. 1987. "Massage for the Masses." *Health* 19: 63–67.

Edmunds, A., and H. Tudor. 1976. *Some Unrecognized Factors in Medicine.* London: Theosophical Society.

Elliott, M. 1999. "Back from Hell: Healing Posttraumatic Stress Disorder." *Massage & Bodywork,* December/January, pp. 13–21.

Feitis, R. 1978. *Ida Rolf Talks about Rolfing and Physical Reality.* New York: Harper & Row.

Feltman, J. (Ed.). 1989. *Hands-on Healing.* Emmaus, PA: Rodale Press.

Field, T. 1989. "Stressors During Pregnancy and the Postnatal Period." *New Directions for Child Development* 45: 19–31.

Field, T. 1998. "Massage Therapy Effects." *American Psychologist,* December, pp. 1270–1281.

Field, T. 2008. Personal communication (email), April 3.

Field, T. 2010. "Pregnancy and Labor Massage." *Expert Review of Obstetrics and Gynecology* 5(2): 177–181.

Field, T., N. Grizzle, F. Scafidi, et al. 1996. "Massage Therapy for Infants of Depressed Mothers." *Infant Behavior and Development* 19(1): 107.

Fisher-Rizzi, S. 1990. *The Complete Aromatherapy Handbook.* New York: Sterling Publishing.

Fox, E., R. Bowers, and M. Foss. 1989. *The Physiological Basis of Physical Education and Athletics.* Dubuque, IA: William C. Brown.

Friz, S. 2000. *Fundamentals of Therapeutic Massage.* St. Louis, MO: Mosby.

Gauthier, P. 1990. "Development of a New Approach to Emotionally Deprived Children and Youth." *Child and Youth Services* 13(1): 71–81.

Goleman, D., and T. Bennett. 1986. *The Relaxed Body Book.* Garden City, NY: Doubleday.

Green, R., and M. Green. 1987. "Relaxation Increases Salivary Immunoglobulin A." *Psychological Reports* 61(2): 623–629.

Gurudas, H. 1983. *Flower Essences and Vibrational Healing.* San Rafael, CA: Cassandra Press.

Harby, K. 1988. "Troubles Float Away." *Psychology* 22(2): 20.

Harrison, A. 1986. "Therapeutic Massage: Getting the Massage." *Nursing Times* 82(48): 34–35.

Havemann, J. S. 1989. "Rubbing out Workday Pain: Massage Rooms Win Departmental Support." *The Washington Post,* February 6.

Hemmings, B., M. Smith, J. Graydon, and R. Dyson. 2000. "Effects of Massage on Physiological Restoration, Perceived Recovery, and Repeated Sports Performance." *British Journal of Sports Medicine* 34(2): 109–114.

Hirsh, J. S. 1989. "Doesn't Everyone Need to Be Kneaded Once in a While?" *Wall Street Journal,* October 17.

Holden, C. 1984. "Human–Animal Relationship Under Scrutiny." *Science* 214(23): 418–458.

Holmes, P. 1995. "Aromatherapy: Applications for Clinical Practice." *Alternative & Complementary Therapies* 1(3): 117–182.

Howdyshell, C. 1998. "Complementary Therapy: Aromatherapy with Massage for Geriatric and Hospice Care—A Call for a Holistic Approach." *Hospice Journal* 13: 69–75.

Hutchinson, M. 1984. *The Book of Floating: Exploring the Private Sea.* New York: Quill Books.

Imamura, M., A. D. Furlan, T. Dryden, and E. Irvin. 2008. "Evidence-Informed Management of Chronic Low Back Pain with Massage." *Spine Journal* 8(1): 121–133.

Jacobs, M. 1960. "Massage for the Relief of Pain: Anatomical and Physical Considerations." *Physical Therapy Review* 40: 93–98.

Jodo, E. R., Y. Yamado, T. Hatayama, et al. 1988. "Effects of Facial Massage on the Spontaneous EEG." *Tohoku-Psychologica Folia* 47(1–4): 8–15.

Johnson, J. 1995. *The Healing Art of Sports Massage.* New York: Rodale Press.

Jones, T. A. 2004. "Rolfing." *Physical and Medicine Rehabilitation Clinics of North America* 15(4): 799–809.

Jorgenson, J. 1997. "Therapeutic Use of Companion Animals in Health Care." *Image: Journal of Nursing Scholarship* 29(3): 249–254.

Kahn, R. 2001. "New Era for Massage Research." *Massage Therapy Journal* 40(3): 104.

Katcher, A. H. 1985. "Physiological and Behavioral Responses to Companion Animals." *Veterinary Clinics of North America: Small Animal Practices* 15: 403–410.

Kaye, A. D., A. J. Kaye, J. Swinford, et al. 2008. "The Effect of Deep-Tissue Massage Therapy on Blood Pressure and Heart Rate." *Alternative Complementary Medicine* 14(2): 125–128.

Kiecolt-Glaser, J. K., J. E. Graham, W. B. Malarkey, et al. 2008. "Olfactory Influences on Mood and Autonomic, Endocrine, and Immune Function." *Psychoneuroendocrinology* 33(3): 328–339.

Kjellgren, A. 2003. "Relaxation in a Flotation Tank Brings Peace and Quiet, Increased Well-Being, and Reduced Pain." *Innovations Report*, May 11.

Kolpakov, S., and S. Rumyantseva. 1987. "Use of a Combined Method of Correcting the Human Psychophysiological State During Work and Constant Vision Strain." *Human Physiology* 13(1): 36–42.

Kotz, D. 2008. "Stressed Out? Try a Flotation Tank." *U.S. News & World Report*, March 12.

Kresge, C. 1996. "Benefits of Sports Massage." *Sports Medicine, Fitness, Training, Injuries*, pp. 43–48.

Lacroix, N. 1990. *Massage for Total Stress Relief.* New York: Random House.

Lippin, R. 1996. "Alternative Medicine in the Workplace." *Alternative Therapies* 2(1): 47–51.

Liu, Y. 2008. "The Role of Massage Therapy in the Relief of Cancer Pain." *Nursing Standards* 22(21): 35–40.

Lundberg, P. 2003. *The Book of Shiatsu: A Complete Guide to Using Hand Pressure and Gentle Manipulation to Improve Your Health, Vitality, and Stamina.* New York: Fireside Books.

Mauskop, A. 2001. "Alternative Therapies in Headache: Is There a Role?" *Medical Clinics of North America* 85(4).

Maxwell-Hudson, C. 1988. *The Complete Book of Massages.* New York: Random House.

McKechnie, A., F. Wilson, N. Watson, and D. Scott. 1983. "Anxiety States: A Preliminary Report on the Value of Connective-Tissue Massage." *Journal of Psychosomatic Research* 27(2): 1245–1249.

Mercati, M. 1998. *Thai Massage.* New York: Sterling.

Mochizuki, S. 2000. "Japanese Chair Massage, Part I." *Massage & Bodywork* 15(1): 98–100.

Moraska, A. 2005. "Sports Massage: A Comprehensive Review." *Journal of Sports Medicine and Physical Fitness* 45(3): 370–380.

Moraska, A., C. Chandler, A. Edmiston-Schaetzel, et al. 2008. "Comparison of a Targeted and General Massage Protocol on Strength, Function, and Symptoms Associated with Carpal Tunnel Syndrome: A Randomized Pilot Study." *Journal of Alternative and Complementary Medicine* 14(3): 259–267.

Muhammad, L. 1999. "Animal Therapy Spurs Human Touch." *USA Today*, May 3, p. 10D.

Muschel, I. J. 1984. "Pet Therapy with Terminally Ill Cancer Patients." *Social Casework* 65(8): 451–458.

Naisbitt, J. 1999. *Megatrends 2000.* New York: Avon.

Naliboff, B. D., and K. H. Tachiki. 1991. "Autonomic and Skeletal Muscle Response to Nonelectrical Cutaneous Stimulation." *Perceptual and Motor Skills* 72(2): 575–584.

Namikoshi, R. 1981. *The Complete Book of Shiatsu Therapy.* New York: Japan Publications.

National Association for Holistic Aromatherapy. https://www.naha.org.

Nixon, T. 1989. "Make Money with Massage." *Fitness Management*, September, pp. 40–42.

Okvat, H., M. C. Oz, W. Ting, and P. B. Namerow. 2002. "Massage Therapy for Patients Undergoing Cardiac Catheterization." *Alternative Therapies* 8(3): 68–77.

Pecher, K. 1985. "Pet Therapy for Heart and Soul." *Prevention*, August, pp. 80–84.

Pelletier, K. R., and D. L. Herzing. 1988. "Psychoneuro-immunology: Toward a Mind-Body Model." *Advances* 5(1): 27–56.

Pitcairn, R. H. 1985. "Why Pets Are Good for Us." *Prevention*, February, pp. 49–51.

Price, S. 1993. *Aromatherapy Workbook.* San Francisco: HarperCollins.

Proulx, D. 1998. "Animal-Assisted Therapy." *Critical Care Nurse* 18(2): 80–85.

Rimmer, L. 1998. "The Clinical Use of Aromatherapy in the Reduction of Stress." *Home Healthcare Nurse* 16: 123–126.

Robinson, I. 1999. "Pet Therapy." *Nursing Times* 95(15): 33–34.

Samples, P. 1989. "Does Sports Massage Have a Role in Sports Medicine?" *The Physician and Sports Medicine,* March, pp. 177–187.

Scafidi, F., R. M. Field, S. M. Schanberg, et al. 1990. "Massage Stimulates Growth in Preterm Infants: A Replication." *Infant Behavior and Development* 13(2): 167–188.

Schatz, B. 2001. *Soft Tissue Massage for Pain Relief.* Charlottesville, VA: Hampton Roads.

Sheldrake, R. 1999. *Dogs That Know When Their Owners Are Coming Home.* New York: Crown Publishers.

Shiina, Y., N. Funabashi, K. Lee, et al. 2008. "Relaxation Effects of Lavender Aromatherapy Improve Coronary Flow Velocity Reserve in Healthy Men Evaluated by Transthoracic Doppler Echocardiography." *International Journal of Cardiology* 129(2): 193–197.

Sims, S. 1990. "Slow-Stroke Back Massage for Cancer Patients." *Infant Behavior and Development* 13(2): 167–188.

Smith, M., M. A. Stallings, S. Mariner, and M. Burrall. 1999. "Benefits of Massage Therapy for Hospitalized Patients: A Descriptive and Qualitative Evaluation." *Alternative Therapies in Health and Medicine* 5(4): 64–71.

Stark, M. A., B. Rudell, and G. Haus. 2008. "Observing Position and Movements in Hydrotherapy: A Pilot Study." *Journal of Obstetric, Gynecololgic, and Neonatal Nursing* 37(1): 116–122.

Steiner, R. 1971. *The Etherisation of the Blood.* London: Steiner.

Stringer, J., R. Swindell, and M. Dennis. 2008. "Massage in Patients Undergoing Intensive Chemotherapy Reduces Serum Cortisol and Prolactin." *Psycho-Oncology,* February 26.

Tignore, S. 2003. "Massage Therapy Research: A Paradigm for Success." *Massage Therapy Journal* 42(2): 80–89.

Toufexis, A. 1987. "Massage Comes out of the Parlor." *Time,* March, pp. 17–20.

Vickers, A., C. Zollman, and J. T. Reinish. 2001. "Massage Therapies." *Western Journal of Medicine* 175(3): 202–204.

Weaver, M. R. 1985. "Acupressure: An Overview of Therapy and Application." *Nurse Practitioner* 10: 38–42.

Weinberg, R., A. Jackson, and K. Kolodny. 1988. "The Relationship of Massage and Exercise to Mood Enhancement." *Sport Psychologist* 2(3): 202–211.

Wilkinson, S., J. Aldridge, I. Salmon, E. Cain, and B. Wilson. 1999. "An Evaluation of Aromatherapy Massage in Palliative Care." *Palliative Medicine* 13(5): 409–417.

Willis, D. A. 1997. "Animal Therapy." *Rehabilitation Nursing* 22(2): 78–81.

Woody, R. H. 1980. *The Use of Massage in Facilitating Holistic Health.* Springfield, CA: Thomas.

Yacenda, J. 1989. "Sport Strokes." *Fitness Management* 5(9): 38–39.

Ylinen, J., and M. Cash. 1988. *Sports Massage.* St. Paul, MN: Hutchinson Educational.

Zimmer, J. 1985. "The Pleasure of Giving a Great Massage." *Health,* April, pp. 52–53.

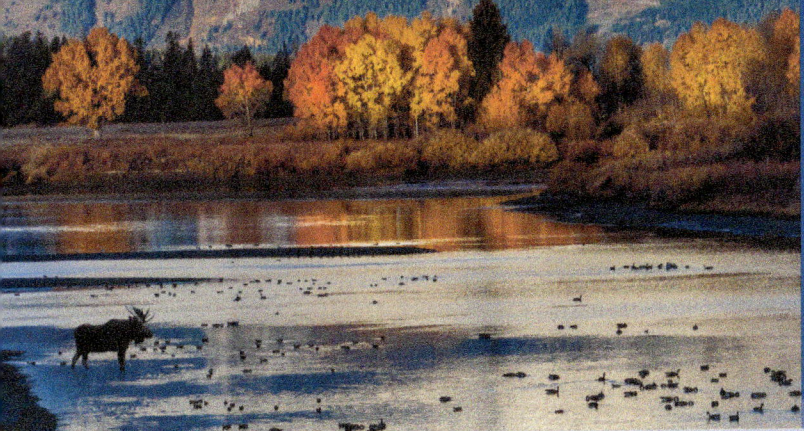

T'ai Chi Ch'uan

Tension is who you think you should be.
Relaxation is who you are.

—T'ai Chi saying

There is a life force or subtle energy that surrounds and permeates us all, which the Chinese call **Chi**. To harmonize with the universe, to move in unison with this energy, to move as freely as running water is to be at peace or one with the universe. This harmony of energy promotes tranquility and inner peace. This is the essence of **T'ai Chi ch'uan**—harmony and balance with the vital life force of the natural world itself. The words *T'ai* and *Chi* can be translated several ways. One is the "supreme ultimate," a meaning symbolic of balance, power, and enlightenment. T'ai Chi, the softest of the martial arts, is also called a moving meditation. Based on concepts similar to Feng Shui and similar to hatha yoga, it is a low-impact exercise that demonstrates unification or harmony of mind and body, and the *Chi* of the universe.

To understand *Chi*, it is helpful to examine the concept in the cultural context where it originated. The Chinese concept of health is quite different from that in Western cultures. Westerners view health as the absence of disease and illness produced by bacteria and viruses, whereas the Chinese see it as an unrestricted current of subtle energy throughout the body. When *Chi*, or subtle energy, which flows through the body in a network of meridians, or energy gates, is restricted or congested, the body is susceptible to physiological dysfunction. In Chinese medicine, it is not necessarily bacteria or viruses that cause physical dysfunction or disease because these are thought to be present everywhere. Rather, poor health is thought to be the result of low resistance, caused by nonharmonious (blocked) energy, to both internal and external factors that ultimately do one in. Stated another way, these pathogens are constantly present; it is low resistance to them that makes one vulnerable to disease. Just as acupuncture is used as a preventive intervention technique to unblock congested meridians to cure ailments, T'ai Chi ch'uan is a type of preventive exercise to maintain the peaceful flow of energy throughout the body and thus maintain good health. From a Chinese perspective, unrestricted flow of energy helps to maintain one's resistance to various influences, be they biological, psychological, or sociological in nature.

It may seem that the practice of self-defense is incongruent with relaxation. Upon closer examination, however, T'ai Chi reveals a profound expression of tranquility. It teaches one to remain calm and centered against

T'ai Chi ch'uan: A relaxation technique originating among the Chinese; a succession of movements to bring the body into harmony with the universal energy (*Chi*); a moving meditation.

Chi: The universal life force of subtle energy that surrounds and permeates everything.

the greatest opposition (stressors), to harmonize with aggression and fear, rather than fight it. As a physical exercise, it teaches how to conserve and concentrate energy rather than to dissipate it randomly. The integration of this life force into this moving meditation of self-defense suggests that T'ai Chi is not a violent exercise. Rather, it is an exercise to maintain balance in one's life. For this reason alone, the practice of T'ai Chi is a wonderful metaphor for conscious relaxation and the ability to move in balance and harmony with the environment. If you were to walk the streets of Beijing or Shanghai in the early morning hours, you would see thousands of people exercising together, practicing T'ai Chi as a mode of physical exercise, much as you would see people in the United States running or cycling.

Historical Perspective

The practice of T'ai Chi dates back thousands of years. Its origins blend the essence of Chinese philosophy with the substance of physical survival. Legend has it that thousands of years ago a man observed a fight between a crane and a serpent. With repeated jabs of his beak, the crane tried to defeat his opponent. But the snake, in a series of calculated maneuvers, shifted its body weight at the right moments and was able to remain free of harm until the crane became tired, gave up, and moved on. Stories have also been handed down through the ages that T'ai Chi developed as a unique style of boxing that emphasized internal strength mixed with flexibility and agility rather than the exhibition of brute force. As the art developed, subtle philosophical concepts were integrated with the movements as a way to teach and emphasize proficiency in mechanical skills, thus lending support to its understanding and mastery (Jou 1988; Lo 1979).

Philosophy of T'ai Chi Ch'uan

What makes T'ai Chi different from all other forms of self-defense, and perhaps unique unto itself, is its basis in philosophy. The practice of its physical movements

> **Yin:** Those complementary components in the Taoist philosophy of yin/yang expressed as dark, feminine, night, soft, etc.
>
> **Yang:** Those complementary components in the Taoist philosophy of yin/yang expressed as light, masculine, day, hard, etc.
>
> **Fasting the heart:** A T'ai Chi expression that explains the flow of one's life energy as a moving essence, and finding comfort in solitude.

is a wonderful metaphor for the essential mental attitude to successfully deal with life's daily stressors. The physical movements are fluid: They move *with* force, not against it. Many times, when we are confronted with situations we perceive to be threatening, our first instinct is to force a change or try to manipulate something we have no control over. T'ai Chi suggests quite literally going with the flow, swimming with the tide, not against it. The philosophy of T'ai Chi involves the manipulation of force by controlling oneself and yielding to become part of it.

As T'ai Chi developed, it quickly assimilated many philosophical concepts from Taoism, and to a lesser extent, Confucianism. Even the symbol used to represent T'ai Chi—a circular mandala of white and black halves with each half carrying a smaller circle of the other inside—represents the balance of opposites (**FIG. 24.1**). These opposites, **yin** and **yang**, symbolize (among other things) the positive and negative aspects in nature. Together, they represent wholeness and essential balance. T'ai Chi strives to attain the harmony of these forces through avoidance of extremes. The philosophical concepts of Taoism are embroidered with metaphorical imagery—light with darkness, good with evil, life with death—all of which express the concept of stillness in motion. Although not every concept can be categorized as "either-or," the theme of yin and yang, or wholeness, is to find peace by acknowledging the duality of these characteristics within yourself.

Four basic philosophical concepts are taught in T'ai Chi: fasting the heart, returning to nature, *Wu-wei*, and winning by losing. **Fasting the heart** is a concept to explain the flow of life's energy, a moving essence. Fasting means silence, the language of the soul. Fasting the heart also means to find comfort in solitude. The

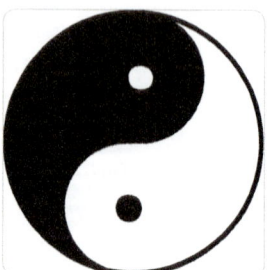

FIGURE 24.1   The Taoist symbol of yin/yang is a circle with two equal and opposite halves.

returning to nature is another way of describing a regression to the joys of childhood, embracing innocence, joy, laughter, and play. These are traits that, as adults, we lose the ability to utilize and appreciate within ourselves. **Wu-wei** is described as the philosophy of nothing-doing, nothing-knowing. It means to act without forcing; to move in accordance with the flow of nature's course. In the words of the great Chinese philosopher Lao Tzu, "Although water is soft and weak, it invariably overcomes the rigid and strong" (Dreher 1991). Often *Wu-wei* is expressed in the comparison of opposites. For example, to shrink, first you must stretch; to enervate, first you must energize; to take, first you must give. Another example is that of a ping-pong ball in water. No matter how many times you push it under, it always comes back up, and does so with little or no effort. The fourth component, **winning by losing**, advocates the success of failure. When failure is acknowledged, it becomes the first step to success. Winning by losing is an expression of unconditional acceptance. An additional concept of T'ai Chi is the realization that true understanding comes from emptying the mind (lowering the walls of the ego). This emptiness allows a liberation of the human spirit to unite with the universal life energy. Although this energy may seem elusive to those who have never practiced T'ai Chi, its effects cascade down through the body to influence the physiological systems as well.

Physiological and Psychological Benefits

Individuals who have practiced T'ai Chi, as well as those who teach this traditional Chinese exercise, make several claims about the wonderful physical and mental benefits it has to offer.

As researchers begin to explore modalities in the cadre of integrative (complementary) medicine, interest in T'ai Chi shows promise for the ancient claims of long ago. Here are some highlights: T'ai Chi is well known for promoting balance, but a study by Michael Irwin and associates (2007) reveals that a 16-week T'ai Chi class can boost the immune system and augment the efficacy of vaccines for influenza. T'ai Chi also was proven to decrease nervous (sympathetic) tension in a group of elderly subjects (Motivala et al. 2006). One study by Jin (1988) investigated both the physiological and psychological effects of T'ai Chi and found effects very similar to those produced by other types of aerobic exercises. In this study, heart rate, norepinephrine, cortisol, and mood

were observed in both beginners and ardent followers (age range 15 to 75 years). These variables were measured three times daily for a period of several weeks. Data analysis showed a marked decrease in postexercise resting heart rate as well as stress hormones over the course of a day. As a result of this technique, subjects reported less physical tension and fatigue, less anger and anxiety, and less mood disturbance. From these observations it was concluded that T'ai Chi does promote a relaxing effect (**FIG. 24.2**). As reported by Koh (1981), a study by Munyi in 1963 indicated that habitual practice of T'ai Chi produced increased measures of muscular strength and flexibility compared to sedentary control subjects. Furthermore, in a study concluded in 1981 by Plummer to compare the effects of T'ai Chi to acupuncture, it was observed that both techniques promoted physical (postural) homeostasis and psychological homeostasis, which together enhanced emotional control and tranquility. T'ai Chi has been recommended as an ideal activity for the actively mobile aged population and is said to be as effective an exercise to promote relaxation as cross-country skiing, swimming, and bicycling (Meusel 1986). Claims from the Far East include that T'ai Chi can cure hypertension, asthma, and insomnia, as well as prevent atherosclerosis and spinal deformity. To date, these claims have not been clinically proven or medically substantiated because they just have not been studied. Although these claims are yet unproven, it is believed by regular practitioners that T'ai Chi may play an important role in the prevention of disorders commonly associated with stress. Researchers also have focused on the effects of T'ai Chi and the prevention and reversal of osteoporosis (Gass 2003).

The topic of T'ai Chi continues to spark much interest in the research community regarding its promising health benefits, particularly for the prevention of falls in elderly people who might fracture their bones in such incidents (Büla et al. 2011; Campbell and Robertson, 2010). T'ai Chi is even thought to help people with Parkinson's disease (Klein 2008). Touch researcher

Returning to nature: A T'ai Chi expression to explain the joys of childhood: innocence, laughter, and play.

Wu-wei: A T'ai Chi term that signifies doing nothing, or action through nonaction, moving with the simple, subtle flow of nature.

Winning by losing: A T'ai Chi expression that explains the benefits of failure as a stepping stone toward success.

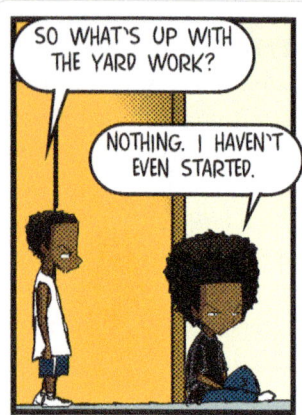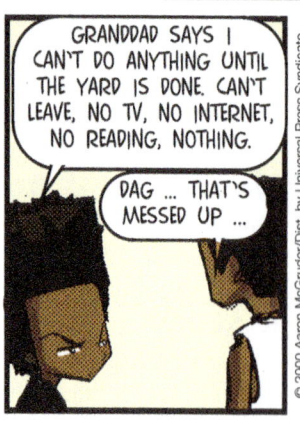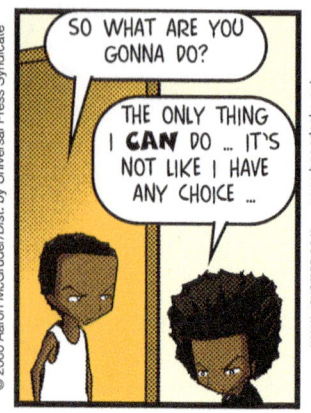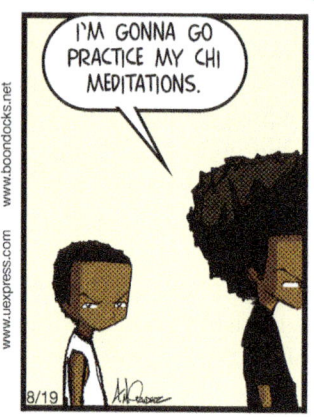

FIGURE 24.2   Practicing T'ai Chi gives a great sense of groundedness. Give it a try.

Tiffany Field studied the effects of T'ai Chi and yoga on anxiety, heart rate, electroencephalogram (EEG) readings, and math computations and noted significant positive effects on promoting relaxation with both modalities (Field 2010). T'ai Chi helped elderly subjects improve their blood flood (Mori et al. 2020). Tufts University professor Chenchen Wang and his colleagues (2010) analyzed more than 40 studies regarding the mental and physiological effects of T'ai Chi. According to their findings, T'ai Chi augments health in so many ways that the question becomes why everyone isn't practicing it.

Although few studies have researched the effects of T'ai Chi on various health parameters, in the past decade numerous studies designed in China and Japan have measured the effects of **Qigong**. Like T'ai Chi, Qigong (pronounced "chee gong") is an energy-based exercise; however, Qigong places no focus or attention on the aspects of self-defense. Rather, the movement of *Chi* throughout the body is the sole emphasis of this practice. In simple terms, energy is moved through the body by meditation and breathing, which, in turn, are combined with a host of physical movements, similar to those observed in T'ai Chi. When practiced regularly, these movements create a sense of balance in the meridian system by opening blocks and clearing congestion in the meridian gates. With regular practice of Qigong, the energy system throughout the entire body operates at its optimal level.

Qigong: A form of Chinese energy exercise and energy healing where *Qi* or *Chi* is directed through the body as a means to balance one's energy.

In an exhaustive literature review on the medical applications of Qigong, Kenneth Sancier (1996) highlights several ways in which Qigong has been used in the clinical setting to improve various aspects of health and wellness. Sancier notes that Qigong has been proven to bring about remarkable and significant results with regards to hypertension, stroke, cardiovascular efficiency, bone density, sex hormone levels, cancer, and even the early stages of senility. Although the majority of these studies have been conducted in China, the statistics indicate that Qigong can be a significant factor in promoting health. Currently, similar studies in the United States are under way, with funding for one study supported by the National Institutes of Health's Center for Complementary and Alternative Medicine.

■ T'ai Chi Ch'uan and Chronic Pain

When engaging in T'ai Chi ch'uan, it is understood that one is employing the use of *Chi* or *Qi*. As such, creating a more harmonious flow of *Chi* through the body is in itself a means to reduce energy blocks, which results in a decrease in pain. Because of the subtleties involved with *Chi*, at first the results may seem less dramatic than those achieved with traditional pain relievers. For those who maintain a regular practice of T'ai Chi or Qigong, however, an obvious change takes place over time to align not only the life force of energy, but also the musculoskeletal structure that houses it. Case studies report that the pain from osteoarthritis is significantly reduced with the practice of T'ai Chi and Qigong (Cohen 2003).

T'ai Chi Ch'uan as a Relaxation Technique

T'ai Chi has more than 100 positions or movements, with several similarities among some of them. Most people who learn T'ai Chi begin with formal lessons, either in a group or with private instruction. The purpose of this chapter is to provide exposure to some of its concepts and movements and to acquaint you with this exercise as an alternative relaxation technique. Keep in mind that initially T'ai Chi can be difficult to learn from reading and studying the movements in a book. It is my hope that this exposure may inspire you to take one or more lessons to further your appreciation of this exercise.

Before T'ai Chi can be practiced effectively, there are some important concepts to understand to make this exercise more enjoyable, which are taken from the *T'ai Chi Handbook* (1974) by Herman Kauz. As with yoga *asanas*, T'ai Chi movements may seem difficult at first. With time and practice, however, they will become so natural they will seem almost effortless. First and foremost, T'ai Chi is an egoless activity. That is, do not compare the precision of your movements with those of others who take part in this exercise for relaxation. And when you try the positions, go for the general movements first and then try to pick up the finer details later. There is no right or wrong, there only is. Keep the following in mind when practicing T'ai Chi:

1. *Breathe effortlessly.* Breathing should be natural. Some teachers instruct students to hold their tongue to the roof of the mouth, breathe through the nose, and allow the abdominal area to expand rather than the chest. When beginning, breathe in whatever fashion is easiest for you. With time you will find your breathing becoming more coordinated with the progression of each movement. Eventually you will probably adopt the suggested breathing style in coordination with the movements.

2. *Free the body of all unnecessary tension.* When watching someone perform T'ai Chi, the first word that comes to mind is *graceful.* When the body is relaxed, the flow of energy will move more freely. Tension in any body region inhibits energy movement. Use only the minimal amount of muscle tension to complete the movement.

3. *Maintain a stance perpendicular to the floor.* With a perpendicular stance, the balance of each position, as well as transition to the next position, is more easily attained. It is important to keep the spinal column completely aligned (perpendicular to the floor). A common metaphor used in teaching T'ai Chi is to move as if you were a marionette suspended by a string from the top of your head. Many instructors teach the 70/30 stance, where in transition from one movement to the next, the forward foot maintains approximately 70 percent of the body weight, with the back foot maintaining 30 percent.

4. *Keep your center of gravity low.* Your center of gravity is approximately an inch or two below your belly button. Stand up, close your eyes, and sense your body's center of gravity. A lower center of gravity means a more stable base to move and position yourself. When performing these movements, bend the knees slightly, especially when shifting your weight from one leg to the other.

5. *Maintain an even speed.* The graceful movements of T'ai Chi are a result of a continuous flow of movement like the gentle flow of water. The progression of these movements should be even, not sudden or jerky. Try to feel the surrounding space with your hands, as if you are swimming in air. Move arms and hands in unison with the body.

6. *Integrate the mind and body as one.* When performing T'ai Chi, the mind should move with the body. Concentration should be sharp. Try not to let your mind wander off to distant thoughts. If this should happen, quickly bring it back to your body movements.

T'ai Chi Ch'uan Movements

The following movements are the first eight positions in this moving meditation as illustrated in Kauz's *T'ai Chi Handbook.* Points of orientation will be north, south, east, and west. For simplicity, the starting position will begin facing north, wherever you decide that to be located. Most people learn T'ai Chi barefoot or in socks because this helps with initial foot placement. The feet also become more relaxed when less confined. The eight positions are as follows:

Position 1: **Starting posture** (**FIG. 24.3**). Stand erect with feet shoulder-width apart, arms by your side,

> **Starting posture:** The stance that begins the first of many positions in the flow of the T'ai Chi exercise; one stands looking straight ahead with one's weight balanced on both feet.

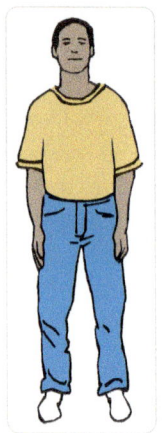

FIGURE 24.3 Starting posture.

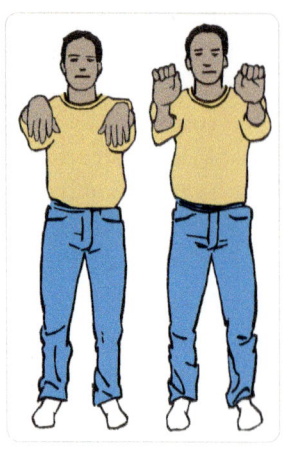

FIGURE 24.4 Beginning position.

palms facing back, chin up, and eyes looking directly ahead.

Position 2: **Beginning position** (**FIG. 24.4**). Raise your arms directly in front to about shoulder level, leading with the wrists. Elbows should be slightly bent, shoulders relaxed. Then, slowly allow arms and hands to return to the starting position below waist level, leading with the elbows.

Position 3: **Left-hand ward-off** (**FIG. 24.5**). Shift weight first to the left foot, allowing the left knee to bend slightly. Next, pivot onto the right foot, slowly rotating the body clockwise about 90 degrees. As you turn east, slowly raise the right hand to mid-chest level, palm facing down, while at the same time raising the left hand to waist level, palm facing up, as if carrying a beach ball in both hands. With completion of the pivot, the majority of your weight now rests on the right foot, and the left heel leaves the ground. Then, rotate the body back (counterclockwise) and

Beginning position: From the starting position, one begins to move the hands upward to eye level, palms facing down.

Left-hand ward-off: The third step in the classic T'ai Chi movement with a specific series of hand motions and feet placement.

Right-hand ward-off: The fourth step in the classic T'ai Chi movement with a specific series of hand motions and feet placement.

return weight to the left foot. (The right foot remains pointed eastward.) Return the right arm to your side, while slowly raising the left arm to mid-chest level, palm facing in. Hips should remain directly under the shoulders.

Position 4: **Right-hand ward-off** (**FIG. 24.6**). With the majority of weight on your left foot, raise your right heel off the ground and turn your body clockwise, to the east. Raise the left hand to mid-chest level, palm facing down, while turning the right palm upward just below the waist. Again, hold the imaginary beach ball between your palms. With your weight on your left foot, raise the heel of your right foot and direct it to the place where the right toe was previously, facing

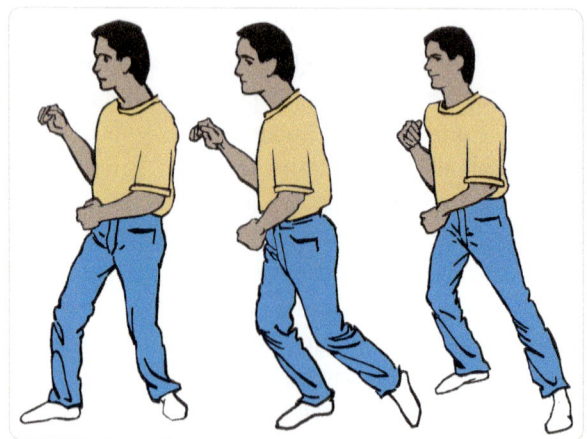

FIGURE 24.5 Left-hand ward-off.

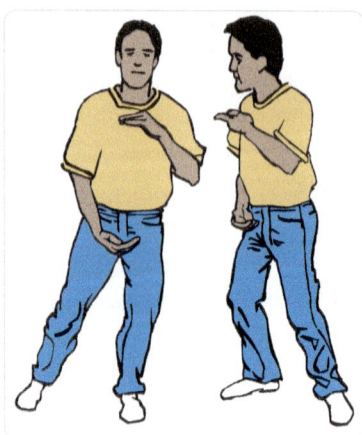

FIGURE 24.6 Right-hand ward-off.

east. As you rotate your body east, shift 70 percent of your body weight from the left foot to the right, keeping knees slightly bent, hips directly parallel to shoulders, and pivoting the left foot east. At the same time, raise the right hand to shoulder level, palm facing toward the chest. Move the left hand with your body at mid-chest level.

Position 5: **Grasp the bird's tail** (*roll back and press*) (**FIG. 24.7**). Now shift your body weight from the right to the left foot (70 percent to 30 percent). With this shift, begin to turn slightly north. Swing the left hand, palm facing in, slowly down past the waist and circle back up and over the left shoulder. Move the right hand, palm facing in, toward the chest. As the left hand comes back to mid-chest level, continue to rotate the body east again and transfer your body weight again to the right foot. Brush the left palm lightly against the right wrist at the same time.

Position 6: Grasp the bird's tail (*push*) (**FIG. 24.8**). Facing east, begin to separate the hands and lower them slowly to upper abdominal level, palms facing out. Shift your weight from the right foot to the left, as if you were slowly backing up. Then, reverse weight back to the right foot and extend your hands out slowly as if you were pushing an object away from your face. As you push, be conscious of directing energy in that direction.

Position 7: **The single whip** (**FIG. 24.9**). Shift your body weight from the right foot to the left, and rotate your body counterclockwise to the north-northwest.

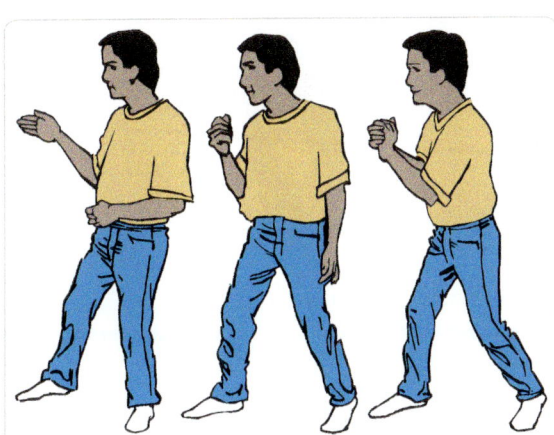

FIGURE 24.7   Grasp the bird's tail (roll back and press).

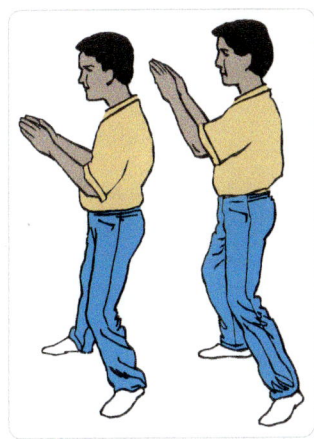

FIGURE 24.8   Grasp the bird's tail (push).

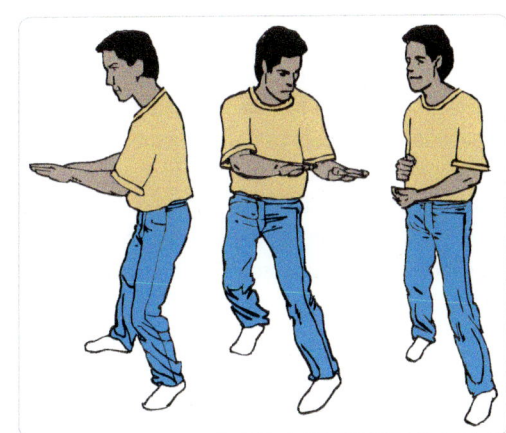

FIGURE 24.9   The single whip.

Swing arms and hands slowly in the same direction, keeping hands directly in front at mid-chest level. Place the right heel where the right toe was, now pointing north. Then, shift weight to the right foot, rotating slightly to the northeast. Swing the left hand slowly to waist level by the right hip, palm

Grasp the bird's tail: The fifth (roll back and press) and sixth (push) steps in the classic T'ai Chi movement with a specific series of hand motions and feet placement.

The single whip: The seventh step in the classic T'ai Chi movement with a specific series of hand motions and feet placement.

Stress with a Human Face

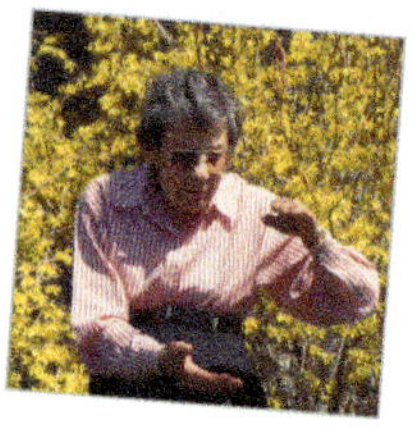

Betty Stewart had heard of T'ai Chi decades ago, but it wasn't until September 1994 that she began to practice it in earnest. In the early 1970s she was intrigued to try this form of relaxation, and even bought a video so she could teach herself, but she said that just didn't work. Then one day she noticed that a class in T'ai Chi was to be offered at the Prestige Club, a unique hospital-based health promotion program for seniors with a special focus on bridging standard and complementary forms of healing. Betty wasted no time in signing up.

What makes Betty's story so remarkable are the changes she saw soon after she began taking the class, as well as those that occurred after the first year. Prior to beginning the course, Betty, at the age of 79, was all of 55 inches tall. To the amazement of her physician, Betty has since added over an inch to her height. And unlike most people her age who lose inches to bone demineralization, Betty's bone density remained unchanged in the 2 years of doing T'ai Chi. Recently she told me, "There was a chance to be involved in a bone demineralization study, but I didn't have time in my life to see if after 4 years of clinical trials, all I got was the placebo. I wanted the real thing—that's why I started T'ai Chi."

Aside from the benefits of bone integrity, Betty says there have been other benefits. "I have a much better sense of balance. Why, one day I tripped on an uneven sidewalk. Because I learned how to shift my weight, all that happened was a little bang, but no fracture. My coordination and concentration skills have also improved, as has my level of energy. You know, you cannot do T'ai Chi if your mind wanders. You lose track of where you are in the progression of movements."

Aside from the physical movements, Betty is attracted to the philosophy of this moving meditation. There is a real poetic quality to T'ai Chi, she says with a smile in her voice. "I can tell you about stress, too! Let's just say that both my husband and I have had our fair share of it these past few years. T'ai Chi has really kept me balanced. I think T'ai Chi is phenomenal and I recommend it to all your students."

facing up. Draw back the right arm to the right hip, leading with the elbow, and close the fingers as if dropping a coin into the palm of the left hand. Next, slowly rotate your body west, shifting weight from the right foot to the left by taking a step with the left foot. At the same time, raise the right hand to about shoulder level, and sweep the left hand slowly in an upward arc from right to left, twisting the wrist to allow the palm to face out as the hand comes to about shoulder level.

Position 8: **Lift hands** (**FIG. 24.10**). Slowly lift your right heel off the floor and place it once again where the right toe was pointing north. As the heel makes contact, begin to shift your weight from the left foot

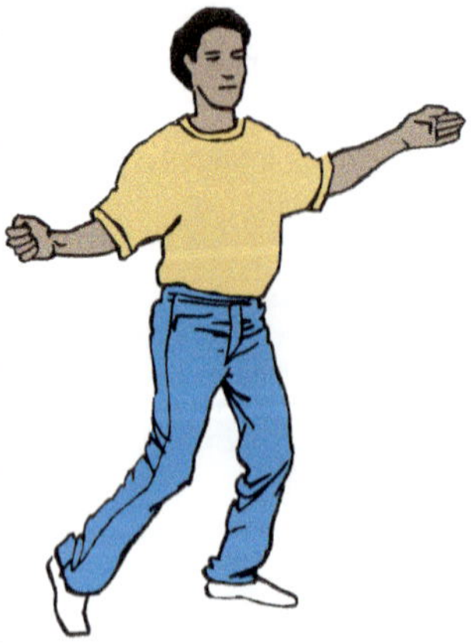

FIGURE 24.10   Lift hands.

Lift hands: The eighth step in the classic T'ai Chi movement, incorporating a series of specific hand motions and foot placement to facilitate optimal *Chi* movement.

to the right, coming back to face north. Starting with hands loosely extended out to the sides, draw palms close together facing inward, and position the left hand near the right elbow.

Additional Comments on T'ai Chi Ch'uan

T'ai Chi is unique unto itself. To feel your body move in a guided motion generates a sense of inner peace that seems unparalleled among relaxation techniques. But to be effective, T'ai Chi takes continual practice, a half hour or so per day. Some advocate early morning practice as a fresh start to the day, while others like to end the day with this exercise. There really is no time that is best; choose whatever time fits into your regular schedule. This technique can certainly be done alone, but group sessions add a whole new element of grace and relaxation. Several YMCA, YWCA, and community programs offer morning sessions open to people of all abilities. Remember not to compare your technique with others: Make it an egoless activity. The practice also may necessitate additional lessons from a qualified instructor. Even the best instructors strive to improve their technique. When looking for a T'ai Chi instructor, be sure that his or her philosophy matches yours. Some instructors see T'ai Chi merely as a form of self-defense and teach it as such. Others teach it as a type of meditation, providing an atmosphere to enhance spiritual well-being as well as physical well-being. Sample several instructors before making a commitment to the advancement of your technique. Trust in the instructor is paramount in learning. Finally, definitely take this advice from my instructor, Steve Pearlman: "T'ai Chi classes should be lighthearted and fun. If you can have fun and be relaxed in a self-defense situation—in a situation of immediate physical harm—and you can learn to go with the flow, you can be relaxed anywhere. T'ai Chi teaches you how to be relaxed in all aspects of your life and how to stay relaxed in the face of stress."

Best Application of T'ai Chi Ch'uan

If you should find yourself getting bored with aerobic exercise or meditation and crave variety, try a session of T'ai Chi. Once you get beyond the idea that you may feel silly, this exercise can be dynamic in its ability to promote relaxation. Some people make T'ai Chi their only method of relaxation, whereas others use it to supplement their repertoire of techniques. When you first try it, remember that the nature of T'ai Chi is calm, not rushed. This moving meditation acts to defuse the emotions that disconnect us from the source of life's energy. To move with the force, not against it, is to abandon emotional attachment to the causes of stress. As a type of physical exercise, T'ai Chi requires its own time and space. Initially, implementation of this technique is not suitable for the overt confrontation of stress. But with practice and understanding, when balance is found, the physical arousal of stress is minimal when faced with a perceived threat.

To practice T'ai Chi, you need some room to move about, approximately 5 feet by 5 feet, although it can be done in less space. Once the movements are committed to memory, they are easy to practice. But like any other skill, the benefits of this technique necessitate regular practice.

SUMMARY

- *Chi* is a Chinese term representing the universal life energy that surrounds and permeates everyone, the life force. T'ai Chi ch'uan is a form of exercise that is thought to help regulate this flow of universal energy.

- The Chinese believe that poor health is a result of blockages and congestion in the flow of internal energy, which, in turn, lowers one's physical resistance and makes one vulnerable to various pathogens.

- T'ai Chi, considered by many to be the softest of the martial arts, is called moving meditation, or a series of movements that act to help unify the life force energy with that of the person.

- T'ai Chi is deeply rooted in philosophy, primarily Taoism, but to a lesser extent, Confucianism. The premise of this exercise is to move with, rather than

against, the flow of universal energy. The positions (more than 100 in all) reinforce the concept of consciously moving with, rather than against, perceived stressors in everyday life.

- The four principles of T'ai Chi are fasting the heart, returning to nature, *Wu-wei*, and winning by losing.

- Studies investigating the physiological effects of T'ai Chi show that this technique is as effective as others in promoting relaxation.

- Qigong, a form of energy work, is often used as a mode of healing for chronic pain.

- When practicing T'ai Chi, breathe effortlessly, hold no excess muscular tension, maintain a perpendicular stance, keep your center of gravity low, move at a continuous speed, and integrate the mind and body as one.

STUDY GUIDE QUESTIONS

1. T'ai Chi is called a moving meditation; explain what this means.

2. Explain the philosophy of Taoism in Western terms as a means to promote relaxation.

3. List and explain the physiological and the psychological effects of T'ai Chi.

REFERENCES AND RESOURCES

Alder, S. S. 1983. "Seeking Stillness in Motion: An Introduction to T'ai Chi for Seniors." *Activities, Adaptations, and Aging* 3: 1–14.

Bolen, J. S. 1979. *The Tao of Psychology*. New York: Harper & Row.

Büla, C. J., S. Monod, C. Hoskovec, and S. Rochat. 2011. "Interventions Aiming at Balance Confidence Improvement in Older Adults: An Updated Review." *Gerontology* 57(3): 276–286.

Campbell, A. J., and M. C. Robertson. 2010. "Comprehensive Approach to Fall Prevention on a National Level: New Zealand." *Clinical Geriatric Medicine* 26(4): 719–731.

Capra, F. 1991. *The Tao of Physics* (3rd ed.). Boston, MA: Shambhala Publications.

Channer, K. S., D. Barrow, R. Barros, M. Osborne, and G. Ives. 1996. "Changes in Hemodynamic Parameters Following T'ai Chi Chuan and Aerobic Exercise in Patients Recovering from Acute Myocardial Infarction." *Postgraduate Medical Journal* 72(848): 349–351.

Cohen, K. 2003. Personal communication, June 23.

Delza, S. 1996. *The T'ai Chi Experience: Reflections and Perceptions on Body-Mind Harmony*. State New York: University of New York Press.

Dreher, D. 1991. *The Tao of Inner Peace*. New York: Harper & Row.

Dunn, T. 1987. "The Practice and Spirit of T'ai Chi Ch'uan." *Yoga Journal*, Nov./Dec.

Field, T., M. Diego, and M. Hernandez-Reif. 2010. "Tai Chi/Yoga Effects on Anxiety, Heart Rate, EEG, and Math Computations." *Complementary Therapy in Clinical Practice* 16(4): 235–238.

Gallagher, B. 2003. "Tai Chi Chuan and Qigong: Physical and Mental Practice for Functional Mobility." *Topics in Geriatric Rehabilitation* 19(3): 172–182.

Gass, R. 2003. "Tai Chi Chuan and Bone Loss in Post Menopausal Women." *Archives of Physical Medicine and Rehabilitation* 84: 621.

Husted, C., L. Pham, A. Hekking, and R. Niederman. 1999. "Improving Quality of Life for People with Chronic

Conditions: The Example of T'ai Chi and Multiple Sclerosis." *Alternative Therapies in Health and Medicine* 5(5): 70–74.

I Ching (Book of Changes). 1950. Translated by R. Wilhelm and C. Baynes. Princeton, NJ: Princeton University Press.

Irwin, M. R., and M. H. Oxman. 2007. "Augmenting Immune Response to Varicella Zoster Virus in Older Adults: A Randomized, Controlled Trial of Tai Chi." *Journal of the American Geriatric Society* 55(4): 511–517.

Jacobson, B. H., H. C. Chen, C. Cashel, and L. Guerrero. 1997. "The Effect of T'ai Chi Chuan Training on Balance, Kinesthetic Sense and Strength." *Perceptual and Motor Skills* 8: 27–33.

Jin, P. 1988. "Changes in Heart Rate, Noradrenaline, Cortisol, and Mood During T'ai Chi." *Journal of Psychosomatic Research* 33: 197–206.

Jou, T. H. 1988. *The Tao of T'ai Chi Ch'uan.* New York: T'ai Chi Foundation.

Kauz, H. 1974. *T'ai Chi Handbook.* New York: Dolphin Books.

Klein, P. J. 2008. "Tai Chi in the Management of Parkinson's Disease and Alzheimer's Disease." *Medicine and Sport Science* 52: 173–181.

Koh, T. C. 1981. "T'ai Chi Ch'uan." *American Journal of Chinese Medicine* 8: 15–22.

Lang, C., J. Lai, and S. Chen. 2002. "Tai Chi Chuan." *Sports Medicine* 32(4): 3217–3224.

Lao Tzu. 1972. *Tao Te Ching One.* Translated by Gia-Fu Feng and Jane English. New York: Random House.

"Learning about Tai Chi Chuan." 2002. *Nursing* 32(12): 86.

Li, J. X. 2001. "Tai Chi: Physiological Characteristics and Beneficial Effects on Health." *British Journal of Sports Medicine* 35(3): 148.

Li, M., K. Chen, and Z. Mo. 2002. "Use of Qigong Therapy in the Detoxification of Heroin Addicts." *Alternative Therapies* 8(1): 50–59.

Lo, B. 1979. *The Essence of T'ai Chi Ch'uan.* Berkeley, CA: North Atlantic Books.

Lordi, J. 2003. "Tai Chi and Its Applications for Massage Therapy." *Massage Therapy Journal* 42(2): 44–53.

Meusel, H. 1986. "Zur Enignung von Sportarten und Ubungsforman fur Altere" (Sport and Exercise Training Suitable for Older People). *Zeitschruift fur Gerontologie* 19: 376–386.

Miller, D., and J. Miller. 1982. "An Ancient Art Can Change Your Running." *Runner's World*, March, pp. 58–61.

Ming-Dao, D. 1996. *Everyday Tao.* San Francisco: HarperCollins.

Mori, K., T. Nomura, Y. Akezaki, R. Yamamoto, and H. Iwakuru. 2020. "Impact of Tai Chi Yuttari-Exercise on Arteriosclerosis and Physical Function in Older People." *Archives of Gerontology and Geriatrics* 10: 87.

Motivala, S. J., J. Sollers, J. Thayer, and M. R. Irwin. 2006. "Tai Chi Chih Acutely Decreases Sympathetic Nervous System Activity in Older Adults." *Journal of Gerontology and Biological Science Medicine* 61(11): 1177–1180.

Perry, P. 1986. "Grasp the Bird's Tail." *American Health* 5: 58–63.

Plummer, J. P. 1981. "Acupuncture and Homeostasis: Physiological, Physical (Postural), and Psychological." *American Journal of Chinese Medicine* 9: 1–14.

Qin, L., S. Au., W. Choy, et al. 2002. "Regular Tai Chi Chuan Exercise May Retard Bone Loss in Postmenopausal Women." *Archives of Physical Medicine and Rehabilitation.* 83: 1355–1359.

Sancier, K. 1996a. "Medical Applications of Qigong." *Alternative Therapies* 2(1): 40–46.

Sancier, K. 1996b. Personal communication, January 24.

Shapira, M., M. Chelouche, R. Yanai, et al. 2001. "Tai Chi Chuan Practice as a Tool for Rehabilitation of Severe Head Trauma: 3 Case Reports." *Archives of Physical Medicine and Rehabilitation* 82: 1283–1285.

Shrier, I. 2003. "Tai Chi Retards Bone Loss and Improves Muscle Strength." *Physician and Sports Medicine* 31(4): 16–17.

Suler, J. R. 1991. "The T'ai Chi Images: A Taoist Model of Psychotherapeutic Change." *Psychologia: An International Journal of Psychology in the Orient* 34(1): 18–27.

Wang, C., R. Bannuru, J. Ramel, et al. 2010. "Tai Chi on Psychological Well-Being: Systematic Review and Meta-analysis." *Complementary and Alternative Medicine* 10: 23.

Wolf, S. L., C. Coogler, and T. Xu. 1997. "Exploring the Basis of T'ai Chi Chuan as a Therapeutic Exercise Approach." *Archives of Physical Medicine and Rehabilitation* 78: 886–892.

Wong, A., Y. Lin, S. Chou, et al. 2001. "Coordination Exercise and Postural Stability in Elderly People: Effect of Tai Chi Chuan." *Archives of Physical Medicine and Rehabilitation* 82: 608–612.

Wu, M. Z. 2006. *Vital Breath of the Dao: Chinese Shamanic Tiger Qigong.* St. Paul, MN: Dragon Door Publications.

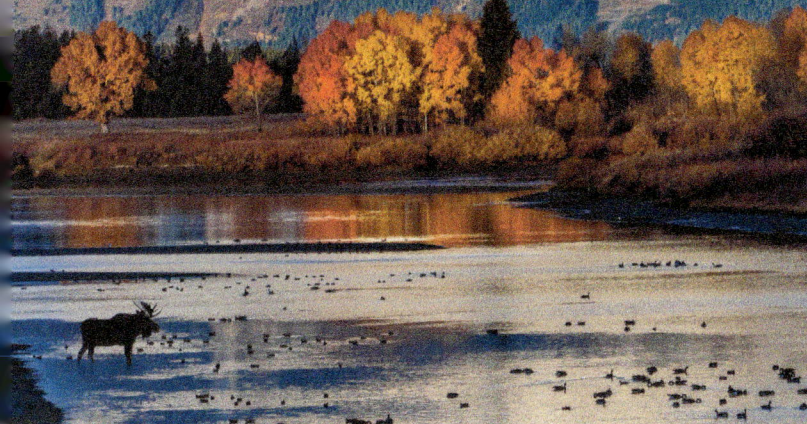

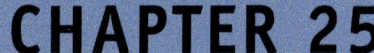

CHAPTER 25

Progressive Muscular Relaxation

Relaxation is the direct negative of nervous excitement. It is the absence of nerve-muscle impulse.

—Edmund Jacobson, M.D.

The body's muscles respond to thoughts of perceived threats with tension or contraction. Muscular tension is believed to be the most common symptom of stress, and although it may not send people to hospital emergency rooms like other stress-related disorders, its cumulative effects can be stiffness, pain, and discomfort. In extreme cases, it can distort and disalign posture and joint stability. The building blocks involved in muscular contraction are a motor end unit, a motor nerve fiber (neuron), a skeletal muscle fiber, and a stimulus from the nerve fiber to the muscle fiber called an action potential. Chemicals called neurotrophic substances are released from these neurons, which then flow from the nerve axon to the muscle fibers. Epinephrine and norepinephrine (neurotransmitters) are secreted to influence muscle contraction.

Quotation Republished with permission from University of Chicago Press from *Progressive Relaxation: A Physiological & Clinical Investigation of Muscular States & Their Significance in Psychology & Medical Practice* by Edmund Jacobson.; permission conveyed through Copyright Clearance Center, Inc.

The word *contraction* is often synonymous with shortening, but this is not always the case. Muscle fibers can, in fact, shorten like the barrel of a telescope, which is called **concentric contraction**. But some actually lengthen, in what is called **eccentric contraction**. Furthermore, muscles can contract without any noticeable motion; this type of contraction is called **isometric contraction**. The degree of intensity may vary considerably in isometric contraction, but tension at some level is exerted. Over time, this can result in stiffness and poor mobility of the joint to which the muscles are attached. It is primarily

Concentric contraction: A muscle contraction during which the length of the muscle shortens.

Eccentric contraction: A muscle contraction during which the size of the muscle lengthens.

Isometric contraction: A muscle contraction during which there is no visible change in the length of the muscle fiber.

isometric contraction that is most commonly associated with the painful muscle tension produced by stress. With repeated excitatory neural stimulation, muscle tension can manifest in various ways, including tension headaches, stiff neck, low back pain, stomach cramps, and some forms of temporomandibular joint (TMJ) dysfunction. Often, muscle tension produced by thoughts in the unconscious mind occurs while we sleep, and it has been known to cause joint stiffness and even damage connective tissue in the jaw, neck, shoulders, and low back. Progressive muscular relaxation (PMR) is a technique specifically designed to help reduce muscle tension.

Historical Perspective

Early in the twentieth century, an American physician named Edmund Jacobson noticed that his patients suffered from a host of physical ailments, but they all seemed to share one symptom—muscle tension. The thought occurred to Jacobson that if muscle tension was reduced or eliminated, these somatic diseases might decrease or perhaps disappear altogether. In questioning his patients, he discovered that they were completely unaware of the levels of muscle tension in their bodies. Moreover, when patients were invited to relax, the suggestion produced only a partial state of relaxation. A slight degree of muscle tension, called **residual tension**, could still be detected.

Jacobson understood that the body cannot be tensed and relaxed at the same time. In an effort to teach his patients how to relax, he created a simple technique to increase physical neuromuscular awareness called **progressive muscular relaxation (PMR)**. In this exercise, patients were led through a series of steps in which they systematically contracted and relaxed each muscle group. Jacobson believed that if a comparison between tension and complete relaxation of muscle fibers could be recognized by the individual, the awareness would promote a deepened sense of relaxation, not only in the muscle itself, but throughout the entire body. This technique, he advocated, could help restore the body's state

> **Residual tension:** A slight degree of muscle tension visible in some people who think they are relaxed.
>
> **Progressive muscular relaxation (PMR):** A relaxation technique; tensing and then relaxing the body's muscle groups in a systematic and progressive fashion to decrease muscle tension.

of physical health, and this turned out to be the case in his patients who began to practice progressive muscular relaxation.

Jacobson presented his technique to the American public in his book *You Must Relax* (1974), one of the first clinical attempts at preventive medicine. He stated that neither the word *stress* nor *relaxation* were part of the American vocabulary prior to World War II. It was Jacobson's work in this field that made *relaxation* a household word. Because of Jacobson's professional background, the medical community unequivocally embraced this technique as its own. For several decades, this was the sole prescribed relaxation technique practiced in the United States, long before the introduction of yoga, Zen meditation, visualization, meditation, and other international techniques now recognized and accepted as bona fide modes of relaxation. In fact, when relaxation courses were first introduced in colleges and universities across the country, progressive muscular relaxation was often the only technique taught. The Jacobson technique proved very easy to learn and teach; in fact, virtually anyone could and did teach it. Consequently, today there are many variations on this theme. Regardless of the variation, the basic process of progressive muscular relaxation remains the same: a progressive series of systematic phases combining isometric muscle contractions with periods of complete muscle relaxation. This technique, perhaps more than any other, illustrates the interception of the stress response by direct, conscious inhibition of the excitatory neural drive to the muscle fibers.

The following are the original steps of Jacobson's progressive muscular relaxation technique:

1. The progression of muscle groups should start with the lower extremities and move up to the head.

2. Muscle groups should be isolated during the contraction phase, leaving all remaining muscles relaxed.

3. The same muscle groups on both sides of the body should be contracted simultaneously.

4. The contraction should be held for 5 to 10 seconds, with a corresponding relaxation phase of about 45 seconds.

5. The individual should focus attention on the intensity of the contraction, sensing the tension level produced.

6. During the relaxation phase of each muscle group, special awareness of the feeling of relaxation should be focused on, comparing it to how the muscle felt when it was contracted.

Physiological Benefits

Research employing PMR has found that this technique is, indeed, beneficial in decreasing levels of muscle tension, as well as increasing overall awareness of muscle tension. This concept has been the premise of investigations measuring electromyographical (EMG) activity, the electrical conductance of muscle tissue. Biofeedback studies (Belar and Cohen 1979; Hayes 1975) in which electrodes were attached to various muscle sites, including the forehead, jaw, neck, shoulder, and low back, to determine neuromuscular tension revealed that tension levels significantly decreased when this technique was practiced. Through biofeedback, individuals proficient in PMR learned to control the extent of neuromuscular electrical conduction and to reach a **zero firing threshold** indicative of complete muscle relaxation. With regular daily practice, neuromuscular awareness developed. People became more attuned to muscular tension as it developed and were better able to release it. Although it may seem incongruent that PMR might be used to reduce the pain of a tension headache, a study by Anderson and Seniscal (2007) revealed that the practice of PMR (with or without osteopathic treatment) showed a significant decrease in headache-free days for 29 patients.

Psychologists also suggest that this technique is effective in controlling muscle tension associated with anger, and some studies suggest cigarette smokers find this technique (without diaphragmatic breathing) more effective than meditation or mental imagery to "kick the habit" (Allen 1983). Jacobson was of the opinion that once the body achieved a state of neuromuscular homeostasis, the mind would follow suit, allowing for a complete state of relaxation and rejuvenation. Currently, PMR is used to effectively intervene in physical disorders such as insomnia, hypertension, headaches, low back pain, and TMJ disorders.

Steps to Initiate Progressive Muscular Relaxation

The purpose of Jacobson's technique is to promote a profound sense of relaxation by comparing the contraction and relaxation phases of each selected muscle group.

What makes this technique different from Eastern-based relaxation techniques is strong body awareness in the absence of internal self-talk or positive thoughts. There is no attempt to expand consciousness with this technique. The following steps can be used to initiate Jacobson's PMR technique:

1. *Position*: Jacobson's relaxation technique can be performed in a comfortable sitting position; however, the best position to learn and practice PMR is lying comfortably on a carpeted floor. Your upper arms should rest on each side and your hands should meet on your stomach (**FIG. 25.1**). Constricting clothing should be loosened around the neck and waist. Jewelry, watches, and glasses should be removed.

2. *Breathing*: The breathing technique with PMR is quite simple. Inhale as you contract the muscles, and then exhale as you release the tension. The release of tension corresponding to relaxation of the diaphragm allows for a deeper sense of relaxation throughout the body.

3. *Concentration and ambiance*: Although concentration is important, interruptions during this technique seem less bothersome than during other meditation-based techniques, when unbroken concentration is more difficult to recapture. Nevertheless, you may wish to minimize distractions by designating a specific time and place to practice. Attention should be given to room temperature, because a cool environment may produce muscle tension (shivering). Once proficient in the technique, you can do it anywhere: while sitting in traffic, standing in line, or lying in bed trying to fall asleep. Benefits may appear soon after the completion of each session, with more profound physiological adaptations evident after prolonged practice (approximately 4 to 6 weeks).

> **Zero firing threshold:** Goal of progressive relaxation; complete muscular relaxation with no tension.

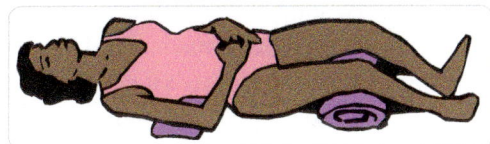

FIGURE 25.1   Starting position.

Jacobson believed the best prescription for this technique was three 5-minute daily sessions on a regular basis.

Alterations of several aspects of this technique have been introduced since its debut in 1929. Variations include (1) starting with the head and working down to the feet, (2) changing the intensity of the contraction phase, (3) diaphragmatic breathing after each muscle group, and (4) sitting instead of lying down. The original premise and process have not changed.

Remember that only the selected muscle group should be contracted, leaving the remainder of the body relaxed. It may seem hard at first not to involve surrounding muscles, but with practice it will come. When finished with the progression, lie still on the floor for a few minutes and internalize all somatic sensations. Enjoy the full sense of relaxation. Then, begin to focus your thoughts on your current surroundings.

The following is a slight variation of Jacobson's original technique, which divides the contraction into three intensities—100, 50, and 5 percent—of 5 seconds each, followed by the relaxation phase after each. I have found this to be the most effective pattern. By sensing the differences between muscle contractions, you become more aware of your muscle tension levels over the course of a day. The following instructions were written to be read yourself before you perform the technique or to be read by a third party. Before you begin, find a comfortable position (preferably on your back on a carpeted floor), loosen any constrictive clothing, kick off your shoes, and begin to unwind:

1. *Face*: Tense the muscles of the forehead and eyes, as if you were pulling all your facial muscles to the center of your nose (**FIG. 25.2**). Pull really tight, as tight as you can, and hold it. Feel the tension you create in these muscles, especially the forehead and eyes. Now relax and exhale. Feel the absence of tension in these muscles, how loose and calm they feel. Try to compare this feeling of relaxation with the tension just produced. Now, contract the same muscles, but this time at 50 percent the intensity, and hold it. Then, relax and exhale. Feel how relaxed these muscles are. Compare this feeling to that during the last contraction. This comparison should make the muscles even more relaxed. Finally, contract the same facial muscles slightly, at only 5 percent the intensity. This is like feeling a slight warm breeze on your forehead

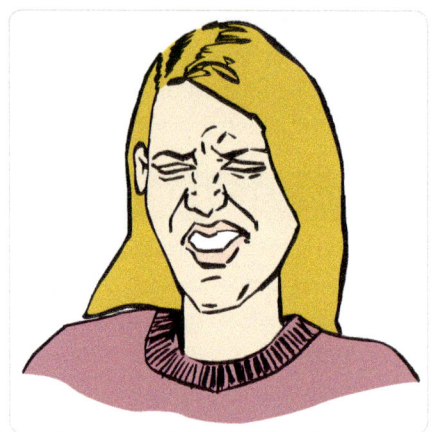

FIGURE 25.2   Facial stretch.

and cheeks. Hold it. And relax. Take a comfortably slow and deep breath and, as you exhale, feel how relaxed the muscles are.

2. *Jaws*: Take a moment to feel the muscles of your jaws. Notice any tension, even the slightest amount. (The jaw muscles can harbor a lot of undetected muscle tension.) Now consciously tense the muscles of your jaws really tight, as tight as you can, and hold it. Now relax these muscles, exhale, and sense the tension disappearing completely. (You may even feel your mouth begin to open a little.) Feel the difference between how the muscles feel now compared to what you just experienced at 100-percent contraction. Feel the absence of tension. Now, contract these same muscles, but at half the full intensity. Hold the tension, keep holding; and now relax again. Feel how relaxed these muscles are. Compare this feeling of relaxation with what you felt at 50 percent the intensity. Once again, contract the same muscles, but with only a 5-percent contraction—just the acknowledgment that these muscles can contract. Now hold it, keep holding, and relax. Release any remaining tension so that the muscles are completely loose and relaxed. Sense how relaxed the muscles are. To enhance this feeling of relaxation, take a comfortably slow, deep breath.

3. *Neck*: Concentrate on the muscles of your neck and isolate them from surrounding head and shoulder muscles. Take a moment to feel the muscles of your neck. Notice any tension. (The neck muscles can harbor a lot of undetected muscle tension.) Now consciously tense the muscles of

your neck really tight, as tight as you can, and hold it, even tighter, and hold it. Now release the tension and completely relax these muscles. Sense the tension disappearing completely. Become aware of the difference between how these muscles feel now compared to how they felt at 100-percent contraction. Once again, contract these same muscles, but at 50-percent contraction. Hold this level of tension, keep holding, and now relax again. Feel how relaxed your neck muscles are. Compare this feeling of relaxation with what you felt at half intensity. Now, finally, contract these same muscles at only 5 percent, a very slight twinge up and down the sides of the neck with no motion whatsoever. Hold it, keep holding, and relax. Release any remaining tension so that the muscles are completely relaxed. Feel just how relaxed these muscles are. To enhance the feeling of relaxation, take a comfortably slow, deep breath and sense how relaxed your neck muscles have become.

4. *Shoulders*: Concentrate on the muscles of your shoulders and isolate these from surrounding neck and upper arm muscles. Take a moment to sense the muscles of the deltoid region. Notice any degree of residual tension. (The shoulder muscles can also harbor a lot of undetected muscle tension, resulting in stiffness. Quite literally, your shoulders carry the weight of all your thoughts, the weight of your world.) Now, consciously tense the muscles of your shoulders really tight, as tight as you can, and hold it, even tighter, and hold it (**FIG. 25.3**). Now relax these muscles and sense the tension disappearing completely. Sense the difference between how these muscles feel now

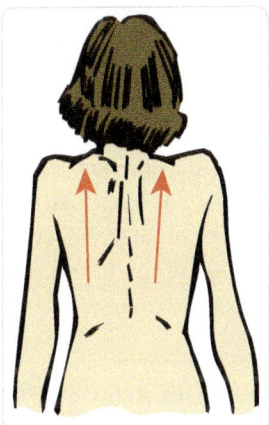

FIGURE 25.3   Shoulder stretch.

and how they felt during contraction. Once again, contract these same muscles, but this time at half the intensity. Hold the tension, keep holding, and then completely relax these muscles. Sense how relaxed your shoulder muscles are. Compare this feeling with what you felt at 50-percent intensity. Finally, contract these same muscles at only 5 percent, only just sensing clothing touching your shoulder muscles. Hold it, keep holding, and relax. Release any remaining tension so that these muscles are completely loose and relaxed. Feel just how relaxed these muscles are. To enhance this feeling of relaxation, take a comfortably slow, deep breath and sense how relaxed your shoulder muscles have become.

5. *Upper chest*: Concentrate on the muscles of your upper chest. Try to isolate these from the muscles of your neck, shoulders, and upper arms. Take a moment to feel these upper chest muscles. Sense the slightest tension these muscles may hold. Now, consciously tense your upper chest muscles really tight, as tight as you can, and hold it, even tighter, and hold it. Now, completely relax these muscles and sense the tension disappearing completely. Sense the difference between how loose these muscles feel now compared with what you just experienced at 100-percent contraction. Contract these same muscles, but at half the full intensity. Hold the tension, keep holding, and now relax again. Feel an even greater sense of relaxation in these muscles. Compare this feeling of relaxation with what you felt at 50-percent intensity. Finally, contract these same muscles at only 5 percent, merely feeling the fabric of clothing over these muscles. Now hold it, keep holding, and relax. Release any remaining tension so that the chest muscles hold absolutely no tension whatsoever. Feel how relaxed these muscles have become. To enhance the feeling, take a comfortably slow, deep breath.

6. *Hands and forearms*: Concentrate on the muscles of your hands and forearms. Take a moment to feel these muscles, including your fingers, palms, and wrists. Notice the slightest bit of tension. Now consciously tense the muscles of each hand and forearm really tight by making a fist, as tight as you can, and hold it as if you were hanging on for dear life. Make it even tighter, and hold it. Now release the tension and relax

these muscles. Sense the tension disappear completely. Open the palm of each hand slowly, extend your fingers, and let them recoil just a bit. Sense the difference between how relaxed these muscles feel now compared with what you just experienced at 100-percent contraction. They should feel very relaxed. Now contract these same muscles at a 50-percent contraction. Hold the tension, keep holding, and relax again. Sense how relaxed these muscles are. Compare this feeling of relaxation with what you just felt. Now, contract these same muscles at only 5 percent, like holding an empty eggshell in the palm of your hand. Now hold it, keep holding, and relax. Release any remaining tension so that these muscles are completely relaxed. Feel just how relaxed these muscles have become. To enhance this feeling of relaxation, take a comfortably slow, deep breath and sense how relaxed your forearm and hand muscles have become.

7. *Abdominals*: Really focus your attention on your abdominal muscles. Take a moment to sense any residual tension in these muscles or the organs they protect. Now, consciously tense your abdominal muscles really tight, as if you have an intense stomach cramp. Contract as tight as you can and hold it, even tighter, and hold it. Now relax these muscles and sense the tension disappearing completely. Feel the complete absence of tension. Compare the difference between how these muscles feel now with what you just experienced at 100-percent contraction. Once again, contract the same muscles, this time at half the full intensity. Hold the tension, keep holding, and now relax again. Feel how relaxed these muscles are. Compare this feeling of relaxation with what you felt at half intensity. When you compare the difference between tension levels and states of relaxation, a greater sense of relaxation will follow. Finally, contract these same muscles at only 5 percent, so that you barely feel the clothing over your stomach area. Just acknowledge that these muscles can contract. Now hold it, keep holding, and relax. Release any remaining tension so that the muscles are completely relaxed. Sense just how relaxed these muscles have become. Take a comfortably slow, deep breath and sense how relaxed your abdominal region has become.

8. *Lower back*: Isolate the muscles of your lower back. These muscles can get quite tense and cause much pain. Now, consciously tense these muscles by trying to press your lower back to the floor. Maintain this posture and hold really tight, as tight as you can, and hold it. Now, relax these muscles, allowing your back to curve naturally, and sense the tension disappearing completely. Sense how relaxed these muscles feel now and compare this with what you just experienced at 100-percent contraction. Once again, contract the same muscles, but at half the intensity. Hold the tension, keep holding, and now relax again. Feel how relaxed these muscles have become. Compare this feeling of relaxation with what you felt at 50-percent intensity. Once again, contract these same muscles, but this time at only 5 percent, a very slight twinge. Now hold it, keep holding, and relax. Release any remaining tension so that these muscles are completely loose and relaxed. Feel just how relaxed your lower back has become. Now, take a comfortably slow, deep breath.

9. *Buttocks*: Concentrate on your buttock muscles. Notice any residual tension and release it. Now, consciously tense these muscles really tight, as tight as you can and hold it, even tighter, and hold it. Now, release the tension, relax the muscles, and sense the tension disappearing completely. Compare the difference between how these muscles feel now and what you just experienced at 100-percent contraction. Now contract these same muscles at 50-percent contraction. Hold the tension, keep holding, and now relax again. Feel how relaxed these muscles are. Compare this feeling of relaxation with what you felt at half intensity. Now, finally, contract these same muscles at only 5 percent, showing no motion whatsoever. Now hold it, keep holding, and relax. Release any remaining tension so that these muscles are completely relaxed. Feel just how relaxed these muscles are. To enhance the feeling of relaxation, take a slow, deep breath and sense how relaxed these muscles have become.

10. *Thighs*: Concentrate on the muscles of your left and right thighs. Try not to involve your abdominal or buttock muscles. Take a moment to sense just the muscles of your thighs. Notice any residual tension

that might be there and release it. Now, consciously contract these muscles as tight as you can and hold it, even tighter, and hold it. Now relax these muscles and sense the tension disappearing completely. Sense the difference between how these muscles feel now and what you just experienced. Once again, contract these same muscles, but at half the intensity. Hold the tension, keep holding, and now relax again. Feel how relaxed these muscles are. Compare this feeling of relaxation with what you felt at 50-percent intensity. Finally, contract these same muscles at only 5 percent. Now hold it, keep holding, and relax. Release any remaining tension so that these muscles are completely relaxed. Feel just how relaxed these muscles have become. Take a comfortably slow, deep breath.

11. *Calves*: Locate and sense the calf muscles of both legs and isolate these from all other leg muscles. Take a moment to sense your calf muscles. Notice if they have any residual tension. (These can be the tightest of all leg muscles.) Now, consciously tense these muscles really tight by pointing your toes (**FIG. 25.4**). (If they should begin to cramp, release the tension by pulling your toes toward your knees.) Contract as tight as you can, and hold it, tighter. Now relax these muscles and sense the tension disappearing. Make a comparison between how relaxed these muscles now feel with the tension you just experienced at 100-percent contraction. Once again, contract these same muscles, but at 50-percent contraction, like tip-toeing on a cold wood floor. Hold the tension, keep holding, and now relax again. Feel how relaxed these muscles are. Compare this feeling of relaxation with what you felt before. Now, contract these same muscles at only 5 percent, a very slight

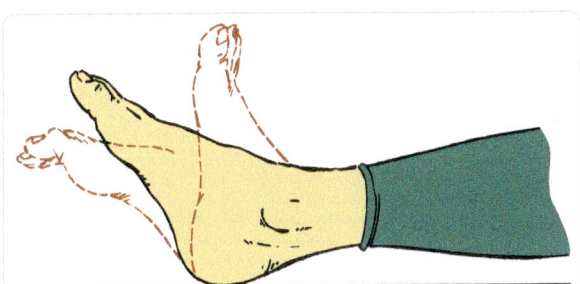

FIGURE 25.4 Pointing the toes to tighten calf muscles.

twinge with no motion whatsoever. Now hold it, keep holding, and relax. Release any remaining tension so that these muscles are completely relaxed. Feel just how relaxed your calf muscles are. To enhance this feeling of relaxation, take a comfortably slow, deep breath and sense how relaxed your calves have become.

12. *Feet*: Focus your attention on the muscles of your right and left feet. (Typically, the muscles of the feet are not tense, but when standing they can produce a lot of tension. In addition, in the confinement of shoes, they can become less than relaxed.) Now, consciously contract the muscles of your feet by scrunching your toes really tight, as tight as you can. Hold it, even tighter, and hold it. Now relax these muscles and sense the tension disappearing completely. (You may even feel your feet become warm as they relax.) Feel the difference between how these muscles feel now and what you just experienced at 100-percent contraction. Once again, contract these same muscles at half the intensity. Hold the tension, keep holding, and now relax again. Feel how relaxed these muscles are. Compare this feeling of relaxation with the tension you felt at 50-percent intensity. Now, contract these same muscles at only 5 percent, a very slight twinge. Now hold it, keep holding, and relax. Release any remaining tension so that these muscles are completely relaxed. Sense how relaxed these muscles are. Finally, take a comfortably slow, deep breath and sense how relaxed your whole body is.

Your face and jaw muscles, your neck, shoulders, upper chest, arms and hands, your stomach and lower back, and your legs and feet—your whole body feels completely relaxed and calm. Now lie still, and enjoy the feeling of complete relaxation.

■ Best Application of Progressive Muscular Relaxation

Although Jacobson's technique was originally developed as a means to prevent the cumulative effects of stress, PMR can also be used as an intervention technique when the body initiates the fight-or-flight response (**FIG. 25.5**). As variations of PMR began to emerge, so, too, did the concept that this technique had the potential to reduce tension on the spot, in the midst of confronting a stressor, such as getting caught in traffic or standing in

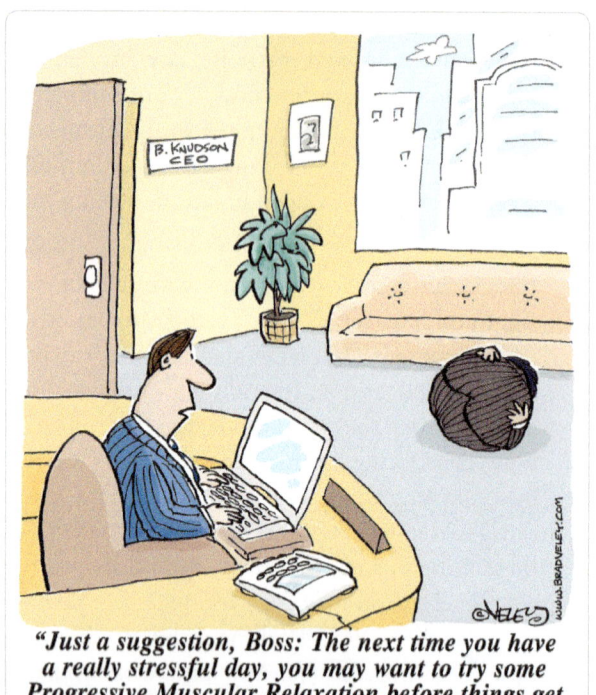

© Bradford Veley, Marquette, MI

"Just a suggestion, Boss: The next time you have a really stressful day, you may want to try some Progressive Muscular Relaxation before things get this bad."

FIGURE 25.5   Progressive Muscular Relaxation. Give it a try.

long shopping lines. As a preventive technique, however, the entire body must be systematically relaxed by progression through all the muscle groups, which may take up to 30 minutes. As an intervention technique, rather than going through the entire sequence of muscle groups, contract the hands or neck and shoulders—whatever muscle groups are tight—instead. This technique should be practiced not only in the morning or evening, but often during short (5-minute) PMR breaks over the course of a day.

Perhaps anger elicits the greatest response of unconscious muscle tension. Research shows that the suppression of anger can manifest itself in tension headaches and TMJ. And conventional wisdom suggests that PMR is one of the best relaxation techniques to deal with symptoms of anger.

However, some cautions should be noted with this technique. The isometric muscle tension used in PMR increases both systolic and diastolic blood pressure, even with contractions of short duration. Individuals with hypertension (elevated systolic and/or diastolic blood pressure) should refrain from using this technique because it will certainly aggravate their condition.

SUMMARY

- Muscle tension is the most common symptom of stress. This is because the initial neural response to stress is the initiation of muscular excitation in preparation for the fight-or-flight response.

- Muscles can contract in one of three ways: concentrically (shortening), eccentrically (lengthening), and isometrically (no visible change in length). Muscle tension produced through the stress response is primarily isometric in that there is very little, if any, noticeable change. Yet, over time, muscles contracted isometrically begin to show signs of shortening.

- In the early twentieth century, Jacobson recognized that virtually all his patients shared the same symptom regardless of illness: muscle tension. He

concluded that if people could reduce muscular tension, their susceptibility to disease would decrease.

- The relaxation technique he created, called progressive muscular relaxation (PMR), involves systematically tensing and relaxing the body's musculature, from the feet to the head.

- PMR was quickly accepted by the medical community in the United States as the best way to promote relaxation. Today, several versions of this technique are practiced, all showing similar positive results.

- Research, specifically biofeedback using electromyography, has proved that this technique indeed helps reduce muscular tension.

STUDY GUIDE QUESTIONS

1. Explain the rationale for PMR as a relaxation technique.

2. Describe in simple terms how to do PMR for relaxation.

REFERENCES AND RESOURCES

Allen, K., and M. Shriver. 1997. "Enhanced Performance Feedback to Strengthen Biofeedback Treatment Outcomes with Childhood Migraine." *Headache* 37: 169–173.

Allen, R. 1983. *Human Stress: Its Nature and Control.* Minneapolis, MN: Burgess.

Anderson, R. E., and C. Seniscal. 2007. "A Comparison of Selected Osteopathic Treatment and Relaxation for Tension-Type Headaches." *Headache* 47(3): 450–451.

Belar, C., and J. Cohen. 1979. "The Use of EMG Feedback and Progressive Muscular Relaxation in the Treatment of a Woman with Chronic Back Pain." *Biofeedback and Self-Regulation* 4: 345–353.

Berkovec, T. D., and D. C. Fowles. 1973. "Controlled Investigation of the Effects of Progressive and Hypnotic Relaxation on Insomnia." *Journal of Abnormal Psychology* 82: 153–158.

Bernstein, D., and T. Berkovec. 1973. *Progressive Relaxation Training: A Manual for the Helping Professions.* Champaign, IL: Research Press.

Caroll, D., and K. Seers. 1998. "Relaxation for the Relief of Chronic Pain: A Systematic Review." *Journal of Advanced Nursing* 27: 467–487.

Charlesworth, E., and R. Nathan. 1984. *Stress Management: A Comprehensive Guide to Wellness.* New York: Ballantine.

Curtis, J., and R. Detert. 1981. *How to Relax.* Mountain View, CA: Mayfield.

Gard, C. 1998. "How Biofeedback May Help You Chill Out." *Current Health* 2(24): 30–32.

Gellhorn, E. 1957. "The Influence of Baroreceptor Reflexes on the Reactivity of the Autonomic Nervous System." *Experientia* 12: 259–260.

Gellhorn, E. 1958. "The Physiological Basis of Neuromuscular Relaxation." *Archives of Internal Medicine* 102: 392–399.

Girdano, D., and G. Everly. 2000. *Controlling Stress and Tension: A Holistic Approach.* Boston, MA: Allyn & Bacon.

Greenberg, J. 2008. *Comprehensive Stress Management* (10th ed.). New York: McGraw-Hill.

Hayes, S. N. 1975. "Electromyographical Biofeedback and Relaxation Instructions in the Treatment of Muscle Contraction Headaches." *Behavior Therapy* 6: 672–678.

Herman, C., E. B. Blanchard, and H. Flor. 1997. "Biofeedback Treatment for Pediatric Migraine: Prediction of Outcomes." *Journal of Consulting and Clinical Psychology* 65(4): 611–616.

Jacobson, E. 1929. *Progressive Relaxation.* Chicago, IL: University of Chicago Press.

Jacobson, E. 1970. *Modern Treatment of Tense Patients.* Springfield, IL: Thomas.

Jacobson, E. 1978. *You Must Relax*. New York: McGraw-Hill.

Marcus, A., and S. C. Smith. 1998. "Biofeedback Helps Heart: A Successful Treatment for Chronic Heart Failure." *Prevention* 50: 149–150.

Miller, E. 1980. *Letting Go of Stress*. (Audio recording.) Albuquerque, NM: Newman Communications.

Mitchell, K., and D. Mitchell. 1978. "Migraine: An Exploratory Treatment, Application of Programmed Behavior Therapy Techniques." *Journal of Psychosomatic Research* 15: 137–157.

Rice, P. 1998. *Stress and Health* (3rd ed.). Belmont, CA: Wadsworth.

Robb, S. 2000. "Music-Assisted Progressive Muscle Relaxation, Progressive Muscle Relaxation, Music Listening, and Silence: A Comparison of Relaxation Techniques." *Journal of Music Therapy* 37(1): 2–21.

Steinhaus, A. H., and J. E. Norris. 1964. *Teaching Neuromuscular Relaxation*. Chicago, IL: George Williams College.

Walker, C. E. 1975. *Learn to Relax: Thirteen Ways to Reduce Tension*. Englewood Cliffs, NJ: Prentice Hall.

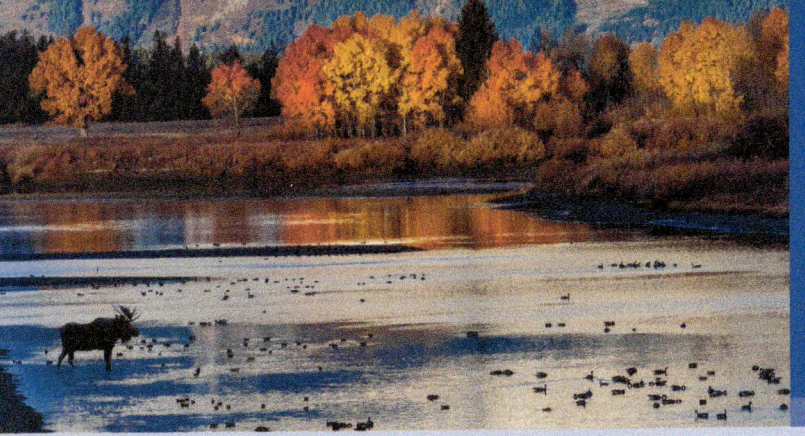

Autogenic Training and Clinical Biofeedback

Open your mind to the power of self-suggestion.

—Johannes Schultz

The ability to control the body's physical reaction to stress is considered the epitome of stress management. Two techniques that specifically focus on this ability are known as autogenic training (AT) and biofeedback. Whereas autogenic training is a technique that can be done practically anywhere without the use of special equipment, biofeedback typically involves a machine of some kind that provides biological metrics. Both relaxation techniques discussed in this chapter highlight the importance of increasing one's awareness of the body's physiology in an effort to return oneself back to homeostasis.

to the ego and identity. So, when mental, emotional, or spiritual concerns threaten the psyche or ego, the body's responses need to be "retrained." By reprogramming the body's responses through self-generated thoughts or passive commands, the physical effects can be lessened considerably. We now know that mind-body integration is so profound that the antiquated fight-or-flight survival mechanism can be overridden, much to our advantage, by conscious thoughts. Thus, the purpose of **autogenic training** is to reprogram the mind so as to override the stress response when physical arousal is not appropriate.

Autogenic Training

During physical arousal, heart rate, blood pressure, ventilation, and muscle tension can all increase in an effort to prepare the body to fight or flee. Although this aroused state is greatly appreciated under the threat of physical harm, it becomes a liability when the threats are

Autogenic training: Introduced by Schultz and Luthe; a relaxation technique where the individual gives conscious messages to various body parts to feel warm and heavy; effects are thought to result from vasodilation to the specified body regions intended for warmth and heaviness.

Historical Perspective

Beliefs regarding the regulation of bodily functions began to change in the nineteenth century, when Europeans traveled the globe and returned recounting stories of human feats in far-off lands. Visitors to the Himalayas reported yogi masters who showed a remarkable ability to control their breathing, heart rate, and blood flow, to the point where they could be mistaken for dead. In a state of profound relaxation produced by meditation, these individuals exhibited incredible control over their body's physiological functions. These yogis appeared to have no magic powers. Rather, they employed exceptional concentration skills to send internal messages from the conscious mind to specific body parts to alter their physiological function. In essence, by believing in the possibility of control, they induced a self-hypnotic state that then produced deep relaxation (**FIG. 26.1**). (These observations were later documented at the Menninger Clinic by Elmer Green, Ph.D., in 1970 with the Hindu yogi Swami Rama.)

Meanwhile, on another continent at the turn of the twentieth century, **self-hypnosis** was being explored by the European brain physiologist Oskar Vogt. Hypnosis, a trancelike state of consciousness, was already commonly practiced by doctors to better understand the relationship between the conscious and unconscious mind in their emotionally disturbed patients. However, Vogt discovered that several of his clients could put themselves into this trancelike state if they relaxed enough. Vogt called this autohypnosis (Greenberg 2010).

Building on this concept, the relaxation technique of autogenic training was introduced by two German physicians, Johannes Schultz and his protégé Wolfgang Luthe, in 1932. Although it was originally designed to calm the mind, patients often remarked on two other distinct physical sensations. The first was increased warmth of the extremities (arms, hands, and feet). The second, which seemed to accompany the first, was an increased sense of heaviness in the extremities. Schultz

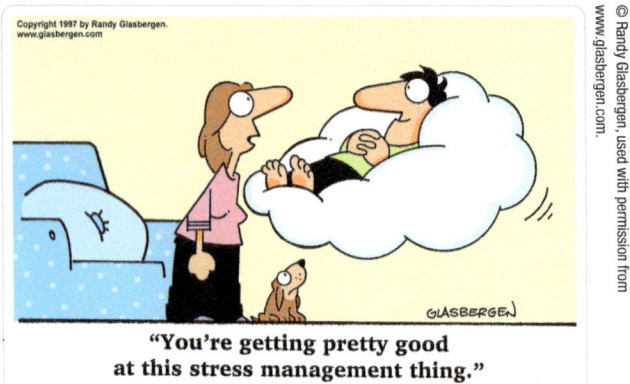

FIGURE 26.1   All relaxation skills take practice. The more you practice, the better they serve you.

speculated that both phenomena were caused by vasodilation of blood vessels to localized musculature. It was this vasodilation that caused a change in the distribution of blood flow, bringing with it warmth from the body's core and a subtle but noticeable perception of heaviness. Although it seems that anyone can reap the benefits of self-hypnosis, Schultz and Luthe discovered several conditions that enhance this autogenic process. The term *training* was added when it was acknowledged that, like other skills, the more the technique was practiced, the better one's command over it, and the greater the relaxation response.

In their work with patients who had mastered the autogenic technique, Schultz and Luthe (1959) concluded that it is most effective when the following factors are taken into consideration:

1. *The individual should be highly motivated and receptive to instructions and suggestions.* To master this technique, one must maintain a strong degree of self-confidence, faith, and willpower, knowing that the thoughts suggested in the conscious state will be passed from the mind through the body to produce the desired relaxation. Schultz and Luthe called this **passive concentration**.

2. *The individual should possess a strong sense of self-direction and control.* When practicing this technique, suggestions must be self-generated. In other words, one must take command or ownership of these thoughts to promote relaxation. Thus, the individual needs to take the initiative to organize thoughts and feed them systematically as the relaxation session unfolds. Individuals can be guided through the process with a series

---

Self-hypnosis: A form of relaxation in which the individual provides him- or herself with suggestions to relax (as with the suggestions of autogenics), as opposed to having someone else provide the suggestions.

Passive concentration: A term coined by the creators of autogenic training to denote the conscious receptivity of self-generated thoughts.

of directions, but ultimately the choice to follow these directions is in the mind of each individual.

3. *The individual should position him- or herself comfortably*. It was noted by Schultz and Luthe that body position is very important to achieve success with this technique. From their observations, they advocated two positions. The most beneficial is lying on one's back on a carpeted surface, with arms resting by the sides and palms facing up. This position is most conducive to feeling the heaviness effects. If this position is not possible, then a comfortably seated position is the best alternative.

4. *The individual should maintain a strong sense of concentration and body awareness*. Loss of mental focus or concentration will impede the flow of messages from the mind to the body. The effectiveness of this technique is enhanced by using both an alert conscious state and imaginative thought processes from the unconscious to focus on specific body regions. Complete attention, like that used by yogis in Nepal, promotes a greater sense of mental control and state of relaxation.

5. *The individual should minimize sensory reception*. Sensory information through the eyes, ears, nose, mouth, and body surface can and will compete for attention at the conscious level. By learning to tune out information from these sources (e.g., closing the eyes), the mind can focus on internal sensations, making them more effective.

6. *The individual should focus on internal physiological processes*. Because the conscious mind normally allows the autonomic nervous system to operate vital body functions, initially the ability to tune into these is embryonic at best. With practice, though, a keen sense of internal physiological processes will develop. Repeated suggestions received by the deeper levels of the mind will eventually transfer to the body through neurobiochemical reactions associated with the relaxation response (**FIG. 26.2**).

Schultz and Luthe strongly believed that when these conditions are met, the stage is set for internal influences of both the conscious and unconscious mind to return the body to homeostasis through a balance of conscious mind-body awareness.

Unlike progressive muscular relaxation, in autogenic training there is no conscious, active effort to relax the

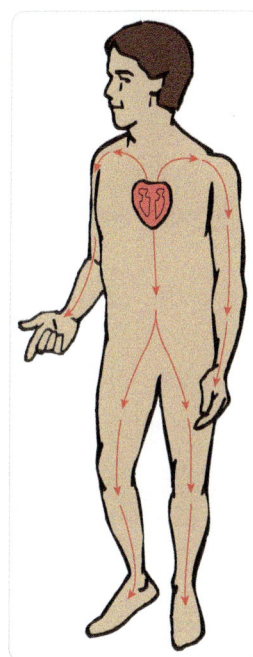

FIGURE 26.2 A person visualizing the flow of blood to the extremities.

muscles. Instead, emphasis is placed on making specific body regions warm and heavy through passive self-suggestions. In addition, greater degrees of body awareness and concentration are required to produce the desired relaxation effect. Because the practice involves a passive attitude, the individual remains in complete control and can stop at any time.

According to the International Committee for the Coordination of Clinical Application and Teaching of Autogenic Therapy (ICAT), the training sequence for autogenic training is a regimented 3-month training program. The systematic and progressive program begins with a breathing warm-up followed by one (or more) of seven phases: (1) heaviness, (2) warmth, (3) calm heart, (4) breathing, (5) stomach, (6) cool forehead, and (7) completion. It is important to note that the suggested affirmations are divided into an inhale phase (e.g., "My right arm is") and an exhale phase (e.g., "limp and heavy"). Once competency is achieved in the first stage, which is 3 weeks in duration, one can then move on to the next phase. Thus, the 3-month training program results in a daily routine that should be maintained to achieve a calm autogenic state under nearly any circumstance (Ernst 2008). The following is a description of the specific step-by-step process for phase 1. (For a complete description of the program, please visit www.guidetopsychology .com/autogen.htm.)

Phase 1: Heaviness Formula (Suggested Practice Time: 21 days). After the breathing warm-up, begin this phase with your right (or dominant) arm. Breathe deeply, and silently repeat the following affirmations six to eight times:

> Inhale: "My right arm is getting," exhale: "limp and heavy."
>
> Inhale: "My right arm is getting," exhale: "heavier and heavier."
>
> Inhale: "My right arm," exhale: "is completely heavy."

Repeat the closing affirmation one time:

> Inhale: "I feel," exhale: "supremely calm."

This segment of this phase should be practiced two to three times a day for 3 days. Then, continue with the following process with each affirmation repeated six to eight times for 3 days:

> Inhale: "My left (or nondominant) arm is getting," exhale: "limp and heavy."
>
> Inhale: "Both my arms are getting," exhale: "limp and heavy."
>
> Inhale: "My right leg is getting," exhale: "limp and heavy."
>
> Inhale: "My left leg is getting," exhale: "limp and heavy."
>
> Inhale: "Both my legs are getting," exhale: "limp and heavy."
>
> Inhale: "My arms and legs are getting," exhale: "limp and heavy."
>
> Inhale: "My arms and legs are getting," exhale: "heavier and heavier."
>
> Inhale: "My arms and legs are," exhale: "completely heavy."

Repeat the closing affirmation one time:

> Inhale: "I feel," exhale: "supremely calm."

> **Selected awareness:** The receptivity of the conscious mind to acknowledge and receive specific thoughts or messages.
>
> **Autogenic discharge:** Physical sensations such as muscle twitching, numbness, and perhaps some emotional responses (tears) released by the unconscious mind from autogenic training sessions.

Psychological and Physiological Responses

The autogenic technique uses what is called **selected awareness**, which refers to the receptivity of the conscious mind to acknowledgment and receipt of specific thoughts or messages. Ideally in the selected awareness process the censorship role of the ego is eliminated and thoughts can travel freely from the conscious to the unconscious. Lack of censorship can dramatically improve the mind's ability to change or alter desired physiological functions. In a state of receptivity, too, sensations of pain are reduced, and sometimes eliminated altogether. In fact, there are volumes of anecdotal stories in newspapers around the world of people who have undergone incredible experiences, which under normal conditions would be impossible. For example, one runner reportedly ran the entire Boston Marathon feeling some pain in his leg, only to cross the finish line and collapse with a broken femur. Although barely understood scientifically, the powerful integration of conscious and unconscious thoughts allows for a greater state of psychic and physiological homeostasis.

Luthe (1969) also suggested that because the barriers between the conscious and unconscious mind are dismantled, there may be what he referred to as **autogenic discharge**; that is, physical sensations such as muscle twitches, numbness, and emotional responses (e.g., crying), all triggered by the release of unconscious thoughts. These are said to be natural and healthy.

In its most characteristic sensations, warmth and heaviness, this technique can be compared to a muscle massage, although in this case, the muscles are massaged internally rather than on the surface of the skin. The body's muscles are connected to a multitude of nerve cells that regularly release catecholamines at their synaptic junctions to produce minimal tension, or optimal tonus. Under hypnosis, however, the muscles become saturated with blood in a resting state, so the tension decreases and a message is sent back to the brain via the afferent nervous system to stop neural firing. It's a win-win situation for both the muscles, which are allowed to relax, and the brain, which has less neurochemical work to do. The overall effect can be quite profound.

Several clinical studies measuring the effectiveness of this technique have revealed that a redistribution of blood flow indeed occurs in autogenic training, as well as many other changes. Decreases in heart rate, respiration, and muscle tension; increases in hemispheric alpha waves indicative of mental calmness; and even

Stress with a Human Face

A good magician never reveals his or her secrets, which is why going to a magic show can be as frustrating as it is entertaining. Trick after trick, you think to yourself, "How did he do that?" And the more amazing the stunt, the more baffled you become.

I once went to a magic show in college. The performer was renowned as an escape artist, and he announced that in the second half of the show he would escape from handcuffs and a locked trunk submerged in water. My friends and I were intrigued, to say the least.

After an amazing first act, I left my seat to stretch my legs. To my surprise, I met the star performer face to face as I walked outside the rear exit of the auditorium. I extended my hand to greet the magician and express my gratitude for a great show. As our hands clasped,

I noticed that his palms and fingers were incredibly swollen, as if he had an acute case of poison ivy. After we exchanged polite comments, he went back to his dressing room and I went back to my seat.

I couldn't get over the feel of that handshake. It was like holding a balloon full of water. The escape act was very impressive and ended with thunderous applause. Walking home that night, I was still perplexed about how he got out of those handcuffs, but I was sure his spongy hands had something to do with it.

Years later, I learned that Houdini practiced a technique similar to autogenic training to effect his escapes. He was not only a master escape artist, but apparently a master of relaxation as well.

decreases in serum cholesterol levels have been clinically observed (Greenberg 2010). Since its introduction, the autogenic relaxation technique has been used successfully in the treatment of several manifestations of physical stress, including insomnia (Coates and Thoreson 1978); migraines (Blanchard et al. 1985); muscle tension; Raynaud's syndrome (Keefe et al. 1980), a chronic condition of poor blood supply to the hands and feet; and perhaps most notably, hypertension (Silver 1979).

But clinical laboratories and counseling centers are not the only sites where this technique has been employed. Houdini and several other magicians are known to have used the autogenic technique to "inflate" the size of their hands and wrists when handcuffed and locked up in a chest, then to reverse the process to escape the trap. National biathlon champion Kari Swenson, who was abducted by two men near Bozeman, Montana, in 1985, used this as a survival technique in an effort to minimize blood loss from her gunshot wound. In his book *Peace, Love, and Healing* (1990), cancer surgeon Bernie Siegel wrote about the use of this technique with his patients during surgical procedures for which they were anesthetized. After giving them a clear understanding of the powers of the conscious and unconscious mind, Siegel asked his patients to shunt the flow of blood away from the operating site. After surgery he asked for their cooperation in healing the site. Siegel found

that, when relaxed, patients can decrease blood flow in the area of the incision. Moreover, he noted that patients who are receptive to this power of suggestion tend to recover much more quickly from their surgery. Siegel also recounted an episode where a patient showed signs of cardiac arrhythmia immediately following surgery. Siegel whispered in the patient's ear to sense his heart contracting in a relaxed rhythm, like a swing moving back and forth on a swing set. Sure enough, the dysrhythmia disappeared.

Since its acceptance as a bona fide relaxation technique, autogenic training has been utilized in many clinical settings and helped a number of patients with a host of stress-related physical problems. As a result of its widespread use, many variations have surfaced in the past 60 years, including its combination with complementary techniques such as diaphragmatic breathing and mental imagery.

Steps to Initiate Autogenic Training

Initiation of autogenic training involves adopting one of the recommended body positions and maintaining concentration and awareness.

Body Position. As Schultz and Luthe suggested, there are two recommended body positions (**FIG. 26.3**). The preferred position is lying on your back on a carpeted

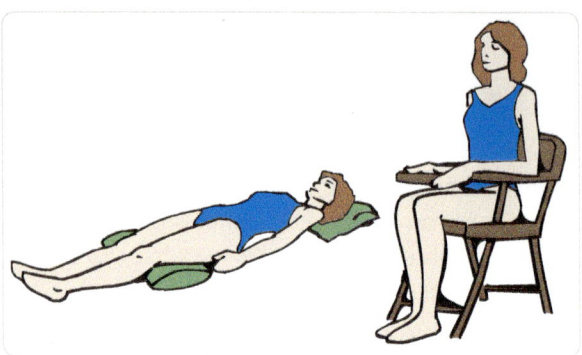

FIGURE 26.3   The two suggested body positions are (1) lying on your back on a comfortable floor surface, or if this is not possible, (2) sitting comfortably in a chair. Once you are proficient, any position will do.

floor or bed with your arms by your sides, palms facing up, and legs straight, heels resting evenly on the surface. Thin pillows or cushions may be used behind the head and knees for support as long as the body remains in comfortable vertebral alignment. If circumstances do not permit lying down, then a seated position in a chair is recommended. While seated, keep your head aligned over your body, with your arms either on your lap or supported by the frame of the chair. It is important to have your limbs supported so that they don't compete with the force of gravity and negate the effects you are trying to produce. Luthe suggests that if your head becomes too heavy, let it hang comfortably. Because several postural muscles are called upon when seated, it may be less effective than the reclining position. With practice, however, sitting will also produce the desired relaxation. It is also recommended to remove jewelry and loosen any restrictive clothing. Perhaps most important, refrain from eating a big meal before practicing this technique. This will compromise its effectiveness because when food is digested, blood concentrates in the gastrointestinal area, and this will compete with the blood flow to the extremities.

Concentration and Awareness. Under normal conditions, attention is easily distracted by interruptions, from

> **Indirect approach:** In autogenic training, when one suggests to oneself that various body parts are warm and heavy.
>
> **Direct approach:** In autogenic training, when one not only suggests the words *warm* and *heavy,* but also imagines the flow of blood to these body regions, such as hands or feet.

phone calls to random thoughts roaming the interiors of our minds. To minimize external distractions, find a quiet place and designate it as your relaxation space. By training your relaxation skills in the same location each time, a comfort pattern is created for both mind and body. Next, control this environment by turning off the phone, closing the door, and making other necessary adjustments such as closing the window or blinds.

Now you can focus internally. When first trying this technique, you may find your mind drifting toward what seems like more important thoughts. But autogenic concentration concerns only the "here and now"—specifically, the present state of your body. If at first you find other thoughts competing for your attention, simply acknowledge them and then redirect your flow of consciousness back to your body. With practice, the frequency of competing thoughts will decrease and concentration will improve.

The concentration for relaxation skills is different from that required for driving a car, listening to a lecture, or watching a movie. Often those events require judgment and analysis. By contrast, during a state of relaxation, particularly autogenic training, concentration involves the ability of the brain's right hemisphere to receive and accept thoughts without judgment. In this technique, you must allow yourself to become open to suggestion and adopt a passive—but not defensive—frame of mind.

Other Suggestions

Despite dogmatic comments from members of the ICAT, the concepts and principles of autogenic training can be learned quickly by most people, and the short-term relaxation effects are often experienced immediately. However, like any skill, it will take several weeks of repeated and disciplined practice to feel the cumulative effects. When learning and practicing this technique, try to practice twice a day for 15 minutes each time so that a training effect does indeed occur.

Over the years, two general approaches to the autogenic relaxation technique have surfaced. The first is the **indirect approach,** wherein one simply suggests to oneself that certain body regions become warm and heavy. The second is a more **direct approach,** wherein one employs a greater sense of mental imagery by making reference to the specific physiological systems responsible for the sensations of warmth and heaviness.

Indirect Approach. As with other relaxation techniques, such as yoga and T'ai Chi, autogenic training has been adapted to meet the needs of particular target audiences. The following is an adaptation from the suggested 3-month intensive training program. This adaptation, the indirect approach, involves very general instructions (affirmations) that you may repeat several times to yourself in an effort to increase body awareness and promote relaxation. There is little detail or internal visual imagery involved. The phases of these instructions are a feeling of heaviness, a feeling of warmth, a calmness of the heart, a calmness of breathing, and even a coolness of the forehead. Attention to each phase should continue for about 1 minute by repeating the instructions until the desired sensation is felt. This whole progression of phases should take approximately 15 minutes. When you are done, remain in position and try to lock the feeling of relaxation into your memory bank so you can recall it during times of stress and tension.

First, take a slow, deep breath and feel the sense of relaxation as you exhale. Do this once more, making the breath even slower and deeper than the last. Then, say the following thoughts to yourself:

Phase 1: Heaviness

"My arms and hands feel heavy."

"My legs and feet feel heavy."

"My arms and legs feel heavy."

Phase 2: Warmth

"My arms and hands feel warm."

"My legs and feet feel warm."

"My arms and legs feel warm."

Phase 3: Heart

"My heart is calm and relaxed."

"My heartbeat is slow and relaxed."

Phase 4: Breathing

"My breathing is slow and relaxed."

"My breathing is calm and comfortable."

Phase 5: Solar Plexus

"My stomach area is calm and relaxed."

Phase 6: Forehead

"My forehead is cool."

"My forehead is calm and relaxed."

"My entire body is calm and relaxed."

Direct Approach. The direct approach, which is also an adaptation of the original 3-month intensive training program, is a more detailed visual interpretation of the general instructions just listed. It is a slight variation on the original technique offering additional instructions for those who need more understanding of how the physiological changes occur. In the direct approach, the specific mechanisms involved in warmth and heaviness are focused on to initiate a stronger sense of relaxation (**FIG. 26.4**). It starts out with diaphragmatic breathing to induce relaxation. When mind and body become relaxed through this technique, the mind becomes more receptive to additional thoughts (warmth and heaviness), and thus the selected awareness process is enhanced. The length of time required for this approach will vary. To begin, you may want to work on only one body region such as the arms and hands. With proficiency, you can add to the duration of each session.

Adding Mental Imagery. As Aristotle once said, "The soul never thinks without a picture." When imagery is combined with autogenic training, it can produce profound physiological effects on the body. Imagery consisting of pictures or symbols that parallel and represent actual physiological responses seems to affect the body's functions in ways that words alone cannot. A host of stories shared in the medical community lend credence to this concept. Hypertensive patients who use mental imagery have shown significant decreases in blood pressure. For example, one client of mine used the image of a bottleneck traffic jam on a highway. By working to clear the jam in his mind and then visualizing only his car on the road, he was able to reduce his resting blood pressure to the point where he was taken off medication by his physician. This phenomenon can be explained through the specific cognitive functions of the right and left hemispheres of the

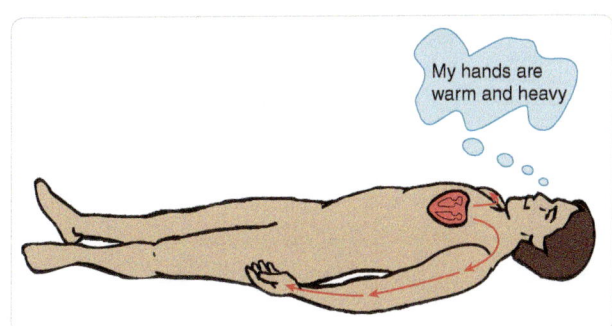

FIGURE 26.4 Visualizing blood flow to the arms and hands, the breath even slower and deeper. With each exhalation, feel how relaxed your body has become.

brain. The left hemisphere, which controls verbal skills, is thought to communicate to the body in words. The right hemisphere, which is quite poor in verbal ability but proficient with symbolic images, appears to communicate to the body visually. The combination of words and pictures seems to have a more profound effect on the body's physiology than do words alone.

The Use of Self-Hypnosis. The use of hypnosis has gained considerable acceptance (and found substantial success) in the field of psychology over the years as a means to enhance health and well-being in endeavors ranging from weight loss to smoking cessation. The premise of self-hypnosis, whether it is used specifically for relaxation, as with autogenic training, or to effect other changes in attitude and behavior, is similar to virtually every relaxation technique: a calm mind and a calm body. Relaxation induced with gentle diaphragmatic breathing sets the stage for a receptive mind, which can then rehearse affirmation statements for the desired attitudinal or behavioral change. Self-generated hypnotic suggestions take root only when the mind and body are calm, because the unconscious mind censors suggestions under any other circumstance (Vickers et al. 2001).

Best Application of Autogenic Training

In its original design, autogenic training was created to be thorough in its attempt to relax the entire body. Sessions would last 20 to 40 minutes and could be done at any time of the day. Today, stress management instructors advocate relaxing all body regions for the entire duration of each session to achieve full effectiveness. With proficiency, however, the ability to relax upon suggestion of warmth and heaviness can be immediate, which is especially useful in situations that trigger the stress response. The autogenic technique is as portable as the thoughts that create it. Some healthcare professionals even suggest periodic short "autogenic breaks" in the course of a busy day as a preventive approach to the cumulative effects of stress. The jury is still out on whether this technique is more advantageous for reducing anxiety or anger. It appears to be effective with both emotional responses, depending on the individual and circumstances. It's best to try it for yourself and find out how it can best work for you (**FIG. 26.5**).

◼ Clinical Biofeedback

Welcome to the techno-nano age of biometrics where anything is possible, and the future is now. Picture this: The shirt or blouse you wear contains thousands

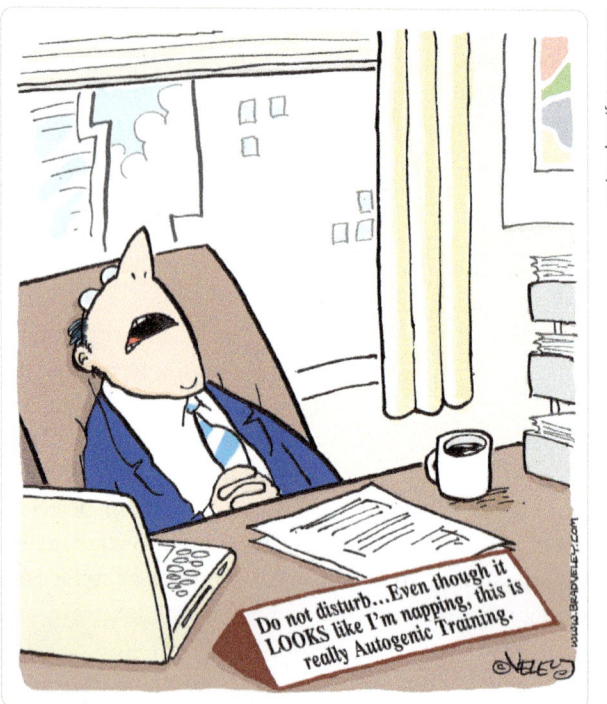

FIGURE 26.5 Autogenic training isn't the same thing as sleeping but it may look like it to some.

of tiny sensors that directly monitor your skin surface temperature, heart rate, blood pressure, muscle tension, and serum levels of cholesterol. The sensor on your computer mouse detects your skin temperature and the slightest beads of perspiration with a mere brush of your thumb. The lower left-hand corner of your computer screen displays a corresponding graph of your stress level with a suggestion to breathe deep to reduce your resting heart rate. Welcome to the age of nanobiofeedback, where your body's physiological parameters are just a mouse click away, giving you more responsibility for your health status. Bed sheets, toothbrushes, bandages, smart wristwatches, and running shoes have all been enhanced with artificial intelligence to help people regulate their physiological stress level and help them achieve homeostasis. Some (like court-ordered ankle bracelets) can even monitor an individual's blood alcohol content and send the information, via Wi-Fi, to a parole officer. Football helmets can transmit head blows and impact tackles to attending physicians. Toilets in Japan are now equipped to determine if a person has diabetes through urine samples. Joysticks, thumb buttons, and eye motion sensors connected to video games are able to determine stress-prone thinking patterns. Even the Wii system is loosely based on biofeedback technology.

Indeed, technology may give you stress, but technology can also provide the means to help you regulate it. The future is now.

These devices may seem like science fiction, but they exist today, funded in large part with your tax dollars for military purposes. Welcome to the age of biofeedback bionics. Although you may not have access to the latest technology, biofeedback is as simple as monitoring your pulse and breaths per minute. When information is accessed through clinical (and now nano) instrumentation, it is referred to as **clinical biofeedback**. With the advancement of computer-interface technology, some researchers now refer to biofeedback as *neurofeedback*.

The big craze these days are apps that monitor various aspects of the body's physiology in order to help individuals regulate their breathing, sleep, blood sugar, and eating habits. All of these apps fall into the biofeedback family, as they offer a way to measure a specific aspect of the body's physiology and help people achieve a sense of inner peace.

What Is Clinical Biofeedback?

Clinical biofeedback can be defined as the use of monitoring instruments to amplify the electrochemical energy produced by body organs. Normally, individuals are not aware of producing this energy, but through biofeedback they can use information to gain voluntary control over various physiological processes. For example, say that you have just learned from your dentist that you apparently grind your teeth at night. Being unaware that your jaw muscles are clenched while you sleep makes the problem difficult to resolve. But the use of instrumentation to measure your physiological responses could show you the tension you produce in your jaw muscles while awake and thus teach you how to reduce it—and eliminate the wear and tear on your teeth.

What distinguishes clinical biofeedback from other techniques is that it allows a person to increase awareness of his or her own physiological responses (breathing, muscle tension, blood pressure, heart rate, and/or body temperature) by learning to monitor them through data gathered by a particular instrument. Through biofeedback training, a person can also learn to recondition the thought processes associated with increased autonomic nervous activity to relax. Some stressors are very obvious, as are our reactions to them. But others

are more subtle, so much so that we condition ourselves to ignore the effects they produce throughout our bodies. Clinical biofeedback has the advantage of magnifying a biological function to give a person immediate evidence of changes in it, which, in turn, allows the person to gain mastery over it as it is happening. And whereas most relaxation techniques are meant to have a general, overall effect, biofeedback is usually specific to one targeted physiological parameter (e.g., tension in your jaw muscles). Athletes (amateur and professional) use all types of biofeedback equipment to enhance their athletic performance.

Clinical biofeedback typically employs sophisticated technological equipment in combination with one or more other relaxation techniques, including meditation, diaphragmatic breathing, mental imagery, autogenic training, and progressive muscular relaxation. When these relaxation techniques are performed in conjunction with data from an instrument revealing what the autonomic nervous system is really doing, the person gains a stronger "feel" for how to relax that body region.

Stress management is not the only area facilitated by this technique. Clinical biofeedback is also used in several types of psychotherapy (e.g., gestalt therapy) and some cases of physical rehabilitation of knee, lower back, and shoulder joints.

Once again, this technique emphasizes the importance of a strong mind-body-spirit connection. Clinical biofeedback is currently used in the treatment of migraine and tension headaches, ulcers, hypertension, bruxism, Raynaud's disease, and a host of other stress-related illnesses. Dr. Edward Blanchard of the Center for Stress and Anxiety Disorders in Albany, New York, has conducted numerous scientific investigations demonstrating the beneficial effects of biofeedback on several different maladies, substantiating the validity of this technique. His work is well respected throughout the allied health fields. But despite the fact that biofeedback is known to be effective in gaining control over specific biological functions, the exact mechanisms involved are as yet not completely understood (**FIG. 26.6**).

Clinical biofeedback: A process using one or more specially designed machines to amplify body signals (e.g., heart rate, muscle tension) and to display them in a way that can be interpreted so that their intensity can be changed for the health of the individual.

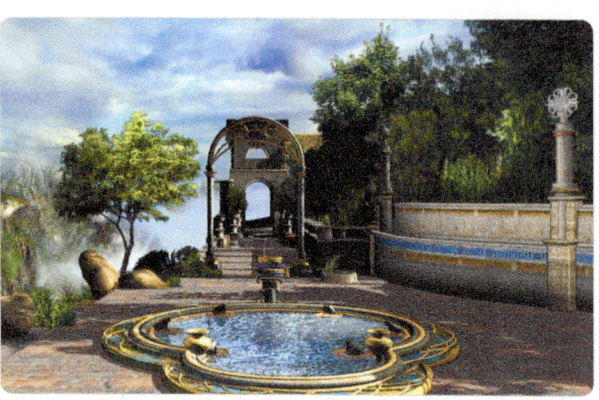

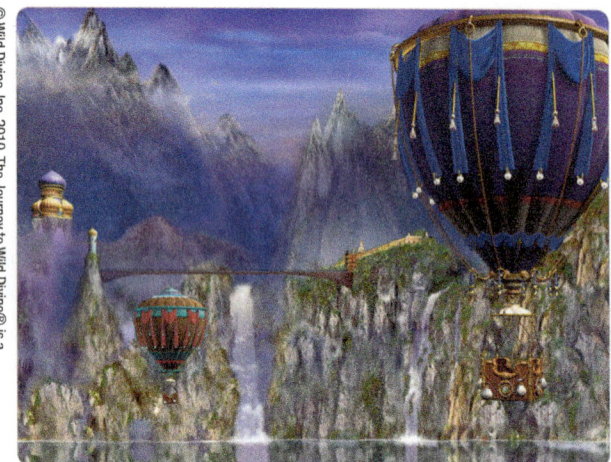

FIGURE 26.6 These two spectacular images are from the Journey to the Wild Divine active feedback and Relaxing Rhythms active feedback programs by Wild Divine. Characters within the Journey help you to control your body's reactions. By increasing, decreasing, or synchronizing your body rhythms, you learn to master the Journey Events and progress through the program.

Historical Perspective

The term *biofeedback* was coined in the late 1960s by researcher Dr. Barbara Brown to describe biological feedback through electrical stimulation. This term was coined just prior to the first annual meeting of the Biofeedback Society in 1969 (Allen 1983). Biofeedback includes information on any physiological parameter that can be electronically detected, amplified, and converted into visual or auditory stimuli. An individual can observe and interpret these stimuli, and thereby make appropriate changes to enhance his or her health. Although the name is rather new, the concepts of biofeedback date back to the classical conditioning theory of Pavlov (every stimulus produces a response through association) and operant conditioning theory of Thorndike (behaviors can be changed by redirected thought processes). Until 1960, it was strongly believed that the autonomic nervous system was reflexive in nature, influenced only by classical conditioning, not conscious thought. Like an autopilot computer program, the autonomic nervous system was thought to be under complete control of the lower brain centers. Basic physiological functions were called "involuntary" because it was believed that they could not be intentionally influenced or manipulated by the individual.

Clinical investigations with the yogi Swami Rama, conducted at the Menninger Clinic, as well as other studies by Miller (1968) began to show that conscious thought really can influence the physiological functions of the autonomic nervous system. In addition to significantly lowering his resting heart rate and breathing well below "normal homeostatic levels," Swami Rama was able to shift blood flow to various regions of his body. Similar studies showed that some people had the ability to change their brain waves at will. In fact, people who were taught autogenic training proved that with practice almost anyone could control these "involuntary" functions. And the more they practiced, the more control they seemed to exhibit. Biofeedback training is now considered a type of operant conditioning wherein, with the help of a trained therapist, an individual can learn to control specific physiological functions by changing the thoughts and perceptions that produced them (**BOX 26.1**).

In his classic book *Mind as Healer, Mind as Slayer* (1977), stress researcher Kenneth Pelletier states that biofeedback comprises three principles: (1) information can be obtained about specific organ activity, meaning that a machine can distinguish electrical conduction of heart muscle from that of brain and skeletal muscles; (2) every physiological change is paralleled by a change in attitude or consciousness, just as a change in feelings will produce a change in some biological function; and (3) people can be taught to control their autonomic nervous systems to influence these physiological changes directly. He adds that individuals must accept responsibility for their own health status—in this case, by learning to recondition thoughts and behaviors away from disease and toward health. This principle is closely related to Rotter's concept of locus of control, where a person learns to shift the focus of control from an external source (a stressor) to

BOX 26.1   Insomnia and Biofeedback

Biofeedback has been used successfully in the treatment of insomnia. Through the use of electroencephalography (EEG), and in some cases electromyography (EMG), patients are shown their brain waves (EEG) and muscle tension (EMG) and then taught how to reduce the neural firing. When this information is combined with other coping skills, including cognitive restructuring, visualization, and diaphragmatic breathing, patients are able to control their thoughts to produce a minimal level of brain activity, indicative of a presleep state. Research studies regarding insomnia and biofeedback include mostly case studies, but the body of evidence yielded by these investigations constitutes a critical mass of data to reveal that the use of biofeedback to train the mind is, indeed, a valuable skill to reduce problems associated with insomnia.

an internal source (his or her thoughts) to take control of physical health.

The HeartMath Institute is world renowned for its well-designed research into heart rate variability. Based on the premise that both emotions and thoughts affect heart rate and other cardiovascular functions, a biofeedback program called the Em Wave PC Stress Relief System was developed by Doc Childre. The Em Wave PC Stress Relief System is an interactive computer learning system (**FIG. 26.7**) designed to teach participants to respond—rather than react—to situations that can promote stress.

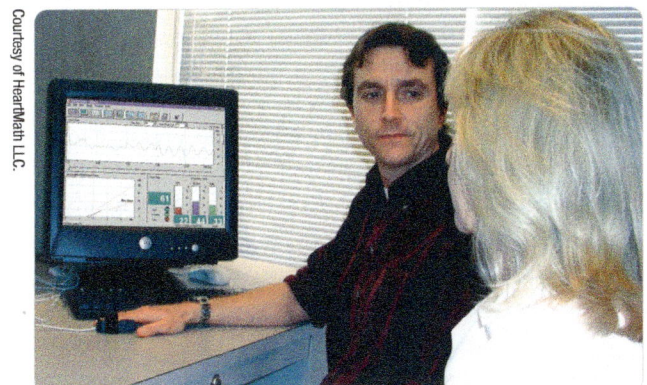

FIGURE 26.7   A client is taught to observe his heart rate activity through the HeartMath Institute's Em Wave PC Stress Relief System program.

Purpose of Biofeedback

To get an idea of our physical appearance, we gaze into a mirror at our hair, our complexion, and the clothing we wear. Mirrors offer a clear reflection of our physical exterior. The many physiological functions that take place inside our bodies are much more difficult to observe, yet equally necessitate our attention. For example, according to the Centers for Disease Control and Prevention (CDC), an estimated 33 percent of the U.S. population has hypertension ("High Blood Pressure Facts" 2019), but blood pressure *cannot* be detected by physical appearance or by simply taking one's pulse. It must be monitored with a blood-pressure cuff, sphygmomanometer, and stethoscope. Physiological functions we cannot see, involving the nervous, endocrine, and immune systems, are strongly activated during the stress response. Whereas some people show the ability to scan their bodies and bring certain functions under control without the aid of a machine, most people need the additional help of biofeedback to do so. With enough practice, these people, too, can attain the ability to perceive and regulate their internal functions without the use of machines, or what is known as a **conditional response**.

Although the technology of clinical biofeedback may seem complex, the concept behind it is quite simple. Biofeedback is a **closed-loop feedback system**, where information taken from the system (the human body) is translated into a language understood by the five senses (**FIG. 26.8**). Biofeedback is like an oval racetrack where the starting and finishing points are the same. In this case, the loop begins with the body, which is connected by wires to some type of electronic machine. The wires receive energy and send it to the machine, where it is converted to recognizable stimuli and then relayed back to the individual through one of the five senses. More technically, biochemical impulses generated by specific body organ tissue are transmitted via one or more electrodes attached to that body region and sent

Conditional response: A learned response (in this case through biofeedback) to control various biological functions such as heart rate and blood pressure.

Closed-loop feedback system: The dynamics of biofeedback with its sensors attached to various parts of the human body. The output (heart rate, skin response, etc.) can be observed by the eyes or ears, which closes the loop so these aspects can be changed.

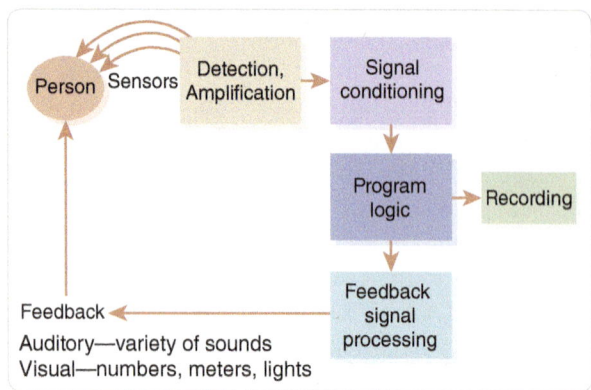

FIGURE 26.8 The biofeedback loop.

to an electronic receiver that converts the impulses to either visual or auditory stimuli. These stimuli can be in the form of colored lights, sounds, and/or parts such as needle pens that chart the data.

Biofeedback has been called an educational tool because it teaches people how to monitor and change the frequency and amplitude of the electronic signals by controlling (relaxing) the body region to which the electrodes are attached. The purpose of biofeedback, therefore, is to teach people how to "tune in" to their bodies so that they can regulate those physiological functions that are susceptible to increased metabolic activity caused by stress.

Biofeedback has three distinct phases:

1. *Awareness of physiological response:* As mentioned before, the sensory stimulation deciphered by the biofeedback machine and decoded by one of the five senses helps one increase awareness of physiological adaptations to stress. A certified

---

Binary biofeedback: One of two categories used to describe biofeedback. Uses instrumentation that provides information that enables a person to know whether he or she is controlling a particular physiological function; an example would be a device that alerts a person to the effect of biofeedback on a specific biological function by a light being lit up on a panel.

Proportional biofeedback: One of two categories used to describe biofeedback. Uses instrumentation that reveals the *amount of change* occurring during a session; an example might be a device that alerts one to the amount of physiological change through the pitch of a noise.

Electromyographic (EMG) biofeedback: Biofeedback that measures the electrical impulses from specific muscles.

---

therapist operates the instrument and teaches the patient to interpret the amplified signals and thereby form an association between the flashing lights or beeping sounds and the body's current state of arousal.

2. *Control of physiological response:* The therapist guides the person through several types of relaxation techniques—meditation, mental imagery, and autogenic training, among others. At the same time, the person attempts to consciously manipulate his or her physiological response to bring a particular body organ or reaction to a state of homeostasis.

3. *Application of reconditioned response in everyday routines:* After much practice with biofeedback instrumentation, the individual then transfers the new skill to the office, home, car, or wherever he or she experiences the sensations of stress, by practicing the relaxation technique without using the equipment. This, of course, is the real test of the effectiveness of biofeedback training sessions.

Types of Biofeedback

Many different types of biofeedback equipment are available. Some are so small you can hold them in your hand, whereas others involve large (expensive) instrumentation in a wall unit. Different machines have been designed to receive the electrical signals from the heart, brain, muscles, skin, back, and so forth. The use of biofeedback is specific to the symptom(s) the patient exhibits in a particular body region. In general, though, biofeedback falls into two categories: binary and proportional. **Binary biofeedback** involves instrumentation that provides information that enables a person to know only whether he or she is controlling a particular physiological function. An example would be a light that is off when a person's systolic blood pressure is above 130 mm Hg and then turns on when his or her blood pressure goes below that number. **Proportional biofeedback,** by contrast, reveals the *amount of change* occurring during a session. An example is a machine that changes the pitch of a sound as a person becomes more relaxed. Because it provides more information to the patient, proportional biofeedback is thought to be more effective as a teaching tool. Regardless of instrumentation, biofeedback is effective because it is accurate and reliable.

Electromyographic (EMG) Biofeedback.

Electromyographic (EMG) biofeedback monitors electrical impulses produced by muscle tissue (**FIG. 26.9**).

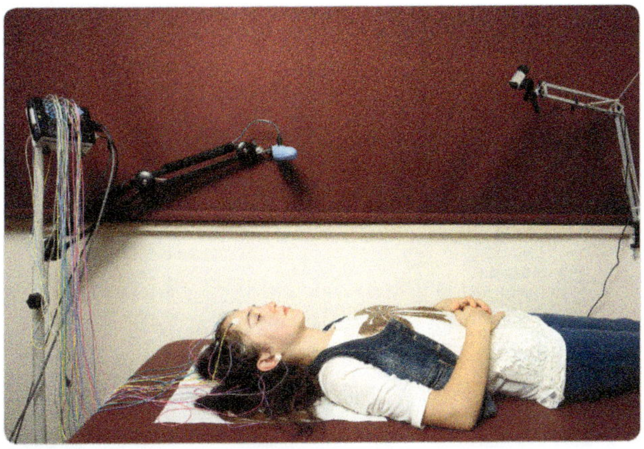

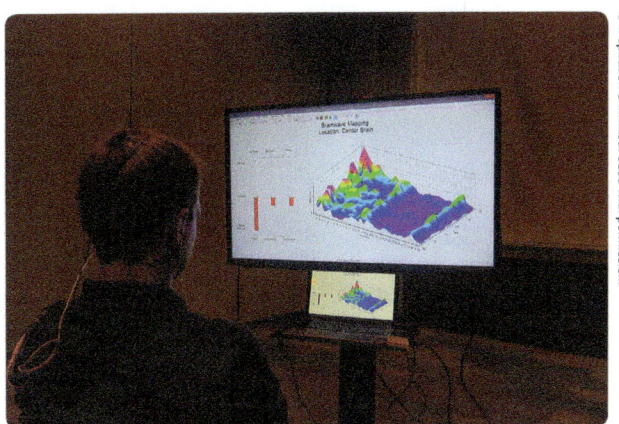

FIGURE 26.9   EMG biofeedback instruments.

FIGURE 26.10   EEG biofeedback equipment.

Electrodes are placed on the skin over specific muscles that are prone to tension, such as the jaw, lower back, neck, and/or shoulders. For overall relaxation, the frontalis muscle on the forehead is used because this muscle has no direct connection to bone. Through the EMG, the patient first becomes aware of the current level of muscle tension by watching visual feedback or hearing auditory feedback. With the aid of the therapist, the subject is then taught to relax the muscles that are diagnosed as tense, and to sense the difference between tension and relaxation, while monitoring visual and/or auditory data produced by the machine. EMG biofeedback is most commonly used for tension headaches, bruxism, or temporomandibular joint (TMJ) dysfunction.

Electroencephalographic (EEG) Biofeedback. Like the heart and muscles, the brain produces electrical impulses. In 1924, Hans Berger created an instrument to detect and monitor brain waves, which he called the electroencephalogram (EEG) (**FIG. 26.10**). An EEG is recorded by applying electrodes to designated points on the scalp, which monitor electrical activity close to the surface of the brain. Through the use of EEG, it has been observed that the human brain produces different electrical rhythms during various states of consciousness. These brain waves are grouped and characterized by oscillations per second and amplitude. The four groups are beta waves (more than 15 cycles per second), which are associated with normal or waking consciousness; alpha waves (7–14 cycles per second), which are produced in an altered or relaxed state of consciousness; and theta (4–7 cycles per second) and delta (0.5–4 cycles per second) waves, which are observed in unconscious and sleeping states. Each type of brain wave is represented by a specific sound or pitch from the EEG. For the purpose of relaxation, the patient is taught to decrease the pitch associated with beta waves and increase the alpha sound. The primary purpose of **electroencephalographic (EEG) biofeedback** is to alleviate the cognitive arousal observed in insomnia. So far, it seems to be of very little help in relieving tension headaches or other stress symptomology.

Cardiovascular (EKG) Biofeedback. Because there appears to be such a strong relationship between stress and coronary heart disease, **cardiovascular (EKG) biofeedback** is often used to augment a patient's ability to control resting heart rate and blood pressure. Portable equipment is now available for cardiac patients so that they can monitor their heart rate on a regular basis. Portable blood pressure kits are also available for people with hypertension. In either case, patients are taught to employ relaxation skills when the biofeedback machine indicates that cardiovascular parameters are above preset resting levels.

However, cardiovascular biofeedback is not used solely by people at risk for cardiac disease. Many Olympic and professional athletes also use portable heart rate monitors to aid their training. Several of these consist of a belt worn around the upper chest and a receiver worn on the wrist like a watch (**FIG. 26.11**). The receiver is set to a

> **Electroencephalographic (EEG) biofeedback:** Biofeedback that measures the electrical activity of the brain.
>
> **Cardiovascular (EKG) biofeedback:** Biofeedback that measures the electrical activity of the heart muscle in terms of amplitude and frequency of each heartbeat.

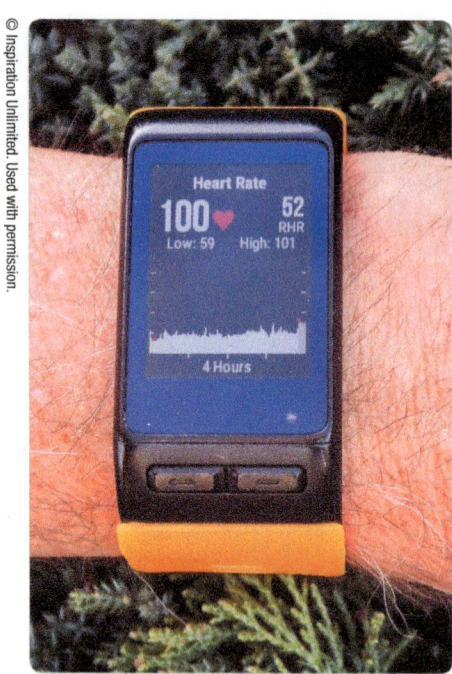

© Inspiration Unlimited. Used with permission.

FIGURE 26.11   A heart rate monitor.

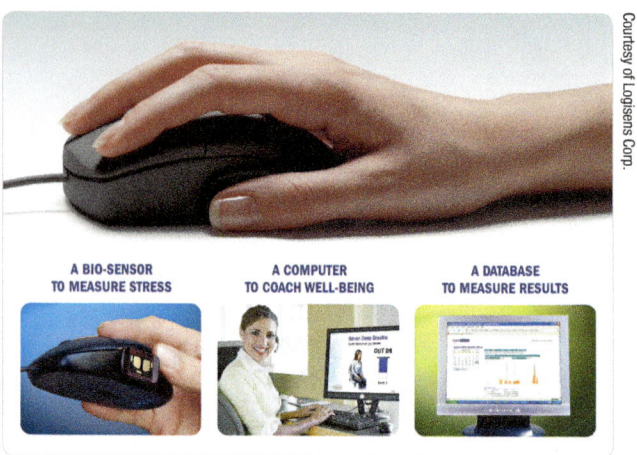

Courtesy of Logisens Corp.

A BIO-SENSOR TO MEASURE STRESS   A COMPUTER TO COACH WELL-BEING   A DATABASE TO MEASURE RESULTS

FIGURE 26.12   The Logisens biosensor (located on the thumb placement of the mouse) detects one's stress level through electrodermal response. The Logisens biofeedback program educates the individual to monitor and control stress levels.

target heart rate range. If the athlete goes below or above this zone, the watch beeps, signifying that the cardiovascular workload needs to be increased or decreased, respectively. In some cases, the receiver records heart rate for up to an hour, and these data can be retrieved and logged into a training diary.

Another type of cardiovascular monitor measures temperature. **Thermal biofeedback**, as it is called, monitors the flow of blood to a specific area by the heat it gives off. Temperature receptors are applied to specific body parts (e.g., fingers and toes) so that changes in blood flow can be detected as changes in temperature. Thermal biofeedback is most often used in the treatment of migraine headaches and Raynaud's disease.

Electrodermal (EDR) Biofeedback. **Electrodermal (EDR) biofeedback** also known as galvanic skin response (GSR), is used to measure electrical conduction in the skin itself (**FIG. 26.12**). The hands and fingers produce beads of sweat under stress, and the fact that water is a good conductor of electricity is the basis of the operation of the EDR instrument. The premise

behind EDR is that electrical impulses produced by the skin are activated by the sympathetic nervous system. In this type of biofeedback, electrodes are lubricated with a conductance gel and placed on the skin, usually the index and ring fingers of the left hand. As in other forms of biofeedback, the patient is then taught to decrease sympathetic activation through relaxation techniques. EDR is employed primarily to detect nervousness, and repeated use can help people learn to decrease anxiety. The same technology, incidentally, is used in polygraph (lie detector) tests.

Biofeedback and Chronic Pain

If you were to do an Internet search on the topic of biofeedback, the vast majority of studies turned up in the search would deal with the beneficial use of biofeedback for pain relief, whether for migraines, TMJ, low back pain, colitis, or a multitude of other chronic symptoms. Because biofeedback is meant to act as an amplification of the body's electrical responses, the regulation of pain is controlled through a conscious decrease of neural firing to the painful area. By using biofeedback technology to increase awareness of self-regulation, pain is brought under control and, in many cases, eliminated. For biofeedback to be fully effective, however, it must do more than simply decrease pain. When used properly with the aid of a certified biofeedback therapist, the causes of stress that manifest themselves as pain are addressed and resolved as well (Norris 2012).

> **Thermal biofeedback:** Biofeedback that measures the response based on skin temperature.
>
> **Electrodermal (EDR) biofeedback:** Biofeedback that measures the sweat response from skin.

Stress with a Human Face

Sara began developing migraine headaches her senior year of high school. Not a week would pass without the effects of a severe migraine. She was placed on a prescription medicine, but it really didn't help much. Some headaches lasted a week, and they felt like they were ripping her skull apart. Her first year in college was worse, sometimes with headaches so bad she curled up in bed for days. It was a program on the Discovery Channel one night that caught her attention. The program featured a technique called biofeedback. Although several people were interviewed for a host of maladies, it was the woman who suffered from migraines that caught her attention. "You become so desperate you are willing to try anything," she said. When the show was over, Sara Googled the word *biofeedback* and the name of her city to see what would show up. After spending an hour reading about biofeedback on the Internet and searching for a well-qualified technician in her area, she made a few phone calls the next day and set up an appointment. "What biofeedback does is put you in touch with your body. In order to listen to your body's signals, you have to pay attention and that's what biofeedback helps you do. Most people are so out of touch with their bodies, and I was one of those people. You can get so caught up in the day-to-day struggles that you lose touch with yourself, until it comes back to bite you in the butt." After several biofeedback sessions, Sara got her migraines under control to where she had only a couple per year, if that. "For me, it worked and I am grateful. Getting in touch with your body is not only beneficial, it's essential if you want to function in the fast-paced world we live in."

Best Application of Clinical Biofeedback

Clinical biofeedback, like muscle massage, is a technique that requires the assistance of a qualified instructor or therapist. The primary organization that certifies therapists in clinical biofeedback training is the Biofeedback Certificate Institute of America (BCIA). Since 1980, all therapists practicing biofeedback are required to have certification. If you are interested in this mode of relaxation therapy because of recurring health problems, contact your primary care physician, local hospital, or psychological counseling center. You can also contact the Association for Applied Psychophysiology and Biofeedback at http://aapb.org. When you meet with a biofeedback therapist, he or she will determine how this treatment can alleviate your stress-related symptoms and which type of biofeedback is best suited to do this. The number of therapy sessions required depends on the type and severity of the symptoms. Once you are familiar with the technique, you will then be given "homework" assignments in which you are to practice the biofeedback therapy on your own for a specified length of time.

One concern that has been raised about biofeedback is that a person may become dependent on biofeedback equipment to obtain a complete state of relaxation. However, if the therapist is good at instruction and the person is conscientious about practicing the relaxation techniques, then there really is no danger of biofeedback dependence. The advent of the smartphone and smart devices has brought with it hundreds if not thousands of apps that fall into the category of biofeedback. These include, but are not limited to, apps that monitor heart rate (e.g., Fitbit) and sleep monitoring apps that help you determine the quality of your sleep (e.g., Headspace, Sleep Cycle, and Sleep Time). Remember, although it's great to use these apps, they are like training wheels on a bike. Once you process the feedback, you don't want to outsource the awareness of your body functions to a device. Use the device to learn how to become self-reliant.

When biofeedback was first introduced into the world of clinical medicine, it was hailed as the most effective of the various relaxation techniques. Since that time, however, experts have learned that this technique holds no superiority over any other relaxation strategies or coping techniques. In many cases, it is effective for people with serious stress-related symptoms for whom meditation or mental imagery alone does not seem to help. In any case, research has shown what many health practitioners and Eastern mystics already knew: We do indeed have conscious control of the autonomic nervous system, and this control can affect health and well-being.

SUMMARY

- The term *autogenic training* refers to the body's ability to regulate specific physiological functions through conscious suggestion. This term is often used synonymously with the clinical term *self-regulation*.

- The autogenic technique was developed by two German physicians, Schultz and Luthe, after learning that some of their patients could hypnotize themselves to achieve a profound state of relaxation. The primary effect was in peripheral body regions, which became warm and heavy. This effect is thought to be the result of changes in blood flow.

- Schultz and Luthe outlined six conditions they felt necessary for this technique to be effective. Among these are receptiveness to the self-suggestion to relax, positioning oneself comfortably, the ability to concentrate, and focusing on internal physiological processes.

- *Selected awareness* is a term used to explain how the mind focuses attention on the self-suggestion and receptivity that produce a sense of relaxation.

- *Autogenic discharge* refers to various sensory sensations and emotional responses triggered by this technique.

- The autogenic technique has been used in hospitals, with patients shunting blood away from surgical sites. It has also been reported to hasten recovery from surgery.

- There are two general approaches to the autogenic technique. In the direct method, the person consciously moves blood to the extremities where warmth and heaviness are desired. In the indirect method, the person focuses only on warmth and heaviness, not blood flow.

- Biofeedback is a process of gathering information about specific physiological functions such as heart rate, respiration, and body temperature. Clinical biofeedback uses sophisticated instrumentation to amplify and measure these functions so that they are easier to detect and interpret.

- The purpose of biofeedback is to teach people with stress-related disorders to recondition their responses so that they gain control over the physiological system responsible for their symptoms.

- Clinical biofeedback combines sophisticated technology with forms of relaxation, including diaphragmatic breathing, autogenic training, progressive muscular relaxation, and mental imagery, to strengthen the conditioned response.

- Several types of clinical biofeedback are available, with each monitoring a specific physiological system. These are electromyography (EMG), electroencephalography (EEG), electrocardiography (EKG), electrodermal (EDR), and thermal biofeedback.

- Clinical biofeedback is widely used and strongly recommended as a modality to decrease episodes of chronic pain.

- Research on the various aspects of clinical biofeedback has produced promising results. Biofeedback is now recognized as one of the most effective methods of relaxation.

STUDY GUIDE QUESTIONS

1. Explain the rationale for autogenic training as a relaxation technique.

2. Describe in simple terms how to do autogenic training for relaxation.

3. Describe the concept of self-hypnosis.

4. Explain the rationale for biofeedback as a relaxation technique.

5. List three types of conditions that can be improved through the use of biofeedback.

6. Describe three types of biofeedback, and explain how each can be used to promote relaxation.

REFERENCES AND RESOURCES

Allen, R. 1983. *Human Stress: Its Nature and Control.* Minneapolis, MN: Burgess Press.

Anderson, N., P. Lawrence, and T. Olson. 1981. "Within-Subject Analysis of Autogenic Training and Cognitive

Coping Training in the Treatment of Tension Headache Pain." *Journal of Behavioral Therapy and Experimental Psychiatry* 12: 219–223.

Basmanjian, J. 1989. *Biofeedback: Principles and Practice for Clinicians.* New York: Williams & Wilkins.

Beech, H. R., L. E. Burns, and B. F. Sheffield. 1982. *A Behavioral Approach to the Management of Stress: A Practical Guide to Techniques.* Chichester, England: Wiley.

Blanchard, E. B., F. Andrasik, D. Devans, and J. Hillhouse. 1985. "Biofeedback and Relaxation Treatments for Headaches in the Elderly: A Caution and a Challenge." *Biofeedback and Self-Regulation* 10(1): 68–73.

Blanchard, E. B., F. Andrasik, D. F. Neff, et al. 1982. "Biofeedback and Relaxation Training with Three Kinds of Headaches: Treatment Effects and Their Predictions." *Journal of Consulting and Clinical Psychology* 50: 562–575.

Blanchard, E. B., and M. R. Haynes. 1975. "Biofeedback Treatment of a Case of Raynaud's Disease." *Journal of Behavioral Therapy and Experimental Psychiatry* 6: 230–234.

Brown, B. B. 1977. *Stress and the Art of Biofeedback.* New York: Harper & Row.

Budzynski, T., and J. Stoyva. 1984. "Biofeedback Methods in the Treatment of Anxiety and Stress." In *Principles and Practices of Stress Management*, edited by R. Wolfolk and D. Lehrer. New York: Guilford Press.

Burish, T. G. 1980. "EMG Biofeedback Transfer of Teaching and Coping with Stress." *Psychosomatic Research* 24(2): 85–96.

Carrol, D. 1984. *Biofeedback in Practice.* New York: Longman.

Carruthers, M. 1979. "Autogenic Training." *Journal of Psychosomatic Research* 23: 437–440.

Coates, T. J., and C. E. Thoreson. 1978. "What to Use Instead of Sleeping Pills." *Journal of the American Medical Association* 240: 2311–2312.

Coutler, I., J. T. Favreau, M. L. Hardy, et al. 2002. "Biofeed-back Interventions for Gastrointestinal Conditions." *Alternative Therapies* 8(3): 76–83.

Danskin, D. G., and M. Crow. 1981. *Biofeedback: An Introduction and Guide.* Palo Alto, CA: Mayfield.

Dhanani, N. M., T. J. Caruso, and A. J. Carinci. 2011. "Complementary and Alternative Medicine for Pain: An Evidence-Based Review." *Current Pain Headache Reports* 15(1): 39–46.

DiCara, L. V. 1970. "Learning in the Autonomic Nervous System." *Scientific American* 222(1): 30–39.

Ernst, E. 2008. British Autogenic Society. https://www.auto-genic-therapy.org.uk.

Everly, G. 2002. *A Clinical Guide to the Treatment of the Human Stress Response.* New York: Plenum.

Fisher-Williams, M. 1986. *A Textbook of Biological Feedback.* New York: Human Sciences Press.

Fuller, G. D. 1977. *Biofeedback: Methods and Procedures in Clinical Practice.* San Francisco, CA: Biofeedback Press.

Gaarder, K., and P. Montgomery. 1977. *Clinical Biofeedback: A Procedural Manual.* Baltimore, MD: Williams & Wilkins.

Glanz, M., S. Klawansky, and T. Chalmers. 1977. "Biofeedback Therapy in Stroke Rehabilitation: A Review." *Journal of the Royal Society of Medicine* 90: 33–39.

Gorton, B. 1959. "Autogenic Training." *American Journal of Clinical Hypnosis* 2: 31–41.

Green, E., and A. Green. 1977. *Beyond Biofeedback.* New York: Delacorte Press.

Green, E., A. Green, and E. D. Walters. 1970. "Voluntary Control of Intense States: Psychological and Physiological." *Journal of Transpersonal Psychology* 2: 1–26.

Greenberg, J. 2010. *Comprehensive Stress Management* (12th ed.). New York: McGraw-Hill.

"A Guide to Psychology and Its Practice." Autogenic Training. www.guidetopsychology.com/autogen.htm.

"High Blood Pressure Facts." 2019. Centers for Disease Control and Prevention. 2019. https://www.cdc.gov/blood pressure/facts.htm.

Keefe, J. F., R. S. Surwit, and R. N. Pilon. 1980. "Biofeedback, Autogenic Training, and Progressive Muscular Relaxation in the Treatment of Raynaud's Disease: A Comparative Study." *Journal of Applied Behavior Analysis* 13: 3–11.

Kirsch, I. 2001. "Altered States." *Social Research* 68(3): 795–809.

Luthe, W. 1962. "Method, Research, and Applications of Autogenic Training." *American Journal of Clinical Hypnosis* 5: 17–23.

Luthe, W. 1969. *Autogenic Theory.* New York: Grune and Stratton.

Marcer, D. 1986. *Biofeedback and Related Therapies in Clinical Practice.* London: Croom Helm.

Middaugh, S., and K. Pawlick. 2002. "Biofeedback and Behavioral Treatment of Persistent Pain in the Older Adult: A Review and Study." *Applied Psychophysiology and Biofeedback* 27: 185–202.

Miller, E. 1980. *Letting Go of Stress.* Albuquerque, NM: Newman Communications.

Miller, N. E. 1968. "Visceral Learning and Other Additional Facts Potentially Applicable to Psychotherapy." *International Psychiatry Clinics* 5: 294–312.

Miller, N. E. 1985. "Rx: Biofeedback." *Psychology Today*, February, pp. 54–59.

Miller, N. E. 1989. "What Biofeedback Does (and Does Not Do)." *Psychology Today*, November, pp. 22–24.

Norris, P. 2012. Personal communication, June 23

Pelletier, K. 1977. *Mind as Healer, Mind as Slayer.* New York: Dell.

Porter, G., and P. Norris. 1985. *Why Me? Harnessing the Healing Power of the Human Spirit.* Walpole, NH: Stillpoint Press.

Robbins, J. 2000. *A Symphony in the Brain: The Evolution of the New Brain Wave Biofeedback.* New York: Atlantic Monthly Press.

Rosenbaum, L. 1988. *Biofeedback Frontiers: Self-Regulation of Stress Reactivity*. New York: AMS Press.

Runick, B. 1980. *Biofeedback: Issues in Treatment Assessment*. Rockville, MD: National Institutes of Mental Health.

Schultz, J. 1932. *Das Autogene Training*. Leipzig: Geerg-Thieme, Verlag.

Schultz, J., and W. Luthe. 1959. *Autogenic Training: A Psychophysiological Approach to Psychotherapy*. New York: Grune and Stratton.

Schwartz, M. S. 1987. *Biofeedback: A Practitioner's Guide*. New York: Guilford Press.

Siegel, B. 1990. *Peace, Love, and Healing*. New York: Perennial Press.

Silver, B. V. 1979. "Temperature Biofeedback and Regulation Training in the Treatment of Migraine Headaches." *Biofeedback and Self-Regulation* 4: 359–366.

Stein, R. 2004. "Number of Americans Who Have High Blood Pressure Up Sharply: 31 Percent of Adults Suffering from Hypertension, Study Finds." *Washington Post*, August 24.

Turk, D. G., D. H. Meichenbaum, and W. H. Berman. 1979. "Application of Biofeedback for the Regulation of Pain: A Critical Review." *Psychological Bulletin* 86: 1322–1338.

Vickers, A., C. Zollman, and D. Payne. 2001. "Toolbox: Hypnosis and Relaxation Therapies." *Western Journal of Medicine* 175(4): 269–272.

Whitman, W. 2000. *Leaves of Grass*. New York: Signet Books.

Whitney, E. 2010. "High-Tech 'Band-Aids' Call Doctors." NPR, July 30. https://www.npr.org/templates/story/story.php?storyId=128877308.

Wisem, A. 2002. *Awakening the Mind: A Guide to Mastering the Power of Your Brain Waves*. New York: Putnam.

Yates, A. J. 1980. *Biofeedback and the Modification of Behavior*. New York: Plenum Press.

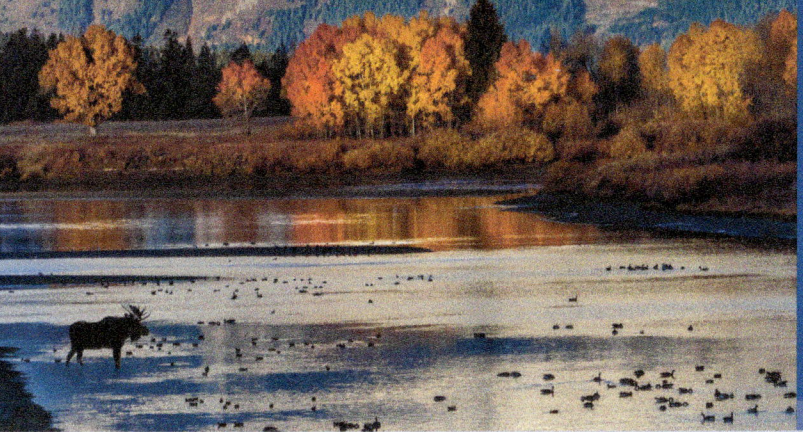

CHAPTER 27

Physical Exercise, Nutrition, and Stress

A sound mind in a sound body.

—Juvenal

Perhaps the most telling sign of stress in the American population is our ever-expanding waistlines. Obesity has reached epidemic proportions. The average American eats a lot more and exercises considerably less than his or her parents a generation ago and far less than his or her grandparents. One of the many examples of the stress–nutrition equation is that children are now being diagnosed with adult-onset diabetes, something unheard of a generation ago. People's lifestyles have changed dramatically over the past few decades, and diseases such as cancer and diabetes and scores of stress-related illnesses have skyrocketed. Sadly, there is no quick fix for optimal health; however, physical exercise and healthy eating habits can help.

Physical exercise not only utilizes the stress hormones for their intended purpose, but the cathartic release of stress is nearly unbeatable. Remember, though, that there is a reason why exercise is called "work." Yet even work can have its rewards, and the health benefits of physical exercise and activity are worth their weight in gold. Let there be no doubt: Physical exercise is stress to the body. It is the fight-or-flight response in motion. Given the promise of physiological homeostasis, physical exercise might just be the closest thing we have to the fountain of youth. According to well-cited research, not only does physical exercise and activity enhance your health and longevity, it appears to increase brain cell tissue associated with memory, multitasking, and attention span (Carmichael 2007; Ratey 2008).

Given what experts call an overweight and sedentary population, one might conclude that Americans are headed down the wrong road. Getting back on track to a healthy lifestyle with a focus on physical activity, however, is just a mindset away, and best of all, the benefits are immeasurable. This chapter highlights exercise and nutrition as stress management relaxation techniques in an effort to maintain physiological homeostasis, physical well-being, and optimal health.

Physical Exercise and Stress

The ancient fight-or-flight response prepares the body for immediate physical movement. An increase in heart rate and blood pressure redistributes blood from the abdominal region to the large muscle groups. Increased ventilation and circulation provide a greater supply of oxygen to the working muscles. The release of catecholamines and stress hormones activates the processes for metabolism of fats and carbohydrates, and these remain elevated long enough to ensure that muscles have adequate energy for contraction. Physical exercise strengthens the integrity of the body's physiological systems. Just as Selye observed physical deterioration from chronic distress, researchers in the field of exercise physiology have observed physical improvement from habitual exercise. There is adaptation to good stress as well as to bad stress.

The human body is a fantastic and complex phenomenon. It has several backup systems to the fight-or-flight response to ensure the best chance of physical survival. For example, there are at least four hormones responsible for increasing blood pressure to shunt blood from the body's core to the periphery. In addition, conversion of proteins to glucose substrates occurs to meet the body's energy demands.

Even though exercise perpetuates the stress response while one is in motion, when physical activity ceases the body returns to homeostasis. In a well-trained individual, the rate of return is not only quicker, but also the degree of homeostasis attained is more complete than before the individual began to exercise. It seems that the body's natural inclination, when confronted with stress, is to move, be active, or exercise. To remain inactive results in an incredible strain on internal systems. When the body stays still, various organ tissues go into metabolic overdrive, like "flooring it" with the car in park for hours at a time. As a case in point, a classic study by Porter and Allsen (1978) showed that head basketball coaches had heart rates well above resting levels during games, in some cases as much as 253 percent (162 beats/minute) above resting pregame levels—for a 90-minute period.

In the past 50 years, since the recognition of coronary heart disease as America's number one cause of death and the factors putting one at risk, the effects of physical exercise on human anatomy and physiology have been studied feverishly. The overwhelming conclusion is that physical exercise is not merely good, but that it is a virtual necessity to maintain proper function of major physiological systems. Just as the body requires a state of calmness or homeostasis, it equally demands physical stimulation or it will go into dysfunction. In other words, use it or lose it. Given what we now know, it is obvious that there must be a balance between physical arousal (activity) and homeostasis (rest) for optimal wellness.

Unless you have been hiding in a cave for the past decade, you cannot help but hear news reports regarding the growing obesity problem in America. Obesity is not only a health issue; it can become a major stressor for those who are overweight and cannot lose those unwanted pounds. Whether the issue takes the form of obese children contracting adult-onset diabetes or news that Fenway Park needs to replace its bleachers with wider seats to accommodate patrons' wider rear ends, obesity and related health problems are clearly at epidemic proportions. Despite the claims made in pending lawsuits against various fast-food outlets, experts like Ken Cooper, M.D., agree that caloric consumption is only half the problem. The human body was not designed to sit lethargically in front of a computer or TV for hours on end. Physical exercise (caloric expenditure) is necessary for physiological homeostasis.

The astonishing benefits of exercise on many aspects of health, from stress and depression (Dahl 2016) to insomnia and longevity, have been researched for decades, and research continues to validate Ken Cooper's classic studies. Recent research by Mark Tarnopolsky at McMaster University in Toronto, Canada, confirms what the landmark studies revealed decades ago—that the combination of cardiovascular exercise and moderate strength training is the closest thing we have to the fountain of youth (Oaklander 2016) with regard to the functioning of the cardiovascular, neuromuscular, immune, and endocrine systems.

Types of Physical Exercise

The six components of fitness are cardiovascular endurance, muscular strength and endurance, flexibility, agility, power, and balance. (Some people include body composition as a seventh component.) **Cardiovascular endurance** is the ability of the heart, lungs, and blood vessels to transport oxygenated blood to the working muscles for energy metabolism. **Muscular strength** is the ability to exert maximal force against a resistance, and **muscular endurance** is the ability to sustain repeated contractions over a prolonged period of time. **Flexibility**

Cardiovascular endurance: The ability of the heart, lungs, and blood vessels to supply oxygenated blood to the working muscles for energy metabolism.

Muscular strength: The ability to exert a maximal force against a resistance.

Muscular endurance: The ability to sustain repeated contractions over a prolonged period of time.

Flexibility: The ability to use a muscle group throughout its entire range of motion.

is defined as the ability to use a muscle group throughout its entire range of motion. These are thought to be the three most important components of fitness. **Agility** refers to maneuverability and coordination of fine and gross motor movements. **Power** is defined as force multiplied by distance over time; **balance** is the ability to maintain equilibrium in motion. Agility, power, and balance supplement the first three components. Some or all of these components are used in every type of physical activity.

Although there are many kinds of exercise (TABLE 27.1)—from swimming, to weightlifting, to golf—exercise physiologists classify all physical activity into two categories: anaerobic or aerobic. These two types of physical exertion nicely parallel the two aspects of the fight-or-flight response as well as the emotions they elicit.

Anaerobic Activities. **Anaerobic exercise** is defined as physical motion that is intense in power and strength but short in duration (**FIG. 27.1**). Theoretically speaking, anaerobic activity is the type of movement or exercise used in the "fight" response. When an expression of anger comes to mind, it is associated with power and strength; that is, when someone becomes angry and attempts to defend self or territory, the corresponding action had better be forceful, quick, and decisive. Without these qualities, this half of the stress response proves ineffective for survival.

The word *anaerobic* means "without oxygen." The body has two anaerobic energy systems: the **adenosine-triphosphate-phosphocreatine (ATP-PC)** system,

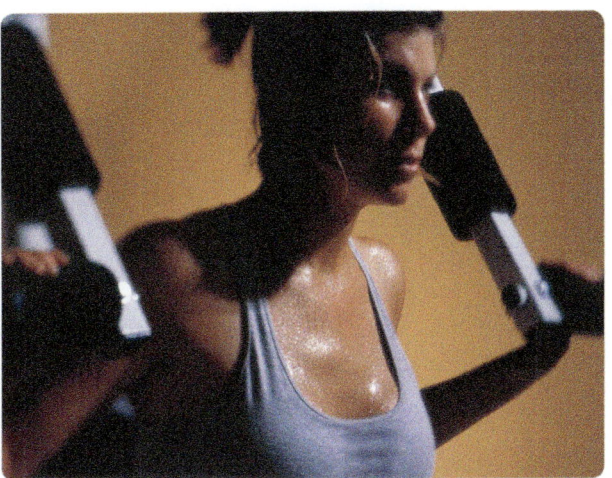

FIGURE 27.1   Anaerobic exercise is important for muscle strength and toning, but a good exercise program should include a balance of aerobic and anaerobic exercise activities to stimulate both the cardiovascular and musculoskeletal systems of the body.

which lasts only 1 to 10 seconds, and anaerobic glycolysis, or the **lactic acid** system, which continues after the ATP-PC system for approximately 5 to 6 minutes. At this point, either activity is suspended because of extreme fatigue or the aerobic energy system kicks in. Lactic acid has an incredibly fatiguing effect on muscle contraction. Because the full redistribution of blood takes 4 to 6 minutes, depending on the individual's physical condition, the initial oxygen supply is minimal, at best. This means that the muscles required to do the work must metabolize energy sources (carbohydrates) using oxygen already stored in muscle cell tissue. Thus, anaerobic exercise involves only short bursts of energy.

TABLE 27.1   Energy Balance

Sport	Calories Burned*
Swimming (freestyle)	249 kcal
Jogging	400 kcal
Golf	129 kcal
Racquetball	348 kcal
Aerobic dance	201 kcal
Cycling	460 kcal
Walking	280 kcal
Snowboarding	250 kcal
Inline skating	345 kcal

*Calories burned during 30 minutes by a person weighing approximately 140 pounds

---

Agility: Maneuverability and coordination of gross and fine motor movements.

Power: Force multiplied by distance over time.

Balance: The ability to maintain equilibrium in motion.

Anaerobic exercise: Physical work done in the absence of oxygen; activity that is powerful and quick but does not last more than a few minutes (e.g., weightlifting).

Adenosine-triphosphate-phosphocreatine: Chemical compound in muscles that produces energy (anaerobically) for muscle contraction.

Lactic acid: A byproduct of the breakdown of ATP that can also be used as a source of energy (anaerobic).

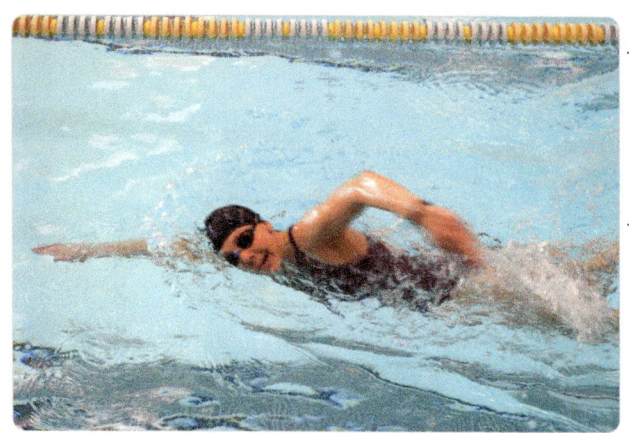

© Inspiration Unlimited. Used with permission.

FIGURE 27.2   Regular rhythmic aerobic exercise (e.g., swimming, jogging, walking) maintains an elevated (target) heart rate for a set duration and can act as a buffer to both physical and mental stress. In essence, aerobic exercise utilizes the stress hormones for their intended purpose rather than becoming a toxic hormonal cocktail in your body. The benefits of aerobic exercise are immeasurable.

Weightlifting is perhaps the most common example of this type of activity. Sprints and some calisthenics also fall into this category. Anaerobic exercise employs the muscular strength and power (force over distance) components of fitness.

Aerobic Activities.   Running, swimming, cycling, cross-country skiing, rhythmic dancing, and walking are examples of aerobic activities (**FIG. 27.2**). **Aerobic exercise**, or cardiovascular endurance activities, are described as rhythmic or continuous in nature. They involve an equal supply and demand of oxygen in the working muscles. Aerobic work involves moderate intensity for a prolonged duration. Intensity is typically measured by heart rate (beats/minute) or volume of oxygen consumed (liters/minute). Aerobic exercise is the "flight" of the fight-or-flight response, and its primary energy source consists of fats. Theoretically speaking, aerobic exercise, as the flight response, is stimulated by fear and anxiety. These emotions make a person want to run for the hills, literally.

The word *aerobic* was coined many years ago to describe biological reactions using oxygen for metabolism.

> **Aerobic exercise:** Rhythmic physical work (e.g., jogging) using a steady supply of oxygen delivered to working muscles for a continuous period of not less than 20 minutes.

The term was adapted by the fitness industry in the early 1970s by physician Kenneth Cooper, whose research on the effects of fitness training (primarily running) set the national standard for fitness programming. Also in the 1970s, with the inspiration of Jackie Sorenson, originator of aerobic dance, the term *aerobics* started being used to describe a new activity—rhythmic (aerobic) dancing. Aerobic dancing soon became a popular alternative to jogging for men and women alike. Since then, *aerobics* has become a household word, not only across America, but also around the world. Today, the big push in aerobic exercise is to get people to move (any way possible). One of the most popular means is to use a Fitbit or exercise app to see if one can pass the sedentary benchmark of 2,000 to 3,000 steps (1 mile) in the course of a day with the goal of reaching about 10,000 steps (5 miles) each day for optimal health.

Whereas anaerobic exercise stimulates muscular strength (hypertrophy of muscle fibers), aerobic exercise challenges the cardiovascular and pulmonary systems to increase endurance (and to some extent muscular endurance, depending on the nature of the activity). Volumes of research support the theory that cardiovascular endurance exercise helps reduce the risk of heart disease by modifying several risk factors. These include (1) reduction of blood pressure; (2) reduction of cholesterol, specifically low-density lipoproteins (LDLs); (3) significant decreases in percentage of body fat; and (4) decreased physical arousal resulting from stress. For this reason, aerobic exercise tends to receive more favorable attention than anaerobic exercise. If it is true that epinephrine, the hormone associated with fear, is released three times as much and lasts much longer than norepinephrine, then perhaps the best technique to deal with fear is aerobic exercise. Note that aerobic exercise provides a great release for all shades of anger as well as anxiety.

The landmark position statement by the American College of Sports Medicine (ACSM) states that for a fitness program to be effective it must integrate all primary components of fitness. Thus, a well-balanced exercise program should incorporate both anaerobic and aerobic exercise, as well as flexibility, in the training regimen.

Physiological Effects of Physical Exercise

Exercise, like money in the bank, can be considered an investment in health. Unfortunately, unlike money, it accrues very little, if any, tangible interest. It is a pay-as-you-go plan. The short-term effects (neural and hormonal) of a single bout of exercise last approximately 36 hours. There are also incredible long-term benefits, but one must continue training to keep them. Studies of inactive astronauts in space (Vailus 1992), deconditioned runners (Coyle et al. 1984), and bed-rest patients (Lenzt 1981) have shown that when a physical training program is interrupted or discontinued for longer than 2 weeks, approximately 10 percent of cardiovascular gains can be lost. In some cases, up to 40 percent is lost after a month's time, depending on the nature of the inactivity (**BOX 27.1**).

On the other hand, clinical studies by Davies and Knibbs (1971) and Shephard (1968) indicate that significant physiological changes begin to become evident between the sixth and eighth weeks of training. And the gains from cardiovascular exercise are quite impressive; they read like a list of who's who in physiological homeostasis. Cardiovascular efficiency can be equated with better health status. The following are some of its benefits:

- Decreased resting heart rate
- Decreased resting blood pressure
- Decreased muscle tension

- Better sleep quality
- Increased resistance to colds and illness
- Decreased cholesterol and triglyceride levels

The following are additional benefits from habitual cardiovascular exercise:

- Decreased body fat, improved body composition
- Increased efficiency of the heart
- Decreased bone demineralization
- Decreased rate of aging (several aspects)
- Increased tolerance of heat and cold through acclimatization

In general, cardiovascular endurance exercise acts as a catalyst to keep the body's physiological systems in balance. Through the multitude of mechanisms involved in energy metabolism, hormones, enzymes, and food substrates are used for their intended purpose. For example, when the body is in a state of balance, minerals like calcium are absorbed by bone tissue where they are needed. However, research has shown that when the body is in a state of imbalance, other organs and tissues, such as the lining of blood vessels or in some cases the mammary glands, begin to absorb these trace minerals and show signs of dysfunction. Just how this unique balance is maintained is still under scientific investigation.

Is cardiovascular exercise a good investment in your health? Apparently so! Research completed at Stanford University by James Fries (Digitale 2008) revealed that, indeed, regular participation in cardiovascular exercise (running) slows the aging process, in essence negating the effect of stress. Tracking over 500 runners, Fries observed that regular exercise led to not only a decrease in disease incidence, but also the ultimate wellness goal: a longer, healthier life span.

Regarding the relationship between physical exercise and the relaxation response, one important concept to remember is **parasympathetic rebound**. In anticipation of movement, seconds before exercise begins, epinephrine and norepinephrine are released by order of the central nervous system. The level of catecholamines

---

BOX 27.1   The Spark That Ignites the Brain

Like Paul Revere riding through the streets of Boston spreading a vital message, John Ratey, M.D., is also hitting the streets across America, spreading an equally important message: Aerobic exercise enhances brain cell activity. The message can be found in his book *Spark* (2008). He can be heard on television and radio talk shows.

National news headlines abound with increased cases of ADHD and Alzheimer's, poor national student achievement scores, and many other factors that hypothesize a decline of cognitive function across all age groups. Ratey explores the remarkable research compiled over the past several years to support the claims that aerobic exercise creates new brain cells, promotes neuroplasticity, increases academic scores, and sharpens mental acuity as well as generally slowing down the aging process. The message in a soundbite: Exercise is not only good for the body—it is great for the brain. The spark that ignites the brain's mental capabilities also helps neutralize the brain's response to stress. People who exercise simply deal better emotionally with stress than those who remain sedentary. This is a message worth paying attention to.

Parasympathetic rebound: The parasympathetic effect of relaxation (homeostasis) after physical exercise. Typically, the response is such that parameters such as heart rate and blood pressure dip below pre-exercise levels.

remains elevated throughout the duration of the activity. Upon completion of physical movement, the secretion of epinephrine and norepinephrine is inhibited by the parasympathetic nervous system, which initiates a calming response. In studies comparing stress-induced arousal (physical exercise) in athletically trained individuals versus sedentary ones, the trained subjects returned to their resting heart rate and serum catecholamine levels sooner than did their nonactive counterparts. In addition, the same values continued to decrease *below* prearousal levels in the conditioned individuals. These results indicate a very efficient calming mechanism by the parasympathetic nervous system.

Based on the landmark work of Bellet et al. (1969), Davies and Few (1974), Galbo et al. (1977), Sutton (1978), Tharp (1975), and Winder et al. (1973, 1982), the following conclusions have been drawn regarding the immediate, short-term, and long-term effects of cardiovascular exercise as a relaxation technique. First, it appears that a single bout of aerobic exercise "burns off" existing catecholamines and stress hormones by directing them toward their intended metabolic functions, rather than allowing them to linger in the body to undermine the integrity of vital organs and the immune system. This in itself can be considered a constructive intervention technique to counter daily stressors. Second, the training effect of aerobic exercise appears to prepare the body for future stressful episodes by decreasing the level of hormonal secretions when feelings of anger or fear manifest. In effect, exercise can be used as a preventive measure with regards to stress because it tends to minimize or neutralize physical arousal to nonphysical threats. Third, the long-term effect of exercise appears to be the prolonged efficient function of several organ systems, including the heart, lungs, blood vessels, kidneys, muscles, and skeletal tissue. Many researchers are of the opinion that although exercise training is not a panacea for the multitude of diseases and illnesses that plague humanity, nor is it a fountain of youth, its cumulative effects do appear to add to both the quality and quantity of life (**FIG. 27.3**).

It has long been thought that keeping in good shape tends to retard the aging process, but research conducted at the University of Illinois (Barlow 2003) confirms that, in terms of cognitive function, this supposition is indeed

> **FITT principle:** A principle of exercise that states that to benefit from physical training one must have the right intensity, frequency, and duration for each component of fitness challenged.

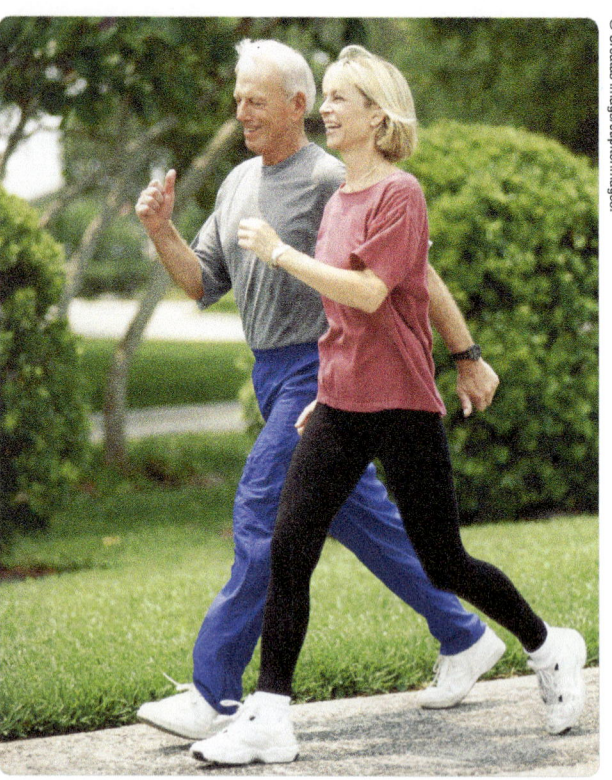

FIGURE 27.3   As we go through the aging process, exercise becomes increasingly more important, not only to maintain a healthy metabolic balance, but also to provide a needed challenge to our cardiovascular and neuromusculoskeletal systems. Exercise may not be the fountain of youth, but it's the closest thing we have to it.

true. Cardiovascular fitness improves cognition in three specific areas of the brain known to be affected by the aging process. Through the use of magnetic resonance imaging (MRI), significant anatomical differences have been observed in the gray and white matter of fit and sedentary individuals, with fit individuals showing less atrophy of these brain regions.

Theories of Athletic Conditioning

Numerous studies have been conducted to determine the minimal amount of exercise needed to maintain its benefits. Studies have investigated the intensity, frequency, and duration of aerobic exercise, specifically, because aerobic activity has the greatest effect on reducing the risks of heart disease. Every possible variable and permutation thereof has been examined, and a formula now accepted by the ACSM has set the standard for exercise programs for virtually all individuals. This is sometimes referred to as the **FITT principle**.

© Creatas Image/Jupiterimages.

FITT Principle. As stated in the ACSM guidelines, four major factors make up what is commonly called the FITT principle: **frequency, intensity, time (duration)**, and **type of exercise**. Let's take a closer look:

- *Frequency*: The number of exercise sessions per week. The minimum number of exercise sessions needed to see physiological benefits is three.

- *Intensity*: The challenge (stress) placed on a specific physiological system involved in an activity. In the case of the cardiovascular system, intensity is measured in terms of heart rate (the number of beats per minute), and it varies with age (**FIG. 27.4**). In a cardiovascular fitness program, the range is between 65 and 85 percent of maximal intensity, with an average intensity of 75 percent for healthy individuals. This is often called the **target heart rate**, or target zone.

- *Time (duration)*: The length of time of one exercise session. An exercise session should be at least 20 to 30 minutes. Less than 20 minutes does not guarantee any benefits.

- *Type of exercise*: The type of activity chosen to challenge a particular physiological system. Walking, running, and swimming, for example, are types of aerobic exercises that adequately challenge the cardiovascular system. Weight training, on the other hand, taxes the anaerobic energy system, despite claims to the contrary by several manufacturers of weight-training equipment.

Only an Olympic-trained athlete could achieve cardiovascular benefits from a circuit weight-training program. Likewise, running will tone and define muscles, but muscle hypertrophy is not of any benefit to cardiovascular endurance, so running is not considered superior to other forms of aerobic work.

Phases of a Workout. Just as there is a formula for maximizing the cardiovascular benefits of exercise, there is also a formula for ensuring safe workouts. The **phases of a workout** are a proper warm-up, a stimulus or conditioning period, and a cooldown:

- *Warm-up*: The **warm-up** is the preparation for exercise. It usually lasts approximately 5 to 10 minutes, during which blood shifts from the gastrointestinal tract to the large muscle groups. Muscles are like sponges. When they are dry, they are difficult to stretch, which is why it is best to stretch at the end of the warm-up.

- *Stimulus*: The **stimulus phase** is the "meat" of the workout, during which physical exertion (intensity) is used to maintain a challenge to the various physiological systems. The stimulus phase should be a minimum of 20 minutes, regardless of which energy system (aerobic or anaerobic) is used (**FIG. 27.5**).

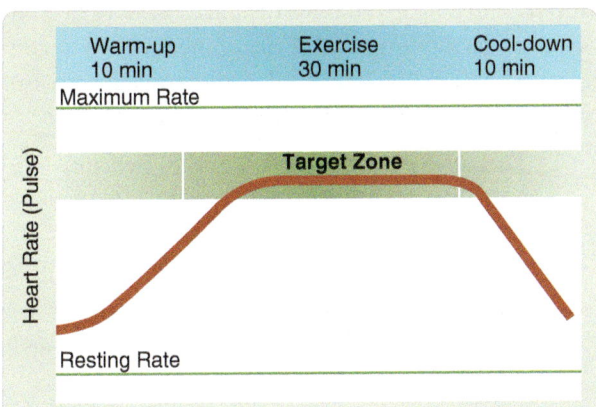

FIGURE 27.4 The target heart rate reflects the intensity of work needed to challenge the heart muscle for a more efficient cardiovascular system. The target heart rate should be maintained for the duration of the workout.

Frequency: The number of exercise sessions per week; the ideal number is three.

Intensity: The physical challenge (stress) placed on a specific physiological system for exercise.

Time (duration): The number of minutes of exercise in one session; the ideal number is 30 minutes in the target zone, not including a warm-up or cooldown.

Type of exercise: The type of activity one chooses to engage in to work one or more physiological systems (e.g., walking, jogging, cycling).

Target heart rate: The recommended heart rate or target zone that reflects the intensity of cardiovascular activity.

Phases of a workout: Warm-up, stimulus phase, and cooldown.

Warm-up: The first phase of a workout involving light exercise and stretching, increasing circulation to the large muscles.

Stimulus phase: The "meat" of the workout, during which one targets the specified intensity toward the heart, lungs, and muscles (e.g., heart rate, sets, reps for weight lifting).

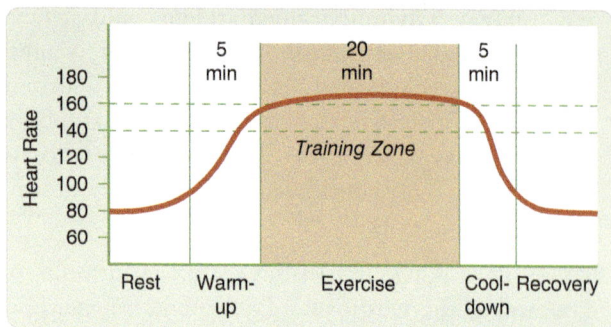

FIGURE 27.5 One's target heart rate should remain elevated during the stimulus phase. The more efficient the cardiovascular system, the sooner the heart rate will return to its resting level during cooldown.

- *Cooldown*: The **cooldown** allows for the body to gradually shift from a stressed state to a relaxation state, during which the blood is directed from the muscles to the body's core, rather than pooling in the extremities. A cooldown begins with decreased intensity of exercise followed by stretching for a total of 5 to 10 minutes.

Fitness Shortcuts to Health?

Let's face it, exercise is work! By and large, people would rather avoid exercise because they are too tired, busy, or lazy. According to recent research, only 20 percent of Americans get the recommended amount of exercise per week. Nearly one-third of Americans over the age of 6 years are completely sedentary (Oaklander 2016). The gold standard for exercise was proven decades ago by Ken Cooper, who popularized the term *aerobics*. That term has now been replaced by the word *cardio*, but the formula hasn't really changed. Enter Martin Gibala, an exercise physiologist from McMaster University who has challenged the gold standard of the FITT principle with his concept of micro workouts called high-intensity interval training (HIIT). Created for people who lack the time, HIIT is said to offer the same benefits as an hour-long Zumba class. Gibala admits that this program is not for everyone (well-trained athletes are too fit to reap any benefits), and other experts cite the dangers of muscle injuries associated with short high-intensity workouts. Is there a shortcut to health? Time will tell. In the meantime, the rest of us mere mortals should consider that there is no shortcut.

> **Cooldown:** A designated time right after the stimulus phase to decrease circulation to the body's periphery and return to a resting state.

Psychological Effects of Physical Exercise

When the fitness movement mushroomed in the late 1970s, the complexity of the many benefits reported caught some in the field of clinical medicine off guard. At the time, the most frequently prescribed drug in the country was the tranquilizer Valium. The Rolling Stones even wrote a hit song, "Mother's Little Helper," satirizing its widespread use.

But as people initiated running programs, they began to talk less and less about muscle soreness, weather conditions, and rude drivers; these concerns seemed to have relatively little importance. Instead, thoughts began to turn inward, and running began to take on a Zen-like quality. Moreover, it became a private time to sort out problems, resolve issues, and reflect about life in general, relationships, and the purpose of life. Running became a time for self-reflection and meditation. Many people stopped taking prescribed sedatives and tranquilizers, and some people even stopped going to their therapists. In time, members of the medical community also took up running. And some psychologists even changed counseling styles, taking their patients off the office couch and onto the sidewalk or high school track.

As an investigative eye was kept on this national activity, reports soon filtered in that running could have an addictive quality. Specifically, it was learned that when running routines were interrupted for more than a few days, some individuals showed signs of withdrawal similar to those observed with chemical addictions. For his book *Positive Addiction* (1976), William Glasser interviewed more than 700 long-distance runners to gain a better understanding of this phenomenon. His analysis revealed six important criteria for a physical activity to take on this addictive nature:

1. The activity must be done for at least an hour per day.

2. The activity must be done on a regular basis.

3. The activity must have a base of 6 months of training.

4. The activity must be well liked by the person doing it.

5. The activity must be noncompetitive.

6. The activity must be done alone or perhaps with one other person.

Just when Glasser was conducting his research, other scientists were investigating the same concept from a physiological approach. In the early 1980s, a new human neuropeptide was discovered, and it showed remarkable morphine-like qualities. Beta-endorphin was soon hailed as the body's own natural opiate. In minute quantities, it significantly reduced sensations of pain and seemed to promote feelings of euphoria and exhilaration. And, like various other chemical substances, beta-endorphin had an addictive quality; many people showed signs of depression after days of inactivity. What's more, this neuropeptide was released by other locations as well as the brain during physical activity, most notably running. Not everyone who ran, however, experienced this effect, perhaps because of the training effect. Today, the research into the "runner's high" not only focuses on endorphins, but also on newly discovered substances called endocannabinoids, neurotransmitters that—unlike endorphins—can pass through the blood–brain barrier to increase pleasure and decrease pain (Ratey 2008).

Although, to date, no songs have been written about **runner's high**, this phenomenon is now commonly accepted as the greatest psychological effect of running. But running is not the only physical activity during which beta-endorphin is released. Many other types of cardiovascular endurance exercises, such as swimming and walking, potentially produce the same effect. What is necessary, regardless of the activity, is that the exercise be egoless, or noncompetitive.

In 2019, researchers Schuch and Stubbs performed a meta-analysis reviewing all studies done on exercise and depression over a 20-year period. Their findings, cited in *Current Sports Medicine Reports*, revealed that, by looking at the experiences of more than 200,000 people, exercise reduced the chance of developing depression by 17 to 41 percent. Simply stated, physical exercise helps prevent depression. In their conclusions they note that although exercise may help, it is not a panacea for everyone.

Although the specific mechanisms of how exercise reduces the risk of depression are not clear, depression is known to be associated with inflammation, and exercise decreases inflammation. Regular exercise is also known to increase levels of a brain chemical, BDNF, that is associated with brain growth. Low levels of BDNF are linked to depression (Stulberg 2019).

Speculation now has it that activities with rhythmic, repetitive motion, such as swimming, running, walking, or cycling, offer a meditative form of conscious awareness. It has been suggested that such rhythmic activities may shift hemispheric dominance from the left to the right brain. Several long-distance runners interviewed by Fixx (1977) and Glasser (1976) stated that running heightened mental receptivity, resulting in greater imagination and creativity to apply to problem solving. Based on this discovery and other positive effects, psychologists took a new interest in cardiovascular exercise as a coping technique to reduce the psychological fallout from stress (**BOX 27.2**). Among the thousands of investigators

> **Runner's high:** The euphoric feeling generated from beta-endorphins released from cardiovascular exercise.

BOX 27.2   Insomnia and Physical Exercise

One of the benefits of exercise that has been touted by exercise physiologists for years is the fact that regular rhythmical (cardiovascular) exercise promotes quality sleep and decreases symptoms of insomnia. The very nature of physical exercise increases one's metabolic activity, thus increasing one's core body temperature. As the body returns to homeostasis after a vigorous workout, core body temperature drops. During sleep, core body temperature is at its lowest point as a result of decreased metabolic activity. Research shows that the drop in core body temperature that occurs when bedtime is 4 to 6 hours after a vigorous workout promotes drowsiness and deeper (delta waves) sleep than in nonactive individuals. For this reason, it is suggested *not* to engage in strenuous physical activity shortly before bedtime. According to *Power Sleep* (2001) author James Maas, the best time to schedule a workout is around the noon hour or late afternoon, with morning exercise having the least effect on sleep quality. The best type of exercise to ensure a good night's sleep is cardiovascular in nature, including vigorous walking, jogging, swimming, or biking that elevates the heart rate to one's specific target zone for the desired duration. All types of rhythmic exercise utilize the cocktail of stress hormones for their intended purposes and help the body metabolize what's not used in this process as waste products for elimination.

Stress with a Human Face

There were basically two types of summer jobs where I come from: waiting tables or lifeguarding. I grew up doing the latter to finance my college education, and I also taught swimming lessons and coached several swim teams over the years. But when I chose a career in academia, lifeguarding and swim lessons became a distant memory—or so I thought. One day on campus, I was introduced to a nationally known figure, and soon found myself agreeing to give swim lessons once again.

At first Dan (not his real name) said his primary goal of getting in shape was to lose weight. Because of a back injury, running and biking were out of the question, so he chose swimming. But after he had progressed from blowing bubbles to swimming a quarter-mile, he confided that getting in shape was really secondary to clearing his mind and coping with stress. He needed not just physical conditioning, but some time alone to think and get his head straight, sort out problems, and access his intuition and creativity on a daily basis. But his fast-paced job in the nation's capital wasn't doing him any good, nor were his coronary risk factors (mainly hypertension). He knew there was only one solution: to take out his aggressions and anxieties in the pool.

Dan is up to a mile a day now, and his physical shape is superseded only by the smile on his face as he gets out of the water and heads for the showers. The risk factors are minimized, and he feels like a new man every day. On numerous occasions he has said that I literally saved his life. I know better than that. How does the expression go? You can lead a horse to water, but ....

to delve into the relationship between exercise and emotional health were Berger (1982, 1983), Berger and Motl (2001), Dishman (1981), Folkins and Sime (1981), Ismail and Young (1977), Morgan (1982), Morgan et al. (1980, 1987), and Gosselin and Taylor (1999). The conclusion drawn from all this research is that athletic training or exercise is viable as both a relaxation technique and a coping technique to deal with stress. The following are the reported psychological benefits of habitual exercise (particularly from jogging):

- Improved self-esteem
- Improved sense of self-reliance and self-efficacy
- Improved mental alertness, perception, and information processing
- Increased perceptions of acceptance by others
- Decreased feelings of depression and anxiety
- Decreased overall sense of stress and tension

Physical Exercise and Chronic Pain

Ten years ago, if you said the word "Pilates," you might have heard someone say, "gesundheit." Today, most people know that Pilates is a form of muscle strength and flexibility exercises (**FIG. 27.6**). What many people don't know is that it is one of the best forms of exercise to help relieve chronic pain associated with the lower back and

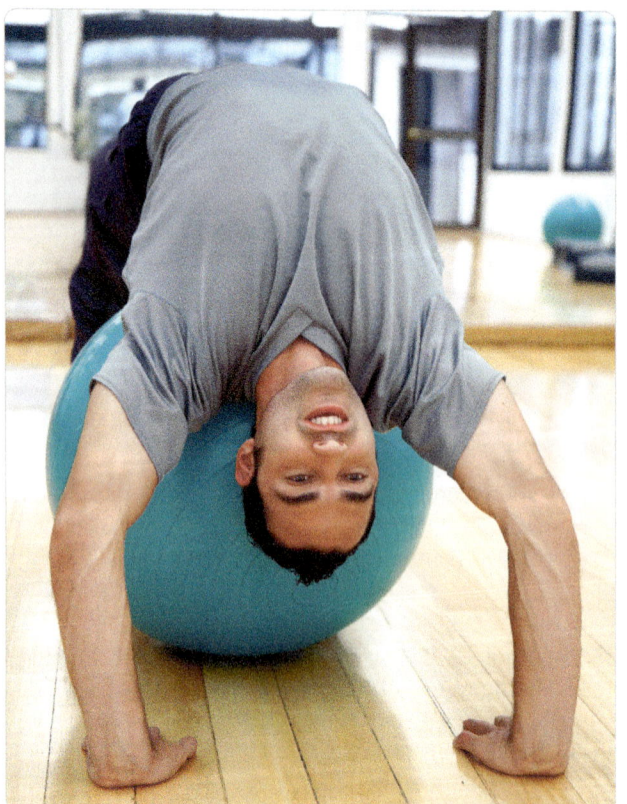

FIGURE 27.6 Pilates exercises have been proven to be quite effective for reducing chronic pain associated with weak muscles and poor posture.

spine area (Stanmore 2002; Ungaro 2002). Developed as a series of exercises to strengthen the core muscles of the body's frame by Joseph Pilates several decades ago, Pilates was originally used by dancers and athletes for both prevention and rehabilitation of athletic injuries. Today, like hatha yoga, Pilates classes are commonly taught at fitness clubs and Pilates centers around the country.

Ironically, many episodes of chronic pain result from physical exercise—specifically, the overuse syndrome (too much, too often), which can lead to joint pain in the area of use. Common sense dictates that acute and chronic joint and muscle pain necessitates taking a break from the exercise that causes the pain. For this reason, it is good to have a complementary exercise or sport, such as swimming or walking, to fall back on if and when your primary mode of fitness is put on hiatus.

Steps to Initiate a Fitness Training Program

Although physical exercise is now praised as the wonder technique for stress reduction, it also poses a threat to physical well-being if not done correctly. The typical way many people approach something can be summarized in four words: too much, too soon (**FIG. 27.7**). Individuals get caught up in the whirlwind of excitement, and as a result often go overboard, thinking that if some is good, more is better. The result is burnout. When too-much/too-soon behavior is applied to physical exercise, it can result in injury, particularly muscle and tendon damage.

Let there be no doubt: Exercise is demanding work. And after cranking out 8 to 10 hours at the office, shop, or other place of business, the last thing a person wants is to go out and do more work. Motivation can be rather elusive at the end of the day. Because the effects of exercise don't occur overnight, people can become quite disenchanted with the concepts of muscle fatigue and sweat. In fact, fitness club owners will tell you that motivation peaks about 3 to 7 days after the start of a fitness program and then rapidly declines. Without internal as well as external reinforcement, most exercise programs peter out before real physiological changes occur.

Exercise specialists and health educators have begun to incorporate goal setting into the design and prescription of exercise programming as a means to maintain motivation during this crucial period. Scientific research has unequivocally proven that physical exercise is necessary for optimal health. It should become a habit in everyone's lifestyle. The following are some suggestions regarding cardiovascular (aerobic) fitness to help guide you through the transition period:

1. *Start cautiously and progress moderately with your program.* The ACSM suggests that every person, particularly those over the age of 35, get a physical examination for medical clearance prior to starting a fitness program. As a part of the physical evaluation, you should be assessed for your fitness capacity and given an exercise prescription. The prescription includes a target heart rate; a mode of exercise; a selected intensity, frequency, and duration; as well as a review of the components of a workout and the design of health and fitness goals. Sometimes it helps to see physical exercise as a process, not an outcome. People who experience a natural high from exercise are in a sense detached from the physical sensations and immediate rewards (e.g., losing weight). One rule of thumb to go by when working out is this: If you can't hold a conversation while exercising, you are pushing too hard. The no pain–no gain approach was discredited a long time ago.

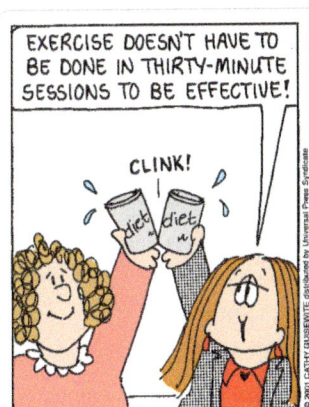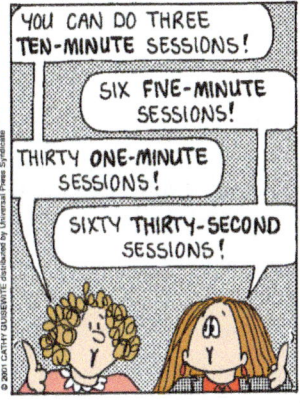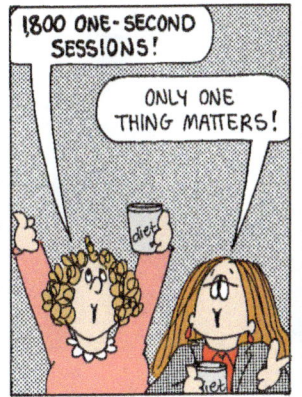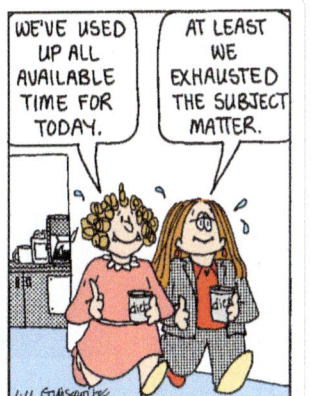

FIGURE 27.7   There is no magic formula for exercise, but you have got to start somewhere.

2. *Pick an activity you really enjoy.* Not everyone is a jogger. If you have tried jogging and found it too difficult or displeasing, there are plenty of other aerobic activities to choose from. Perhaps the most underrated exercise is walking. Walking provides the same benefits as running if an adequate heart rate is maintained. Likewise, swimming is one of the best choices because it not only improves cardiovascular endurance, muscular endurance, and flexibility, but it also is the least likely to result in overuse injuries to muscle tissue and joints. Sometimes alternating activities is a great way to avoid burnout or staleness from the same sport (**FIG. 27.8**). Most important, pick an activity that doesn't involve the ego and is noncompetitive. Many people find that when the ego gets involved, the activity promotes, rather than reduces, feelings of stress.

3. *Select a time of day to exercise.* Make a commitment to allocate a special time each day just for this purpose, and make this time yours and yours alone, with no other responsibilities and commitments to take this time away from you. Mornings before work or school are often the easiest times to schedule exercise, and the immediate physiological effects certainly help meet the challenges of the day. Sometimes early morning workouts mean sacrificing badly needed sleep; in this case, afternoon

> **Chondromalacia:** Chronic knee pain, typically from excessive running and improper foot placement.

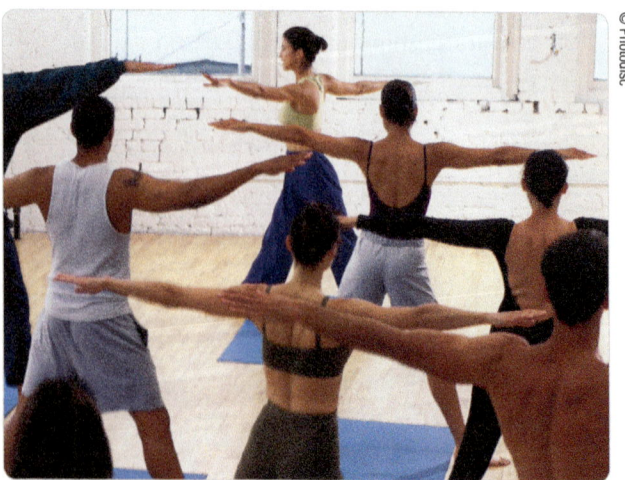

FIGURE 27.8   Noncompetitive exercising with a group of people serves as a great motivation factor to continue the activity.

or evening is a good option. After a long and perhaps busy day, exercise is a great way to unwind and literally release pent-up energy. If neither of these options is workable, the lunch hour (the new executive recess) is always an alternative. And to be realistic, if you are like many people with busy schedules and no two days alike, the time for exercise may have to vary from day to day. Remember, you only need three days a week, half an hour each day to achieve and maintain the benefits of exercise. That is a total of one and a half hours per week.

4. *Exercise using the right clothes and equipment.* Perhaps the most important piece of equipment is a good pair of athletic shoes. The cost may be rather high, but quality shoes serve as a good insurance policy against injuries to the lower back, shins, ankles, feet, and most notably, knees. The knees are the weakest joint in the body. Poor shoes can decrease the stability of the tendons and ligaments supporting the knee, resulting in chronic knee pain known as **chondromalacia**. Also, cardiovascular exercise tends to significantly increase core body temperature, so clothing should be layered so that it can be "peeled off" if you get overheated in the cool months.

5. *Initiate a support group.* Although exercise is not always considered miserable, at times it does love company. There may be times when you would like nothing better than to exercise alone, but a companion certainly serves as a motivator for those days when the thought of exercising is not appealing.

6. *Set personal fitness goals for yourself.* Do you want to lose weight? Would you like to decrease your cholesterol levels? Would you like to have a "washboard" stomach? Do you want to reduce your resting blood pressure? Would you like to run a 10K road race? These are some commonly heard goals. Progression toward and accomplishment of health and fitness goals can be wonderful means of motivation. It is easy to see the progress you have made when you keep track of it. The most popular method for doing so is jotting a short note on a calendar. The companion to goal-setting is reward: When you accomplish a goal, treat yourself to something special.

7. *Care and prevention of injuries.* The best way to treat an injury is to prevent it, but if you encounter pain along the way, treat the injury immediately. The most common injuries occur to joints, where

tendons begin to pull away from bone. If you feel pain in a joint, you should stop the activity and put ice on the joint as soon as possible. Some injuries, if caught early, may not need immediate medical attention. If pain persists after a day or two, however, see a physician. Not long ago, physicians knew very little about sports medicine, but today it is easier to find qualified care in this area. Please don't take an injury lightly.

These are some of the basic guidelines to follow when initiating a personal fitness program. But above all, use common sense. If you would like assistance in developing your personal fitness program, health clubs, community recreation centers, and YMCAs and YWCAs have qualified personnel to help you design a safe, quality program. Good luck and have fun!

Best Application of Physical Exercise and Activity

To get the most benefits from physical exercise, there must be the right intensity, frequency, and duration as well as the best mode of exercise for the individual involved. Physical activity of any type is best used as a postponed response to stress, unless the situation is right to put on your exercise clothes and run out the door. Exercise—both aerobic and anaerobic—provides a wonderful catharsis of emotional frustrations. This includes both anger and anxiety. It is best to schedule a time to work out, and stick to it. Because injury or burnout can occur with a once-favorite activity, it is a good idea to have a backup sport.

How can you best find the means to balance your caloric intake and expenditure? Like most everything else in this book, it comes down to your attitude. Experts in the field of exercise physiology will tell you any activity is ideal, whether it's walking up stairs a few flights rather than taking the elevator, parking farther away from the entrance to the nearest store, or taking a Pilates class. Finding the balance between keeping active and sitting still transfers to the balance between a calm mind and a healthy body. Ultimately, the best application of physical exercise is to do some type of activity every day to flush the stress hormones out of your body (**BOX 27.3**).

BOX 27.3   Cortisol and Weight Gain

Is there a connection between chronic stress and obesity? Perhaps! There is speculation that cortisol, a hormone released from the adrenal gland during the stress response, may be related to the steady accumulation of body fat in one's lifetime. Given the amount of chronic stressors each American has today, and the incredible rate of obesity, there may indeed be a connection. Cortisol is responsible for a number of metabolic activities for fight or flight, including ensuring the release of glucose and free fatty acids into the blood for short- and long-term energy. If a person chooses not to fight or flee (anaerobic or aerobic exercise), watching hours of television instead, then the body may redistribute these energy nutrients as adipose tissue (fat). Additional speculation suggests that cortisol may be a principal hormone to regulate appetite under stress, to ensure that there is an adequate supply of both short- and long-term energy. It is well known that stress (acute and chronic) raises blood glucose levels in people with type 2 diabetes, hence making an exercise program all the more important for this target population.

Human physiology is much more complex than a single cause-and-effect scenario when it comes to cortisol, weight gain, and obesity, experts say. The combined effect of insulin and cortisol may be the culprit. Is cortisol the primary hormone responsible for weight gain? The jury is still out on this (Chang 2006); however, given the dynamics of stress and the mind-body-spirit connection, one cannot understate its importance.

A training program that includes regular cardiovascular exercise helps to ensure that the hormones synthesized and released as a result of chronic stress are used for their intended purposes and then flushed out of the system with other metabolic waste products. Exercise also burns calories, making this a desired health package for everyone. It's no secret that the marketplace is becoming flooded with drugs and herbal products to minimize or block the effect of cortisol on appetite and weight gain. However, drugs and supplements can have several side effects, throwing the body's biochemistry out of balance. When performed correctly, the short- and long-term effects of exercise restore balance to mind, body, and spirit with no harmful side effects—and it's free.

Nutrition and Stress

Like millions of Americans, no doubt you take great pleasure in sitting down to a good meal. Food not only provides necessary nutrients to our body, but also provides emotional pleasure to the mind, particularly when these morsels taste really good. Experts have recognized for eons that food serves as a pacifier to calm nerves; as such, eating not only is a means for physical survival, but also is considered a popular relaxation technique (hence the expression "comfort food"). Yet for many people, eating as a coping technique is often abused. We eat to celebrate, we eat to relax, we eat out of frustration and boredom, and we eat to satisfy our hunger. Food and mood go together like peanut butter and jelly.

It is impossible to talk about proper nutrition without addressing the issue of stress. The two are inextricably linked. For that matter, it is impossible to talk about proper nutrition and ignore the issue of politics of special-interest groups and the power of the Food and Drug Administration (FDA) that work diligently to control the dissemination of information, leading to much inconsistent factual reporting, and thus to even more stress for the consumer who tries to make sense of it all. One day there is a study reporting a particular finding, and the next day another study refutes the findings of the first study. It's no exaggeration to say that many people are confused and frustrated about the controversies in the field of nutrition—not to mention the ever-increasing number of popular diets, which in itself can prove stressful, especially in our weight-conscious culture. This section attempts to clarify some of the concepts regarding sound nutritional habits, how stress affects diet, and how diet affects stress and mood. In addition, this section contains information on an Eastern approach to eating called "spiritual nutrition."

It is fair to say that the quantities of food in America are the envy of the world, yet the quality of our food choices is abysmal: High sugar, high fat, bleached flour, genetically modified organisms (GMOs), hormones, antibiotics, and untold amounts of petrochemicals introduced by means of fertilizers, herbicides, fungicides, and pesticides on and in our foods make healing more challenging today and give a whole new meaning to saying grace before a meal. Toxins (bioecological stressors) in our foods become stored in the body (now known as *bioaccumulation*) and compromise the immune system, leading to a plethora of health-related problems. When emotional stress is added to the equation, all of these health-related problems are magnified, with dire consequences. Specifically, stress compromises the ability to digest, absorb, metabolize, and eliminate nutrients (e.g., carbohydrates, fats, proteins, vitamins, minerals, and water) because the body's wisdom overrides these processes during fight or flight. By now, you should know the basics of nutrition (or can find this information easily elsewhere), but let's take a closer look at the relationship between nutrition and stress.

If we examine the dynamics of food, stress, and health, we see a confluence of factors that directly affect the immune system. In simplest terms, the relationship among nutrition, stress, and the immune system might best be illustrated through the use of four dominos (**FIG. 27.9**).

- *Domino 1*: Stress tends to deplete nutrients in the body. Water-soluble vitamins and several essential minerals are used for energy production in preparation for fight or flight, even if you sit still in front of a computer screen all day.

- *Domino 2*: The stressful American lifestyle does not promote or reinforce good eating habits. Consequently, the nutrients depleted under chronic stress are not restored. (Comfort foods, junk foods, fast foods, and processed foods are high in calories and low in nutrients [empty calories]. This is often cited as a leading cause of obesity.) The body will do all it can to compensate for the lack of nutrients, but eventually various aspects of health are compromised.

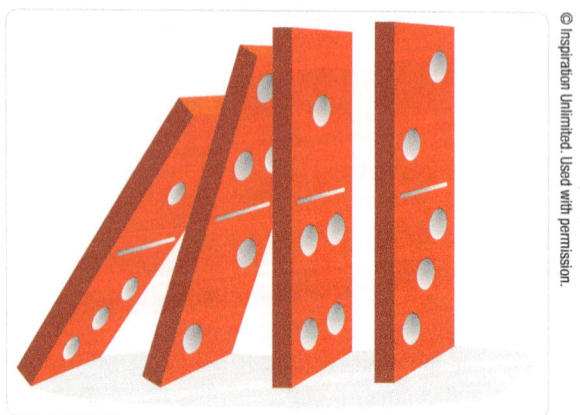

FIGURE 27.9 Dominos illustrate the delicate balance of stress and nutrition. When the first domino falls, it is typically not long before the others also tumble, compromising one's health.

■ *Domino 3*: Some food substances are known to increase sympathetic drive or other physiological responses that keep the stress response elevated. These include caffeine, processed sugar, processed flour, and salt. Some people use alcohol to relax, yet beyond moderation, alcohol presents many problems itself, including tilting this domino to fall on the next one.

■ *Domino 4*: Many foods that are processed contribute to a cumulative effect of toxins. For example, residues of synthetic or petroleum-based fertilizers, herbicides, pesticides, and even mold found in many foods hinder the immune system from doing its job effectively. When this domino falls, one's health is greatly compromised (e.g., cancer, diabetes, colds, flus, etc.).

The fall of each domino increases the chance of health-related problems as a result of the confluence of stress-prone eating habits. This section highlights important aspects of these factors so that you can make choices about what you put in your mouth to nourish mind, body, and spirit.

Diet for a Stressed Planet

Because of the global economy and trade among nations, the choices of foods available today are unparalleled. At a grocery store it is not uncommon to see strawberries, grapes, and a whole host of vegetables available year-round, not to mention a selection of meats, fish, and other foods imported from states and countries thousands of miles away. Quantities of food are abundant as well, but this does not necessarily mean the quality of food is superior to that of our grandparents. Across the planet, there is an alarming concern that the soil used to grow crops is severely depleted of its nutrients, resulting in a loss of nutrient density in foods and people experiencing the effects of malnourishment, even though the caloric intake is much greater than in the days of our grandparents.

The biggest nutrition problem in the United States is overconsumption, yet overconsumption does not necessarily mean an overabundance of the various nutrients that the body requires for optimal functioning (Taubes 2007; Wansink 2006). Foods high in fat and simple sugars (i.e., empty calories) tend to rob the body of essential nutrients. Consequently, the body is operating under a nutritional deficiency, not nutritional abundance. Under these conditions, the body is stressed to maintain its integrity for metabolic functioning. Over time, one

or more physiological systems may go into a state of dysfunction. In addition, it is no secret that when people are stressed, their eating habits are greatly compromised, perpetuating an already compromised condition. Stated simply, a person under stress is extremely vulnerable to nutritional deficiency (**BOX 27.4**).

Under the most optimal conditions, stress can cause problems with the body's ability to digest and absorb nutrients, thus impeding the availability of the essential nutrients, particularly vitamins and minerals. As you will see, the physiological system most seriously affected by a poor nutritional state is the immune system. Following is a description of how stress affects our absorption of essential nutrients and, ultimately, our susceptibility to a wide range of illnesses (**BOX 27.5**).

Stress and Mineral Depletion. Research conducted by the U.S. Department of Agriculture (Sizer and Whitney 2007) has revealed that, despite what appeared to be an adequate dietary intake, intake of several minerals has decreased by as much as 33 percent in the past 20 years across people of all ages. A depletion of minerals decreases the integrity of the immune system, making one more susceptible to disease and illness. The following minerals are in deficit under conditions of chronic stress: magnesium, chromium, copper, iron, and zinc.

Stress and Vitamin Depletion. Four vitamins are known to be greatly affected by chronic stress: the antioxidant vitamins A, C, and E and vitamin B complex.

The Antioxidants. The body encounters many environmental stressors in the course of a day, including particles known as free radicals. **Free radicals** are highly reactive oxygen particles most commonly found in air pollution, tobacco smoke, radiation, herbicides, and rancid fatty foods. Free radicals are also produced in the body under normal metabolic functioning. Left uncontrolled, free radicals will destroy various constituents of cells they come in contact with, including:

■ *The cell membrane*: Free radicals change the permeability of the cell membrane, disturbing the transportation of essential nutrients into the cell as well as byproducts out of the cell.

Free radicals: Highly reactive oxygen molecules with an aberrant electron that can cause damage to cell membranes and DNA.

BOX 27.4   Eat for a Healthy Immune System

An old proverb states, "Let food be your medicine, and let medicine be your food." Unfortunately, rather than eating food as medicine, the vast majority of people today eat food as poison. Like toxins dumped into a river, the human body can take only so much before signs of disease and illness become manifest. The following is a list of suggestions to tip the scale back into balance and to promote a sense of health and well-being by engaging in a combination of behaviors that (1) enhances the natural abilities of the immune system and (2) decreases the amount of toxins that the immune system must assist in eliminating.

1. Consume a good supply of antioxidants (beta-carotene, vitamins C and E, and selenium). These fight the damage of free radicals, which destroy cell membranes, DNA, RNA, and mitochondria. Antioxidants can be found in fresh fruits, vegetables, and fresh herbs.

2. Consume a good supply of fiber (30 to 40 grams/day with organic vegetables). Fiber helps clean the colon of toxic materials that might otherwise be absorbed into the bloodstream. Fiber is found in fresh fruits, vegetables, and some grains.

3. Drink plenty of fresh, clean (filtered) water. (A good goal is nearly clear urine.) Being properly hydrated is essential for the elimination of toxins and metabolic byproducts.

4. Decrease consumption of pesticides, fungicides, herbicides, and fertilizers found on and in produce, many of which are toxic or carcinogenic. (Eat organics whenever possible.)

5. Consume an adequate supply of complete proteins to ensure intake of essential amino acids. (White blood cells are made up of amino acids from protein sources.)

6. Decrease or eliminate the consumption of processed foods (e.g., junk food, fast food). Think "outside the box" to avoid overconsumption of additives and preservatives that are used merely to extend the shelf life of a product.

7. Decrease consumption of antibiotics and hormones (e.g., found in dairy, beef, and chicken products). These can have a negative effect on your body's physiology, including the elimination of the intestinal flora *Lactobacillus acidophilus*, leading to *Candida* infection.

8. Consume a good supply (and balance) of omega-3 fatty acids (cold-water fish and flaxseed oil) and omega-6 fatty acids (vegetable oils).

9. Decrease intake of saturated (solid) fats (meat and dairy products).

10. Eat a variety of food colors (fruits and vegetables with bioflavonoids).

11. Consume a good balance of foods with proper pH. (Many processed and pasteurized foods are acidic, tipping the scales by creating a hospitable breeding ground for diseases such as cancer.)

12. Decrease intake of total percentage of fats. (High fat intake compromises the integrity of the lymphatic system, the highway taken by the immune system's cells.)

13. Replenish nutrients consumed by the stress response (e.g., B-complex vitamins, minerals).

14. Decrease consumption of simple sugars, including high-fructose corn syrup. (This not only takes a load off of the pancreas, but also is good for the immune system because cancerous tumors appear to like sugars.)

15. Decrease or avoid excitotoxins (aspartame, Nutrasweet, and MSG), which are believed to inhibit brain function.

16. Moderate your consumption of alcohol. (High alcohol intake compromises liver and immune system function.)

17. Prepare food in the best way possible (e.g., steam veggies, no microwave ovens).

18. Eat organic produce and free-range meats whenever possible.

19. Avoid GMOs (Frankenfoods), which are known to promote allergy problems.

20. Use herbal therapies to boost the immune system (e.g., astragalus, echinacea, shiitake mushrooms, milk thistle).

Tip: Eat at least one meal a day for your immune system.

It's not uncommon to see students burning the midnight oil with a cup of coffee or caffeinated soda in hand. Perhaps more than any other foodstuff, caffeine intake greatly affects one's physiology—making it the number one thing to avoid if you are plagued by insomnia. Research reveals that caffeine intake decreases the amount of REM sleep, which has been noted as the most essential phase of each 2-hour sleep cycle.

Why is drinking a glass of milk thought to send you trundling off to la-la land? The answer resides in the amino acid found in milk, called tryptophan. Tryptophan (also found in high concentrations in turkey meat) is known to induce sleep. For this reason, it is often used as a bedtime snack. With the popularity of natural remedies, the following herbs are renowned for their ability to decrease neural firing, thus relaxing the body in preparation for a good night's sleep: valerian, ginseng, passion flower, and kava kava (please take as directed). Finally, it should be noted that most processed foods contain a plethora of chemicals that undoubtedly have some impact on brain chemistry, including aspartame and MSG, and these should be avoided.

- *The mitochondria*: Free radicals destroy the constituents of the mitochondria (where cell respiration occurs) and compromise the energy capabilities of the cell.

- *DNA*: Free radicals attach to the DNA structure and inhibit the genetic code process that regulates cell reproduction and function.

- *RNA*: Free radicals distort the ability of the RNA to transmit messages throughout the central nervous system.

Under normal, healthy conditions, free radicals are removed (metabolized by beta-carotene and vitamins C and E). Under bouts of chronic stress, these vitamins are depleted or, in many cases, not even absorbed into the body so that free radicals are not destroyed. It has been noted that free radicals are often associated with the development of several diseases, including coronary heart disease and cancer.

Vitamin C. In addition to acting as an antioxidant, vitamin C is known to aid the immune system in battling colds and flu. Current estimates are that it takes about 200 milligrams (mg) of vitamin C to maintain the integrity of the immune system under stressful conditions. As a rule, people consume less than half that amount (about 60 mg per day, which is the Dietary Reference Intake [DRI]).

Vitamin B Complex. Vitamin B requirements are known to increase during prolonged bouts of stress because they aid primarily in the function of the central nervous system, which is in a high state of arousal during periods of stress. The vitamin B complex includes thiamin (B_1), riboflavin (B_2), niacin (B_3), B_6, folate, biotin, pantothenic acid, and B_{12}. According to studies at Loma Linda University in California, decreases in B_6 vitamin levels correlate with decreased immune function (Webb 2001).

A Word About Supplements. Years ago, when the soil used to grow crops was rich in nutrients, supplements were not necessary. Those who took them were looking for quick cures, trying to lose weight, or, in many cases, taking them in place of regular meals. For the average person, though, it was widely believed that if you ate well-balanced meals, there really was no need to take supplements. The same cannot be said today! Because of soil depletion, combined with the rushed pace of life leading to greatly compromised dietary habits, taking supplements is not only recommended, it is often required to maintain optimal health (**FIG. 27.10**). Some

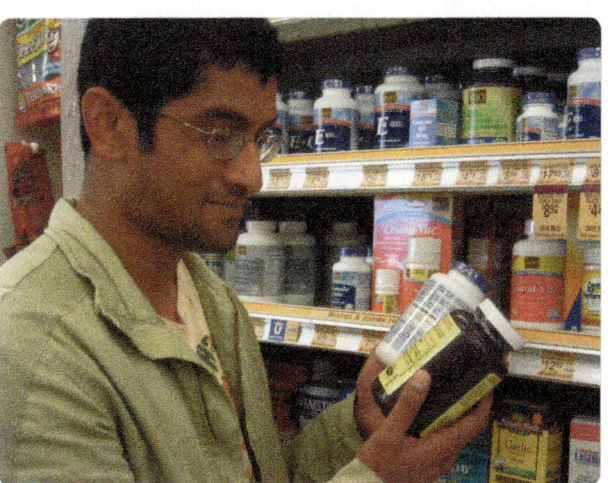

Courtesy of Jesse Geraci.

FIGURE 27.10 The best source of vitamins is unprocessed food. Vitamin supplements are recommended for people who may not get essential nutrients, but vitamins should not be taken in place of a meal.

facts to be aware of when choosing dietary supplements include the following:

- Not all **vitamin supplements** are created equal. Vitamin sources are either extracted from their original food sources or chemically synthesized. In the act of processing, vitamins may be synthesized, crystallized, lyophilized (freeze-dried), or whole-food supplements. In the first two processes, extreme heat is used and, as a result, any beneficial qualities once present are most likely lost. In addition, the substance used in the process of binding the vitamins in a tablet is so strong that the body's enzymes cannot dissolve it. Consequently, the tablet is passed through the gastrointestinal tract without ever being absorbed. Therefore, it is recommended that any vitamin supplement taken be lyophilized or made from whole-food extracts and that it be in the form of a powdered substance in a gel capsule for easy digestion and absorption.

- Taken in concentrated form, vitamin, mineral, and protein supplements can actually block the absorption rate (decrease bioavailability) of other essential nutrients (other vitamins and minerals), thereby negating any positive effect. Consult a certified nutritionist about taking supplements.

- In large doses, the fat-soluble vitamins (A, D, E, and K) are toxic. Because vitamins B and C are water soluble, excess amounts of them will be excreted—making for very expensive urine.

Nutritional Shortcuts for Health?

Since this textbook was first published there have been countless fad diets, including the Beverly Hills diet, the grapefruit diet, the Atkins diet, the cookie diet, the South Beach diet, the vegan diet, the Zone diet, the paleo diet, and now the ketogenic diet. Each diet tweaks the percentages of carbohydrates, fats, and proteins for optimal health. Because everyone differs with regards to their metabolism and microbiome, as well as with their calorie expenditures, it is nearly impossible to create a diet that works for everyone, offering promises of decreased weight, decreased body fat, and better body composition. Currently, new studies are looking at intermittent fasting as an alternative to fad diets, with

> **Vitamin supplements:** Processed pills containing various vitamins (e.g., A, B complex, C, E).

more research needed in this area before positive conclusions can be reached. Currently there are *no* shortcuts to health regarding a special diet.

Additional Stress and Nutritional Factors to Consider

Nutrition plays a crucial role in both minimizing and increasing the physiological arousal of the stress response. The stress response increases the rate of metabolism by activating the mobilization of carbohydrates and fats into the bloodstream for energy production. Additionally, several substances, when ingested, tend to mimic or induce the stress response or decrease the efficiency of the body's metabolic pathways, thus setting the stage for a more pronounced physiological reaction to stress. Likewise, the stress response can deplete necessary nutrients, vitamins, and minerals, creating a cyclical process of poor health. The relationship between stress and nutrition is profound for many reasons, including the following:

- Stress increases the production of cortisol, which, in turn, increases the production of the chemical neuropeptide Y (NPY) in the brain. NPY is thought to be responsible for people craving carbohydrate-rich foods, particularly sweets (possibly a reason for weight gain). NPY levels are normally high in the morning. This, coupled with a stress-filled day, can create the urge for sweets all day long. Eating a good breakfast is believed to help maintain levels of NPY and keep it in balance (Sommer 1999).

- According to nutritionist Elizabeth Sommer (1999), a low-fat diet stimulates the immune system, whereas a high-fat diet increases the risk of illness. Therefore, eating foods with high fat content may be convenient during a long working day, but the long-term effects are quite detrimental to optimal health.

- An excess of simple sugars tends to deplete vitamin stores, particularly vitamin B complex (niacin, thiamin, riboflavin, B_6, and B_{12}). White sugar (even bleached flour), flushed of its vitamin and mineral content, requires additional B-complex vitamins to be metabolized. These and other vitamins are crucial for the optimal functioning of the central nervous system. A depletion of the B-complex vitamins may manifest itself in fatigue, anxiety, and irritability. In addition, increased amounts of ingested simple sugars may cause major fluctuations in blood glucose levels, resulting in pronounced fatigue, headaches, and general irritability. *New York Times Magazine* investigative reporter Gary Taubes, author of the best-seller *Good Calories, Bad Calories* (2007), notes that refined sugars (not saturated fats) are the primary factor associated with obesity and many other chronic diseases.

■ Caffeine is a stimulant that arouses the sympathetic nervous system—most likely the reason people drink coffee in the morning to help wake up and get a start on the day (**FIG. 27.11**). Caffeine is quickly absorbed in the bloodstream and delivered to all parts of the body, with a direct effect on the brain. It is a well-known fact that caffeine is a diuretic. Also eliminated are various minerals such as calcium and magnesium. Food sources with caffeine that trigger the sympathetic nervous system are referred to as sympathomimetic agents. The substance in caffeine responsible for this effect is called **methylated xanthine**. This chemical stimulant with amphetamine-like characteristics triggers the sympathetic nervous system for a heightened state of arousal as well as stimulates the release of several stress hormones. The result is a heightened state of alertness, which makes the individual more susceptible to perceived stress. Caffeine is found in many foods, including chocolate, coffee, tea, and several types of soft drinks. According to current estimates, the average American consumes three 6-ounce cups of coffee per day. A 6-ounce cup of caffeinated coffee contains approximately 250 mg of caffeine, half the amount necessary to evoke an adverse arousal of the central nervous system. The body takes about 8 hours to metabolize one cup of coffee (Cherniske 1998).

■ Chronic stress can cause a depletion of several vitamins necessary for energy metabolism, as well as a depletion of constituents required by the stress response itself. The synthesis of cortisol requires the presence of vitamins. The stress response activates several hormones responsible for mobilizing and metabolizing fats and carbohydrates for energy production. The breakdown of fats and carbohydrates requires the involvement of vitamins—specifically, vitamin C and B-complex vitamins. An inadequate supply of these vitamins may affect mental alertness and promote depression and insomnia. Stress is also associated with a depletion of calcium and the inability of bones to absorb calcium properly. This sets the stage for the development of osteoporosis, the demineralization of bone tissue. Vitamin supplementation is a controversial issue. When a balanced diet is consumed, there is typically an adequate supply of vitamins and nutrients for energy metabolism. However, a balanced diet is not the rule for the majority of Americans. Vitamin supplements may be recommended for individuals who are prone to excessive stress.

■ It seems that Americans have a love affair with salt. Some people even add salt to their food without tasting it. High sodium intake is associated with high blood pressure because sodium acts to increase water retention. As water volume increases in a closed system, blood pressure increases. If this condition persists, it may contribute to hypertension.

■ The excessive consumption of alcohol is thought to suppress the immune system by depleting water-soluble vitamins and minerals (primarily potassium, magnesium, calcium, and zinc) that

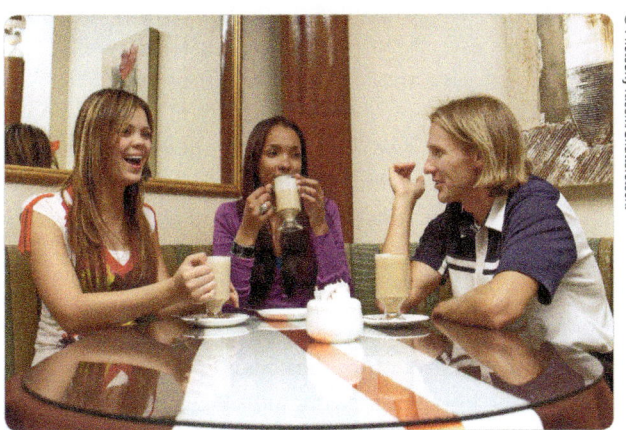

© PhotoSky4t.com/Shutterstock.

FIGURE 27.11 You may consider coffee to be one of your essential food groups, but research reveals that more than two 8-ounce cups per day contains enough caffeine to trigger the fight-or-flight response. Caffeine is also found in tea, sodas, and chocolate. If you are stressed, coffee, tea, or soda is not a recommended beverage, despite cultural trends reinforcing this habit.

Methylated xanthine: The active ingredient in caffeine, which triggers a sympathetic response.

are involved in the synthesis of components for the immune system. What is excess consumption of alcohol? Although this may vary from person to person, nutritionists suggest that more than one 8-ounce drink per day is excessive.

- For years scientists have warned against the dangers of eating too many foods with cholesterol and saturated fat (**FIG. 27.12**), but the choices of foods that are offered as substitutes are proving to be no better and, in some cases, perhaps worse. Margarine is a processed form of corn oil; it is produced by changing the molecular structure through *hydrogenation*, in which the empty bonds are filled to turn the liquid oil into a solid at room temperature. Recently, scientists have observed an association between the hydrogenation process and the loss of integrity of the cell wall (through free radicals), setting the stage for the development of cancer and coronary heart disease. As of November 2013, the FDA banned all foods with trans fats (hydrogenated oils) because of the chronic health risks associated with them.

- People who are constantly on the go rarely have time to prepare their own meals and may not eat regularly (**FIG. 27.13**). On average, many people

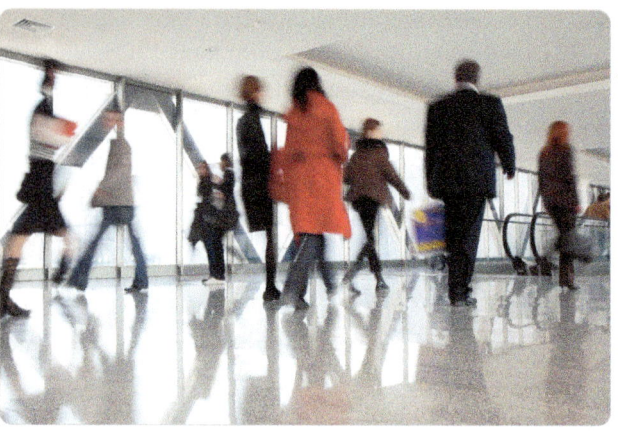

FIGURE 27.13 A stressed lifestyle can produce poor eating habits, which, in turn, can leave you with a nutrient deficiency and a compromised immune system. Get in the habit, no matter how busy your day, to eat one meal a day for your immune system.

eat one or two meals a day outside the home, which frequently leads to some rather unhealthy eating habits that will, over time, be the cause of stress and illness. If you tend to eat out frequently—whether as a matter of convenience or social habit—you should be aware of these facts. Food prepared in restaurants is generally high in sodium and sugar, and is particularly high in saturated fats. People like fatty foods because they taste good, and many of the selections on a menu are created with this in mind. Appetizers that are fried, salad dressings made with heavy oils, and rich desserts with heavy creams are where the fat calories are hidden. Fast food is even higher in fat, sodium, and sugars. If you must eat out, make a habit of skipping appetizers, soft drinks, and salad dressings; choosing fresh fruits and vegetables over fried foods; and passing on dessert.

A Word about Genetically Altered Foods

Research into various hybrids of plant species, such as peas, oranges, and lettuce, has been conducted for centuries, in the hopes of making more delicious and nutritious food. The line between science and science fiction became rather fuzzy in 2000 when it was reported that food scientists were splicing a unique gene from flounder (a saltwater fish) into the DNA of tomatoes, and the genes of Brazil nuts into the DNA of corn. Scientists proceeded to alter the genetic makeup of corn by splicing Roundup, a synthetic pesticide, into the DNA of corn, which resulted in the mysterious death of thousands of

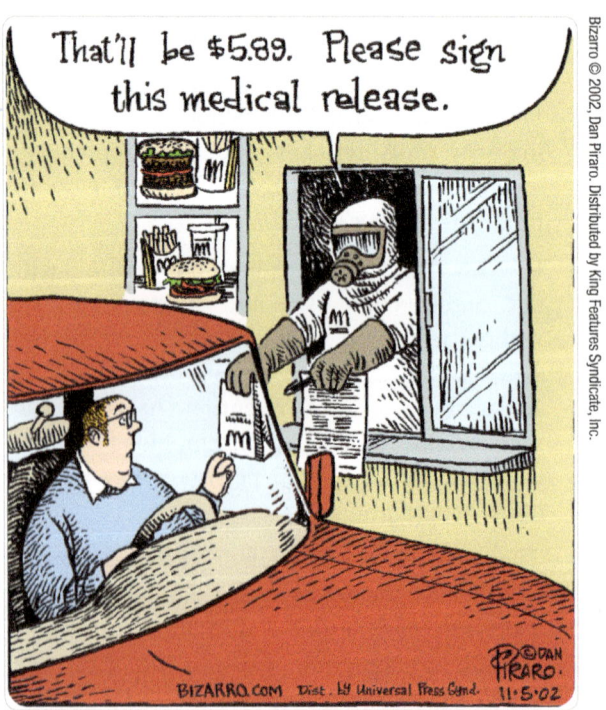

FIGURE 27.12 Think twice before you eat processed food.

migrating monarch butterflies (Teitel and Wilson 1999). In the fall of 2000, corn taco shells were recalled from Taco John restaurants and corn flakes were recalled from grocery store shelves by Kellogg Corporation because of consumer alarm over **genetically modified organisms (GMOs)**, or what some have labeled as **Frankenfood**. GMOs are considered by some people to be a bioecological stressor to the body. Over 65 percent of foods found in the grocery store are genetically modified (Glave 2004; Mercola 2008). Commercial foods and food products may not be labeled as containing "genetically altered" ingredients. Because of the possibility of severe allergic reactions to such foods, it is best to avoid them and choose whole foods with "certified organic" labels (**FIG. 27.14**) (**BOX 27.6**).

Spiritual Nutrition

What does nutrition have to do with spirituality? On the surface, perhaps not much, but upon closer examination we learn that some aspects of nutrition have a very strong spiritual and energy component. For instance, in some Eastern cultures it is believed that there are several energy centers (called chakras) that run from the top of the head to the base of the spine. Each of the seven energy centers is associated with a color: red (base of spine), orange (navel), yellow (spleen), green (heart), aqua-blue (throat), indigo blue (forehead), and violet (crown). It's not a coincidence that women are advised to drink cranberry juice for a urinary tract infection or that diabetics are advised to consume bilberries for their eyes to minimize the effects of retinopathy. The Ayurvedic principles from India suggest that people eat

foods, specifically fruits and vegetables, that correspond to the colors of the energy centers. New research into light and color therapy suggests that every color has a vibrational frequency, and that when people or animals are denied full-spectrum lighting, the effects are evident in the functions of various organs. Eating foods that contain a specific frequency may, indeed, replenish what is not available through exposure to natural light. New research suggests that **bioflavonoids**, the "nonnutrients" in fruits and vegetables that are responsible for food color, act like antioxidants and seem to have an anticancer action (Kale et al. 2008; Simone 1994).

The Taoist philosophy of the Chinese culture also advocates finding balance in the foods we eat, specifically in terms of acid (yin) and alkaline (yang) substances. Grains and animal foods (acids) should be balanced with seeds, vegetables, and salt (alkalines). According to this approach, the correct alkaline/acid balance is 80/20. The Chinese believe that a diet consisting of food heavy in acids creates an energy disturbance, resulting in poor health and disease.

In his book *Spiritual Nutrition and the Rainbow Diet* (1986), Gabriel Cousens, M.D., highlights several ways to make our nutrition and eating habits more conducive to healthy living and more harmonious with the planet. His suggestions include the following:

1. Eat a great variety (full spectrum) of foods, noting color (outside), to nurture the care of specific organs associated with each chakra.

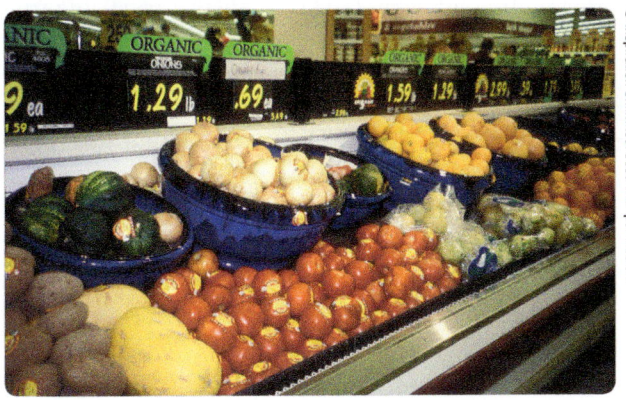

© Inspiration Unlimited. Used with permission.

FIGURE 27.14 Organic foods that contain no herbicides, fungicides, pesticides, or synthetic fertilizers are highly recommended, particularly for anyone with a compromised immune system.

Genetically modified organisms (GMOs): Manipulated foods in which genes from one species are spliced into the DNA of a different species to enhance quality or shelf life, such as taking the genes from a flounder and splicing them into the DNA of a tomato. They are currently associated with a host of food allergies.

Frankenfood: A name coined in Europe to promote the hidden dangers of genetically modified organisms (GMOs). GMOs are currently banned in Europe.

Spiritual nutrition: A term to suggest that the colors of specific fruits and vegetables augment the flow of subtle energy to the respective chakras represented by these colors (e.g., foods with the color red are beneficial for the root chakra and organs associated with this area).

Bioflavonoids: Nonnutrients that provide the colors in foods (fruits and vegetables); contain antioxidants and seem to provide a means of fighting cancer and other illnesses.

BOX 27.6   Food Allergies and GMOs

On Saturday, May 22, 2013, millions of people around the world gathered in a unified demonstration to protest against the American company Monsanto, which is notorious for its efforts to produce genetically modified foods (e.g., splicing the herbicide Roundup into corn). Cross-species tinkering with DNA has harmful consequences. With the rise in GMO foods, there has also been a rise in food allergies. The proverbial question becomes this: When you place a gene of a flounder fish into a tomato plant, is it an animal or a vegetable? Less than a week after the global protests, scientists were quite surprised to find genetically modified wheat in a field in Oregon. Although genetically modified corn and soy are permitted by the U.S. government, genetically modified wheat is not. Wheat that is high in protein creates bigger yields for farmers and is considered more drought resistant. It also is considered harder to digest and absorb. It is estimated that over 30 percent of Americans are now gluten intolerant. (Gluten is the protein source in wheat, rye, and barley.) The Mayo Clinic estimates that 1 in every 110 people have celiac disease (dire wheat intolerance). Wheat products include more than slices of bread and hamburger buns. They can be found in breadcrumbs in hamburgers, meatballs, cereals, soups, imitation crab, mashed potatoes, some spices, and many sauces (Rizzo 2013). Well beyond eggs, peanuts, and milk, people today suffer from a great many food allergies. GMO foods may be to blame, as these genetic "creations" are considered by some to be a foreign pathogen (a stressor) to the human immune system. It is estimated that over 65 percent of foods sold in grocery stores are genetically modified, yet not labeled as so due to powerful corporate lobbying efforts.

2. Avoid eating big meals prior to meditation because the stomach and the brain compete for blood flow, and when the stomach is full, more blood is needed for digestion. As a rule, undereat.

3. Drink plenty of clean/fresh water to cleanse the body of nutrients and toxins that are no longer needed.

4. In addition to digesting quality foods, good nutrition includes adequate sunlight (vitamin D), plenty of fresh air (oxygen), and plenty of fresh water to drink.

5. Learn what foods are associated with the acid/alkaline balance, and make an effort to achieve this balance in your daily diet.

6. Learn to concentrate on the foods you are eating, noting the taste, texture, and temperature, and even the origin. According to the Eastern tradition, being mindful of the food we eat (mindfulness) is a spiritual experience.

Psychological Effects of Food

Brian Wansink begins his book *Mindless Eating* (2006) by describing a culture under the hypnotic effect of mass marketers vying to undermine good eating habits by influencing people's subconscious with subliminal messages to eat and eat and eat. When emotional stress is combined with the marketing of unhealthy foods, the results can be alarming. It would be a simple world if eating were done solely to meet nutritional needs, but this is not the case. Often the act of eating is done for emotional reasons that have nothing to do with the body's nutritional needs. Food is often used as a means to pacify our minds and hearts, a behavior learned from day one at a mother's breast or with a bottle (**FIG. 27.15**). This pattern continues from infancy well into adulthood as we stuff our faces in an attempt to stuff our feelings or control them at some level. The consequences are serious, if not fatal. Experts in dietary behaviors will tell you that the problem of being overweight may look like a problem of overconsumption, but a closer examination reveals that there are some serious emotional issues under the surface. Likewise, eating disorders such as anorexia and bulimia may appear to suggest a problem with malnutrition, but the truth is that eating disorders are symptoms of much more serious unresolved emotional problems. Eating can be an outlet for unresolved anger or guilt (e.g., the self-punisher or even the underhander who eats and drinks on an employer's expense account to seek revenge for working extra hours). But anger alone is not the cause of eating problems. Boredom, loneliness, procrastination, anxiety, and poor willpower also contribute to the blend of psychological and physiological interactions. In essence, food becomes a tranquilizer that calms the nerves.

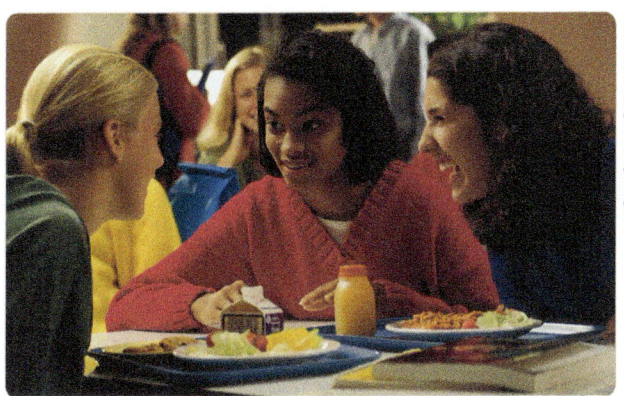

FIGURE 27.15 Eating a healthy meal can be considered a form of relaxation, particularly when done in the company of good friends. When dining with others, relax and enjoy the experience, keeping in mind that a strong social support group augments the relaxation potential.

Cravings. The average person tends to gravitate toward one or more foods when feeling depressed or lonely. Food can become a "friend" when there are no other friends around. If at first we become acquainted with a particular food at a low point, we can become conditioned to return to that type of food when the situation arises again (i.e., comfort foods). Chocolate, French fries, diet sodas, potato chips, candy bars, popcorn, and ice cream are some foods people crave in times of stress. If you are like most people, you also crave a particular food or foods when you are stuck at the end of your emotional spectrum. What is your particular craving? What specific food calms your nerves or gives you a lift when things are not going as expected? Although it is acceptable to seek simple pleasures in food, problems arise when the occasional craving becomes a habit. An occasional craving is not bad, but it can become self-destructive if the behavior is not stopped or if help is not sought to regain emotional balance.

Eating Disorders. There is no simple solution to eating disorders because they involve various eating habits, perceptions of foods, personal history, social pressures, and personality—all of which add up to the monumental task of aligning these factors long enough to make some positive changes. Three of the most common eating disorders are anorexia, bulimia, and overeating:

Anorexia. Anorexics are classified into two groups: (1) those who restrict food intake and starve themselves and (2) those who run through cycles of gorging and then purging (i.e., bulimia). Typically, anorexics are

described as well-educated females with a middle- to upper-class background. The issue of starvation is centered on control—there is something the anorexic feels helpless about, and self-starvation is a way to appease this condition, however remote or tangential. Anorexics have a very distorted body image, often seeing themselves as fat when they have little or no body fat. Aside from the obvious characteristic of extreme weight loss, anorexics are prone to insomnia, obsessive-compulsive disorder, stoicism, perfectionism, introversion, and, frequently, emotional inhibition. Statistics reveal that 1 out of every 100 adolescent girls is diagnosed with this condition (Gordon 2000; Levenkron 2000).

Bulimia. In the American culture, thinness is an obsession. This fact is validated by the plethora of women's magazines that feature thin models on the covers and convey the subliminal message that, unless you look like this, you are not pretty. Women who fall prey to the whims of these marketing attempts and social mores are often confronted with a dilemma, and food becomes the vehicle to control feelings of self-image, self-worth, and self-esteem. In an effort to control body weight, bulimics binge on an assortment of foods (typically junk food) and then purge (either by vomiting or using laxatives) in an attempt to satisfy the need to eat and also satisfy the need to control their weight. Bingeing efforts can be quite extreme—eating a whole gallon of ice cream or consuming an entire pizza or an entire box of cookies. The result of such behavior is the loss of control over caloric balance and the beginning of a cycle of bingeing and purging that frequently leads to malnutrition. Continued bulimia may result in tooth enamel erosion from vomiting, bowel problems, constipation, irregular menstruation, electrolyte imbalance, and rips and tears in the gastrointestinal tract.

Overeating. Excessive overeating may be a result of many factors, including guilt, loneliness, or nervousness. The use of food as a pacifier to calm the nerves becomes ingrained in the daily lifestyle. Overeating can also be a means to create a protective shell in an effort to keep people at a distance. This is often the case with people who were sexually abused or violently attacked as children. In many cases of overeating, low self-esteem is observed.

Is there a physiological explanation for eating disorders? Perhaps not, but there are links between eating and personality that can lead to a better understanding of how to deal with the problem. For example, there is a direct link between the mind and the body, as evidenced by the hypothalamus. The hypothalamus, which registers emotional feelings, also controls appetite—the desire to consume food. When food is placed in the stomach, a calming message is sent to the hypothalamus to decrease the intensity of neural stimulation throughout the rest of the body. There is a profound connection between food and stress. Eating to pacify the nerves is such a common behavior that it is often overlooked in the field of stress management. But what is considered normal is not necessarily healthy. Take note (perhaps in a journal) of your eating behaviors in times of stress. From there, ask yourself whether eating is something you feel you have control over, or whether eating is something that is controlling you.

Recommendations for Healthy Eating Habits

Experts agree that the following dietary practices can minimize the body's arousal to stress and enhance optimal functioning (**BOX 27.7**).

Eat a Well-Balanced Diet. The typical American consumes too many fats and proteins and, frequently, not enough carbohydrates, specifically complex carbohydrates (Sizer and Whitney 2007). An unbalanced diet leads to poor physical and mental performance. At a young age it can retard the physical growth process. During the college years, both men and women seem to function at an acceptable level with an unbalanced diet, but if poor eating habits are not corrected, the foundation is laid for a series of health-related problems later in life. **TABLE 27.2** compares the typical American diet versus the DRI recommendations set by the federal government.

Eat a Good Breakfast and Space Meals Evenly Throughout the Day. Americans typically skip breakfast, with college students being the worst offenders. The body operates on carbohydrates, and this is usually what breakfast foods consist of: breads, cereals, and fruits. When the body is not refueled after 8 to 10 hours

of sleep, it doesn't function well. Symptoms of shortened attention span, early fatigue, and depression are common. When the mind is not alert, the body does not respond well to stress—it typically overreacts. Poor cognitive functioning can result in poor decision making, which can perpetuate the stress cycle. Some experts suggest that we should eat six small meals a day rather than three large ones for better metabolism. Regardless of the number, meals should be spaced evenly throughout the day. An irregular eating schedule interrupts the body's natural rhythms.

Avoid or Minimize the Consumption of Caffeine and Sugar. Overconsumption of caffeine is unhealthy on many fronts. In the short term it can cause headaches, irritability, nervousness, sleeplessness, and in some cases gastrointestinal irritation. Caffeine should be avoided when you know you may encounter a stressor, and caffeine consumption is not recommended when performing relaxation techniques. Refined sugar can also lead to problems. Research indicates that individuals consume their body weight in refined sugar each year (Sizer and Whitney 2007). For reasons explained earlier, this is extremely unhealthy. Efforts should be made to decrease consumption of refined sugar.

Eat a Diet That Provides Adequate Levels of Vitamins and Minerals That Are Potentially Vulnerable to Stress. Vitamins are classified as either fat soluble (A, D, E, and K) or water soluble (B complex and C). The water-soluble vitamins tend to be targeted for destruction during the stress response. A well-balanced diet should exceed the minimum requirements of all of these vitamins, as well as the RDA of essential minerals. Poor nutritional habits compounded by chronic physical stress set the stage for vitamin depletion and deficiency. Caution is advised with vitamin supplementation. An overabundance of fat-soluble vitamins can lead to vitamin toxicity, whereas an excess of vitamins C and B complex is usually excreted, making for very

TABLE 27.2 Typical American Diet vs. DRI Recommendations

Nutrient	Typical American Diet	DRI Recommendation
Carbohydrates	30–40%	55–70%
Fats	40–50%	20–30%
Proteins	20–30%	15–20%

BOX 27.7   Food Label Warning

The following items have been noted to be dangers to your health and should be minimized or completely avoided in your diet:

Artificial flavors and colorings

Artificial preservatives

Aspartame (Nutrasweet and AminoSweet)

Caffeine

Foods with more than 30 percent simple sugars or high-fructose corn syrup

Hydrogenated oils (trans fatty acids)

Monosodium glutamate (MSG)

Nitrates

Nitrites

Nonorganic homogenized milk (contains hormones and steroids)

Olestra

Partially hydrogenated oils (trans fatty acids)

Red and blue dyes

Saturated fats

Sodium

Steroids, pesticides, and hormones in meats and chicken

The bottom line is that if you can't pronounce it, you probably shouldn't eat it.

---

1. Aim for a healthy weight.

2. Be physically active each day.

3. Let the MyPlate food guidance system guide your food choices.

4. Choose a variety of grains daily, especially whole grains.

5. Choose a variety of fruits and vegetables daily.

6. Keep foods safe to eat.

7. Choose a diet that is low in saturated fat and cholesterol and moderate in total fat.

8. Choose beverages and foods to moderate your intake of sugars.

9. Choose and prepare foods with less salt.

10. If you drink alcoholic beverages, do so in moderation.

Additional Tips for Healthy Eating

Many of our eating habits were formed years ago and have become ingrained. When it comes to nutrition, there is no shortage of ideas and suggestions to follow to get back on the right track to eating better. Here are some additional tips:

- Thoroughly wash all pesticides from fruits and vegetables before eating. Studies show that, individually, these pesticides are not harmful, but no studies have looked at the cumulative effects of various pesticides. It's a good idea to rinse all produce well. Eat organic produce whenever possible.

- Avoid canned fruits and vegetables when possible. By the time they are eaten, the vitamins and minerals have been absorbed into the water used to package the goods and are often discarded in preparation.

expensive urine. Eat a well-balanced diet with whole and fresh foods and add a quality vitamin supplement (Sizer and Whitney 2007).

Follow the U.S. Dietary Guidelines. Unlike developing nations that struggle to feed their citizens, the United States suffers from a problem of overconsumption. According to federal government sources, we as a nation overconsume calories in general, and especially fats, simple sugars, salt, and alcohol. These trends in the American diet are closely associated with 6 of the 10 leading causes of death in this country, including coronary heart disease, diabetes, and cancer. Based on a review of these national eating behaviors, the following Dietary Guidelines were established by the U.S. Departments of Agriculture and Health and Human Services:

Aspartame: Two amino acids that combine to make an artificially sweet taste, including one that is documented to affect brain chemistry and cognitive function. Like MSG, this substance is known as an excitotoxin. It is also marketed as Nutrasweet.

Monosodium glutamate (MSG): A food brightener that is documented to affect brain chemistry and cognitive function. Like aspartame, this substance is known as an excitotoxin. Listed as "spice" on many condiments.

- Avoid nutritional supplements that advertise "time released." This phrase is a marketing gimmick that does not hold up under the constraints of human physiology.

- Consider alternative options for healthier meals when you are away from home. It is just as easy to go to a grocery store and pick up some produce as it is to pull into a fast-food restaurant.

- If you do choose to take a nutritional supplement, take it with food and water, not on an empty stomach.

- Eating a high-carbohydrate meal can make your blood glucose levels soar, only to fall down below resting levels soon thereafter. Eat some protein with the carbohydrates so that fatigue will not set in.

- If you are in the habit of eating while watching TV and you are hoping to lose weight, make a new habit to eat only in the kitchen area. TV commercials often send a message to eat even when you are not hungry. Hold fast to this rule: No eating in front of the TV.

- The DRIs were designed to inform the general public about nutritional needs, yet these recommendations were not established for optimal levels; rather, they list average amounts. Without pushing the limits of toxicity, you should consider slightly increasing your levels of nutrients, specifically vitamins and minerals.

- Switch from diet drinks that contain aspartame and caffeine to caffeine-free herbal teas or water when looking for a beverage and rehydration.

- If you are having problems sleeping at night, be careful to avoid foods that contain caffeine, and avoid eating a meal or snack before bedtime.

- Don't try to make several dietary changes all at once. Try making one change at a time (perhaps one each week) until you are at a level where it is comfortable to adopt a new eating behavior that will become part of your lifestyle.

SUMMARY

- Physical exercise is a form of stress; it is the enactment of all the physiological systems that the fight-or-flight response triggers for physical survival.

- Physical exercise is classified as either anaerobic (fight) or aerobic (flight). Anaerobic (without oxygen) is a short, intense, and powerful activity, whereas aerobic exercise (with oxygen) is moderately intense activity for a prolonged period of time. Aerobic exercise is the better type to promote relaxation.

- The body adapts, either negatively or positively, to the stress placed upon it. Proper physical exercise will cause many adaptations that in the long term are thought to be effective in reducing the deleterious effects of stress by returning the body to a profound state of homeostasis. Physical exercise allows the body to use stress hormones for their intended purposes, detoxifying the body of stress hormones by utilizing them constructively.

- To get the benefits of physical exercise, four criteria must be met: intensity, duration, frequency of training, and type of exercise. Together they are called the FITT principle, meaning that without meeting all four requirements, few if any benefits will be gained. It takes between 6 and 8 weeks to see significant benefits in the body.

- The positive effects of physical exercise are lower resting heart rate and resting blood pressure, decreased muscle tension, and improvement in a host of other functions that help one to maintain or regain physiological calmness.

- Exercise evokes not only physiological changes, but also various psychological changes (e.g., runner's high), again suggesting that mind and body act as one entity. Habitual physical exercise produces both physiological homeostasis and mental homeostasis. Individuals who engage in regular physical exercise report higher levels of self-esteem and lower incidences of depression and anxiety.

- Although the primary purpose of food is as a source of nutrients, many people use food as a means to fill an emotional void created by stress.

- Because of the global condition of soil depletion, even a healthy diet is considered deficient in the essential vitamins and minerals; therefore, supplementation is encouraged.

- A malnourished diet—one that is deficient in essential amino acids, essential fats, vitamins, and minerals—is itself a stressor on the body.

- Research has shown that some foods actually induce a state of stress. Excess amounts of sugar, caffeine, salt, and foods poor in vitamins and minerals weaken the body's resistance to the stress response and may ultimately make a person more vulnerable to disease and illness.

- Not all supplements are created equal. Check to see that the processing does not destroy what it is intended to promote. Taken in excess, supplements can do more harm than good by inhibiting the proper digestion and absorption of essential nutrients.

- Food can either boost or suppress the immune system.

- Food affects not only the physical body, but the mental, emotional, and spiritual aspects as well. The concept of spiritual nutrition suggests eating a wide variety of fruits, vegetables, and grains that nurture the health of the seven primary chakras. In addition, spiritual nutrition suggests ensuring a balance in all aspects of food, including the acid/base balance.

- Eating disorders are emotionally rather than physiologically based, ranging from bulimia and anorexia to overeating—all of which have serious consequences if not resolved.

- Change various aspects of your diet, including reducing or eliminating the consumption of caffeine, refined sugar, sodium, and fats, to reduce the risk of stress-related problems.

STUDY GUIDE QUESTIONS

1. Explain how physical exercise is stress but also helps reduce stress.

2. How does anaerobic exercise differ from aerobic exercise?

3. List five physiological effects of cardiovascular exercise.

4. List and explain the proven steps to begin and continue a successful exercise program.

5. How does stress affect eating habits?

6. How does stress affect digestion, absorption, and elimination?

7. How does stress affect the body's nutrients?

8. What foods trigger the stress response?

9. List three recommendations for healthy nutrition.

REFERENCES AND RESOURCES

American College of Sports Medicine. 1990. *Recommended Quantity and Quality of Exercise for Developing and Maintaining Cardiovascular and Muscular Fitness in Healthy Adults.* Indianapolis, IN: ACSM.

American College of Sports Medicine. 2000. *Guidelines for Exercise Testing and Prescription* (6th ed.). New York: Lippincott.

Anoja, S., J.-T. Xie, and C.-S. Yuan. 2000. "Treatment of Insomnia: An Alternative Approach." *Alternative Medicine Review* 5(3): 249–259.

Aronson, D. 2003. "Taking the Right Vitamins for You." *Natural Health*, August, pp. 67–77.

Aronson, V., and B. Fitzgerald. 1990. *Guidebook for Nutrition Counselors.* Upper Saddle River, NJ: Prentice Hall.

Artal, M., and C. Sherman. 1998. "Exercise and Depression." *Physician and Sports Medicine,* October, pp. 55–60.

Barlow, J. 2003. "Study Is First to Confirm Link Between Exercise and Changes in Brain." News release, University of Illinois Champaign-Urbana. https://www.news.uiuc.edu/scitips/03/0127exercise.html.

Bartholomew, J. B. 2000. "Stress Reactivity After Maximal Exercise: The Effect of Manipulated Performance Feedback in Endurance Athletes." *Journal of Sports Science* 18(11): 893.

Bein-Ari, E. T. 2000. "Take Two Exercise Sessions and Call Me in the Morning." *BioScience* 50(1): 96.

Bellet, S., L. Roman, and F. Barham. 1969. "Effect of Physical Exercise on Adrenocortical Excretion." *Metabolism* 18: 484–487.

Berger, B. G. 1982. "Facts and Fancy: Mood Alteration Through Exercise." *Journal of Physical Education, Recreation, and Dance* 53(9): 47–48.

Berger, B. G. 1983. "Stress Reduction Through Exercise: The Mind-Body Connection." *Motor Skills: Theory into Practice* 7(2): 31–46.

Berger, B., E. Friedmann, and M. Eaton. 1988. "Comparison of Jogging, the Relaxation Response, and Group Interaction for Stress Reduction." *Journal of Sport and Exercise Psychology* 10(4): 431–447.

Berger, B. G., and R. Motl. 2001. "Physical Activity and Quality of Life." In *Handbook of Sport Psychology*, edited by R. Singer, H. A. Hausenbals, and C. M. Janelle. New York: Wiley and Sons.

Blackburn, G. 1991. "Nutritional Medicine: Eating Under Stress." *Prevention* 43(6): 104.

Blaylock, R. 1994. *Excitotoxins: The Taste That Kills.* Santa Fe, NM: Health Press.

Carmichael, M. 2007. "Stronger, Faster, Smarter: Exercise and the Brain." *Newsweek*, March 26, pp. 38–55.

Chang, L. 2006. "Stress Hormone: No Link to Obesity?" MedicineNet.com, February 3. https://www.medicinenet.com/script/main/art.asp?articlekey=57726.

Cherniske, S. 1998. *Caffeine Blues: Wake Up to the Hidden Dangers of America's #1 Drug*. New York: Grand Central Publishing.

Colcombe, S. J., K. I. Erickson, N. Raz, A. G. Webb, et al. 2003. "Aerobic Fitness Reduces Brain Tissue Loss in Aging Humans." *Journal of Gerontology* 58(2): 176–180.

Collingwood, T. 1971. "The Effects of Physical Training upon Behavior and Self-Attitudes." *Journal of Clinical Psychology* 28: 583–585.

Colt, E., S. L. Wardlaw, and A. G. Franz. 1984. "Effect of Running on Plasma B-Endorphin." *Life Science* 28: 1637–1640.

Cooper, K. 1970. *The New Aerobics*. New York: Evans.

Cooper, K. 1985. *The Aerobics Program for Total Wellbeing*. New York: Bantam Books.

Cousens, G. 1986. *Spiritual Nutrition and the Rainbow Diet*. San Rafael, CA: Cassandra Press.

Cousens, G. 2000. *Conscious Eating*. New York: North Atlantic Books.

Cowley, G. 1998. "Cancer and Diet." *Newsweek,* November 30, pp. 60–68.

Coyle, E. G., W. H. Martin 3rd, D. R. Sinacore, et al. 1984. "Time Course of Loss of Adaptations After Stopping Prolonged Intense Endurance Training." *Journal of Applied Physiology* 57(6): 1857–1864.

Dahl, M. 2016. "How Running and Meditation Change the Brains of the Depressed." *Science of Us*, March 24. http://nymag.com/scienceofus/2016/03/how-running-and-meditation-change-the-brains-of-the-depressed.html.

Davies, C., and J. D. Few. 1974. "Effects of Exercise on Adrenocortical Function." *Journal of Applied Physiology* 35: 887–891.

Davies, C., and A. Knibbs. 1971. "The Training Stimulus: The Effects of Intensity, Duration, and Frequency of Effort on Maximum Aerobic Power Output." *Internationale Zeitschrift für angewandte Physiologie, einschliesslich Arbeitsphysiologie* 29: 299–305.

DeBenedette, V. 1988. "Getting Fit for Life: Can Exercise Reduce Stress?" *The Physician and Sports Medicine* 16: 185–200.

Digitale, E. 2008. "Running Slows Aging and Postpones Disability, Study Finds." *Stanford Report*, August 20. https://news.stanford.edu/news/2008/august20/med-aging-082008.html.

Dishman, R. K. 1981. "Biological Influences on Exercise Adherence." *Research Quarterly for Exercise and Sport* 52(2): 143–159.

Dishman, R. K., W. Ickes, and W. P. Morgan. 1980. "Self-Motivation and Adherence to Habitual Physical Activity." *Journal of Applied Social Psychology* 1: 115–125.

Dotson, G. 1986. "Food in Treatment: Education for Self-Nurturance of the Body/Mind/Spirit." *Journal of Traditional Acupuncture,* Summer, pp. 35–38.

Dragland, S., H. Senoo, K. Wake, et al. 2003. "Several Culinary and Medicinal Herbs Are Important Sources of Dietary Antioxidants." *Journal of Nutrition* 133(5): 1286–1290.

Egoscue, P. 1998. *Pain Free*. New York: Bantam Books.

Farrell, P. A. 1985. "Exercise and Endorphins: Male Responses." *Medicine and Science in Sports and Exercise* 17: 89–92.

Fixx, J. 1977. *The Complete Book of Running*. New York: Random House.

Folkins, C. H. 1972. "Psychological Fitness as a Function of Physical Fitness." *Archives of Physical Medicine and Rehabilitation* 53: 503–508.

Folkins, C. H., and W. E. Sime. 1981. "Physical Fitness Training and Mental Health." *American Psychologist* 36: 373–389.

Galbo, H., E. A. Richter, J. J. Holst, and N. J. Christensen. 1977. "Diminished Hormonal Responses to Exercise in Trained Rats." *Journal of Applied Physiology* 43: 953–958.

Getchel, B. 1983. *Physical Fitness: A Way of Life*. New York: Wiley.

Glasser, W. 1976. *Positive Addiction*. New York: Harper & Row.

Glave, M. P. 2004. "Most Food in U.S. Grocery Stores Will Be Organic by 2020." *The Santa Fe New Mexican*, July 9. https://www.organicconsumers.org/organic/most071904.cfm.

Gordon, R. 2000. *Eating Disorders: Anatomy of a Social Epidemic*. New York: Blackwell Publishing.

Gosselin, C., and A. Taylor. 1999. "Exercise as Stress Management Tool." *Stress News* 11(4). https://www.isma.org.uk/stressnw/exercise.htm.

Grossman, A. 1985. "Endorphins: Opiates for the Masses." *Medicine and Science in Sport and Exercise* 17: 74–80.

Husband, A. J., and W. L. Bryden. 1996. "Nutrition, Stress and Immune Activities." *Proceedings of the Nutrition Society of Australia* 20: 60–70.

Ismail, A. H., and R. J. Young. 1977. "Effect of Chronic Exercise on the Personality of Adults." *Annals of the New York Academy of Sciences* 301: 958–969.

Kale, A., S. Gawande, and S. Kotwal. 2008. "Cancer Phytotherapeutics: Role for Flavonoids at the Cellular Level." *Phytotherapy Research* 22(5): 567–577.

Kemper, K., A. Amata-Hynvi, L. Dvorkin, et al. 2003. "Herbs and Other Dietary Supplements: Healthcare Professionals' Knowledge, Attitudes, and Practices." *Alternative Therapies* 9(3): 42–49.

Kesten, D. 1997. *Feeding the Body, Nourishing the Soul: Essentials of Eating for Physical, Emotional, and Spiritual Wellbeing*. Berkeley, CA: Conari Press.

Kirby, J. 1997. "Eat to Beat Stress." *American Health*, December, p. 81.

Kozak, D. 2001. "Keep Moving—Stay Happy." *Prevention* 53(2): 39.

Lamb, D. 1984. *Physiology of Exercise*. New York: Macmillan.

Langer, S. 1998. "Stressless: Natural Strategies to Help You Cope." *Better Nutrition* 60(11): 38.

Lenzt, M. 1981. "Selected Aspects of Deconditioning Secondary to Immobilization." *Nursing Clinics of North America* 16(4): 729–737.

Levenkron, S. 2000. *Anatomy of Anorexia*. New York: W. W. Norton.

Lyon, L. S. 1978. "Psychological Effects of Jogging: A Preliminary Study." *Perceptual and Motor Skills* 47: 1215–1218.

Maas, J. 2001. *Power Sleep*. New York: Quill Books.

McCaleb, R. 1993. "Research and Reviews." *HerbalGram* 29: 19–22.

Mercola, J. 2008. "Genetically Modified (GM) Foods Prepare a Takeover." http://articles.mercola.com/sites/articles/archive/2005/04/06/gm-foods-part-eight.aspx.

Mikevic, P. 1982. "Anxiety, Depression, and Exercise." *Quest* 33(1): 140–153.

Mobily, K. 1982. "Using Physical Activity and Recreation to Cope with Stress and Anxiety: A Review." *American Corrective Therapy Journal* 36(3): 77–81.

Morgan, W., and Goldstein, S. (eds.). 1987. *Exercise and Mental Health*. New York: Hemisphere.

Morgan, W. P. 1982. "Psychological Effects of Exercise." *Behavioral Medicine Update* 4: 25–30.

Morgan, W. P., D. H. Horstman, A. Cymerman, and J. Stokes. 1980. "Exercise as a Relaxation Technique." *Primary Cardiology* 6: 48–57.

Morse, A., R. Walker, and D. Monroe. 1994. "The Effect of Exercise on a Psychological Measure of the Stress Response." *Wellness Perspectives* 11(1): 39–46.

Moss, M. 2013. *Salt, Sugar, Fat*. New York: Random House.

National Dairy Council. 1977. *Statement of Dietary Goals for the United States Submitted to the Select Committee on Nutrition and Human Needs, U.S. Senate*. Rosemont, IL: National Dairy Council.

Nieman, D. C. 1997. *The Exercise–Health Connection*. Champaign, IL: Human Kinetics.

Oaklander, M. 2016. "The New Science of Exercise." *Time*, September 12, pp. 54–60.

Pizzorno, J. 1994. "Pow! Supercharge Your Immune System." *Natural Health*, September/October, pp. 81–85.

Porter, D. T., and P. E. Allsen. 1978. "Heart Rates of Basketball Coaches." *Physician and Sports Medicine*, October, pp. 84–90.

President's Council on Physical Fitness and Sports. 1980. *Introduction to Running: One Step at a Time*. Washington, DC: President's Council on Physical Fitness and Sports.

Ratey, J. 2008. *Spark: The Revolutionary New Science of Exercise and the Brain*. New York: Little Brown.

Reid, T. R. 2005. "Caffeine—What's the Buzz." *National Geographic*.

Rizzo, J. 2013. "Gut Reactions." *National Geographic*, April.

Robbins, J. 2001. *The Food Revolution*. Berkeley, CA: Conari Press.

Rubin, J. 2003. *Patient Heal Thyself*. Topanga, CA: Freedom Press.

Sachs, M., and G. Buffone (eds.). 1984. *Running as Therapy: An Integrated Approach*. Lincoln, NE: University of Nebraska Press.

Schuch, F., and B. Stubbs. 2019. "The Role of Exercise in Preventing and Treating Depression." *Current Sports Medicine Reports* 18(8): 299–304.

Shephard, R. 1968. "Intensity, Duration, and Frequency of Exercise as Determinants of the Response to a Training Regimen." *Internationale Zeitschrift für angewandte Physiologie, einschliesslich Arbeitsphysiologie* 26: 272–278.

Shephard, R. 1987. *Exercise Physiology*. Toronto: Decker.

Simone, C. 1994. *Cancer and Nutrition: A Ten-Point Plan to Reduce Your Risk of Getting Cancer* (rev. ed.). New York: Avery Books.

Sizer, F., and E. Whitney. 2007. *Hamilton and Whitney's Nutrition: Concepts and Controversies* (11th ed.). Belmont, CA: Brooks Cole.

Sleep Foundation. https://www.sleepfoundation.org.

Smith, L. 1985. *Dr. Lendon Smith's Low-Stress Diet*. New York: McGraw-Hill.

Sobel, D., and R. Ornstein. 1997. "Exercise Improves Sleep." *Mind/Body Health Newsletter* VI: 1–2.

Sommer, E. 1999. *Food and Mood* (2nd ed.). New York: Henry Holt.

Stamford, B. 1987. "The Adrenaline Rush." *The Physician and Sports Medicine* 15: 205–212.

Stanmore, T. 2002. *The Pilates Back Book: Heal Neck, Back and Shoulder Pain with Easy Pilates Stretches*. Gloucester, MA: Fair Winds Press.

Steinman, D. 1990. *Diet for a Poisoned Planet*. New York: Random House.

Stulberg, G. 2019. "Everything We Know About Exercise and Depression." *Outside*, September 9. https://www.outsideonline.com/2401557/exercise-depression-research.

Sutton, J. R. 1978. "Hormonal and Metabolic Responses to Exercise in Subjects of High and Low Work Capacity." *Medicine and Science in Sport* 10: 1–6.

Taubes, G. 2007. *Good Calories, Bad Calories*. New York: Knopf Books.

Teitel, M., and K. Wilson. 1999. *Genetically Engineered Food: Changing the Nature of Nature*. Rochester, VT: Park Street Press.

Tharp, G. D. 1975. "The Role of Glucocorticoids in Exercise." *Medicine and Science in Sports* 7: 6–11.

Townsend Letter for Doctors and Patients. www.tldp.com.

Ungaro, A. 2002. *Pilates: Body in Motion*. New York: DK Publishing.

Vailus, A. 1992. "Effects of Weightlessness on Aerobic and Anaerobic Capacity." Unpublished paper, Department of Health Fitness, American University, Washington, DC.

Wansink, B. 2006. *Mindless Eating: Why We Eat More Than We Think*. New York: Bantam Books.

Waterman, R. *Nutrition and Stress*.

Watson, T., and C. Wu. 1996. "Are You Too Fat?" *U.S. News and World Report* 120(1): 52–61.

Webb, D. 2001. "Can B Vitamins Ease Holiday Nerves?" *Prevention*, pp. 64–65.

Weil, A. 1995. *Spontaneous Healing*. New York: Fawcett Books.

Weil, A. 2000. *Eating Well for Optimal Health: The Essential Guide to Food, Diet, and Nutrition*. New York: Knopf.

Willett, W., and P. J. Skerett. 2005. *Eat, Drink and Be Healthy*. New York: Free Press.

Wilson, V., N. Morley, and E. Bird. 1980. "Mood Profiles of Marathon Runners, Joggers, and Nonexercisers." *Perceptual and Motor Skills* 50: 117–118.

Winder, W. W., M. A. Beattie, and R. T. Holman. 1982. "Endurance Training Attenuates Stress-Hormone Responses to Exercise in Fasted Rats." *American Journal of Physiology* 243: R179–R184.

Winder, W. W., and R. W. Heinger. 1973. "Effect of Exercise on Degradation of Thyroxine in the Rat." *American Journal of Physiology* 224: 572–575.

Wolfe, K., and D. Kern. 2003. *Create the Body Your Soul Desires*. Duluth, GA: Southern Century Press.

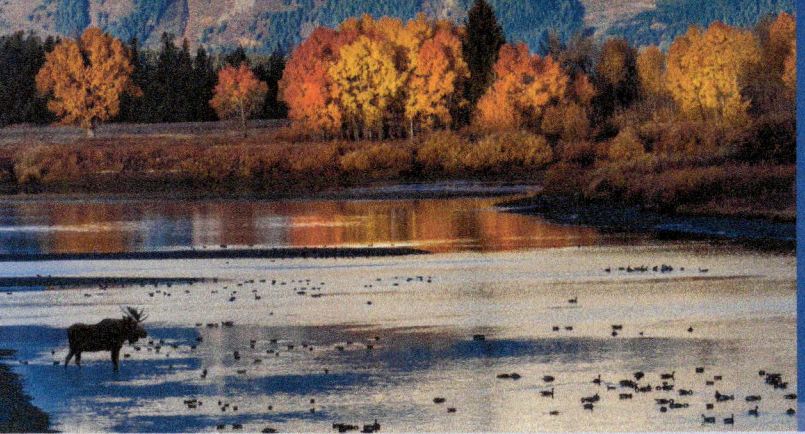

CHAPTER 28

Ecotherapy: The Healing Power of Nature

I go to nature to be soothed and healed and to have my senses put back in order.

—John Burroughs

The COVID-19 pandemic did many terrible things to the American culture, but there were also a few good things that came from it. Being stuck inside under lockdown for weeks on end gave people a much greater appreciation for the outdoors. Self-imposed quarantine measures, followed by recurring government-imposed lockdowns, proved to be a surefire recipe for cabin fever. Even before these restrictions were lifted, people from all demographics made a beeline for parks, beaches, forests, city parks, state parks, and national parks in droves. For the first time in years, kids were playing outside in the streets. Noticing birds for the first time in their backyards and neighborhoods, people took up bird watching as a hobby like never before (some even discovered ebird.com). The Neowise comet that graced our summer skies became a fascination for millions, as photos on social media revealed. Across the country bicycle sales skyrocketed, with many bicycle shops quickly becoming empty of inventory. Park pass applications exceeded previous years' numbers, and people overall spent more time outdoors, breathing fresh air, getting doses of vitamin D with natural sunlight, and forest bathing (a newfound concept for many). What you will read in this chapter may seem a bit dated, but take it as a warning not to take the natural world for granted, as was so easily done before the pandemic. Nature has been regarded as a panacea for ages; our time now is no different.

To smell the fragrant scent of pines as you breathe in the fresh air on a morning hike exhilarates the senses. To feel the warm sunlight on your face as you stroll on a beach and gaze over the ocean fills your heart with a sense of wonder. And no words can adequately describe what you see and feel as you stand atop a mountain before you make your descent on groomed-powder ski slopes. Ageless wisdom reminds us time and again that nature in all her glory is a remarkable healing force of homeostasis for mind, body, and spirit. Yet what seems like common sense has become lost in the madness of our current love affair with a 24/7, on-demand, instant-gratification world teeming with technology. With every click of a mouse, text message, Facebook update, Instagram post, and downloaded app, we are losing our inherent connection to the natural world. If Henry David Thoreau, author of the literary classic *Walden* (first published in 1854), were alive today, he would cover his face with disbelief. He's not alone. Experts from all corners of the world believe that our disconnect from nature has become a serious health problem (Sifferlin 2016).

Consider this: Various estimates suggest that people today spend less than 5 percent of their day outdoors—a remarkable, if not drastic, change from the agrarian society of many decades ago. Moreover, studies investigating the impact of our highly industrialized environment on physical and mental health show that repeated exposure to artificial light, office noise, poor indoor air quality, chemical particulates from photocopiers, and electromagnetic pollution all have a harmful effect on wellness. These variables are thought to be directly tied to the related epidemics of stress and chronic disease (Chalquist 2009).

The abyss separating humankind from nature, however, didn't begin with the invention of the desktop computer or the Internet. For centuries, influential members of Western civilization have advocated a sense of superiority to and dominion over nature. This philosophy continues today, from genetically modified crops and cloning of cows for beef steaks to the installation of bright city lights, but now there are serious unintended health consequences.

Although the negative health consequences of our withdrawal from nature are well documented, they can be counteracted. Enter ecotherapy, one of the newest (yet perhaps oldest) means of relaxation to be (re)introduced to humanity in the twenty-first century. **Ecotherapy** is a method of restoring optimal health and well-being through routine exposure to and experience in the natural world.

> **Ecotherapy:** A method of restoring optimal health and well-being through routine exposure to and experience in the natural world.

A Historical Perspective on Ecotherapy

For millennia, health experts of all kinds have known of and promoted the benefits of nature as healer, from ancient Zen gardens to European mineral baths. Frederick Law Olmstead specifically designed New York City's Central Park in 1858 to erase the ills of modern civilization from its citizens. Moreover, the establishment of our national park system was not merely to protect the wilderness, but to ensure our healthy relationship with it. The word *vacation* (to vacate one's urban home) entered the American lexicon after the Civil War, when an 1869 best-selling book written by William H. H. Murray titled *Adventures in the Wilderness* encouraged city slickers from Boston and New York to leave their rushed urban lifestyles and head to the Adirondack Mountains in upper New York state as a tonic for mind, body, and spirit (Perrottet 2013).

It wasn't until the early 1990s, however, that the field of psychology took a deeper look at the effects of nature on mental health and the connection between psychology and environmentalism. This awareness first began in the city of San Francisco, which is named after St. Francis, the patron saint of nature and animals. Therapists began getting their clients off the couch and into the woods and parks for walks and precious moments of solitude. Before long an emerging field of psychotherapy developed under the umbrella term *ecotherapy*. Deep ecology, ecopsychology, green therapy, terra-psychology, and wilderness therapy fall under this umbrella, and the latest research in this area has given way to a few other related therapies: forest therapy, nature therapy, and even "avatar therapy" (a name based on James Cameron's mega-hit movie, *Avatar*). A quick Google search of the term "ecotherapy" (and related terms) highlights the significance—if not the immensity—of this topic as it relates to stress levels and the personal health of human beings.

Several people have made significant contributions to the field of ecotherapy, including Theodore Roszak, Joanna Macy, Bill McKibben, Craig Chalquist, Elizabeth Roberts, Larry Robinson, and Linda Buzzell. These and other professionals showed great interest in the connection between the psyche and the natural world. They began to track patients' anxiety levels, grieving process, fear of death, and other spiritual concerns against rising concerns of deforestation, global warming, animal extinction, and other environmental problems. They found that worrying about environmental problems exacerbated patients' psychological conditions.

Although individuals alone cannot solve global environmental problems, they can influence their immediate environment. It became quite evident to these early researchers that bringing our relationship with nature back into balance can help the psyche. Everything from worksite infrastructure and hospital settings to school classroom environments, backyard gardens, animal therapy, and home design can be part of ecotherapy for people of all ages and demographics. Ecotherapy was first used among professionals in psychology, but this umbrella term now extends well beyond the domains of mental health to physical health and optimal well-being. Ecotherapy, as it turns out, is not merely a cognitive therapy recommended by counselors, therapists, and psychologists. Experts from a great many disciplines, including psychology, immunology, anthropology, outdoor recreation, and even theology, have come to the same conclusion: People need to get outside and expose themselves to nature regularly to reach optimal health. What was once taken for granted (spending time outdoors) is now recognized as an essential part of living a balanced life (**FIG. 28.1**). As emerging research in this new field suggests, the relaxing mind-body effects of being in nature cannot be understated. Simply stated: We are a part of nature, and it is a part of us.

Up until the coronavirus outbreak in 2020, the vast majority of Americans didn't spend much time outdoors. But when forced to stay in their homes under a lockdown quarantine, many people soon saw the merits of getting out in nature. People took walks and strolls in their neighborhood parks (many with dogs on leashes). Despite the fact that local governments closed city parks, local playgrounds, and even some national parks, people snuck outside, most in their backyards, to feel sunlight on their face or a warm breeze on their skin. As winter turned to spring, a new interest in birding was noted by the Audubon Society as people filled up their bird feeders and rehung bird houses, with birds of all kinds stopping in for frequent visits, migrating back from southern climates. Some people noted that with the streets empty, some wildlife, such as bears, deer, and even mountain lions, came out of the woods, forests, and nature preserves to explore a wider habitat with an urban flare. Kids across the country who were often tethered to their smartphones and gaming devices before the virus lockdown were seen playing outside, riding bikes, skateboarding, and playing hoops. Many people started a new hobby of gardening as well. Sadly, it took a pandemic to make people realize how important a connection to nature really is.

A Nature-Deficit Disorder?

Several years ago, a serious revelation came upon author and journalist Richard Louv. He realized that many kids of today's generation simply don't go outside to play, something that every kid did in his generation, and perhaps hundreds of generations before him. (If kids do play outside, it's often through structured enrichment programs like soccer, rather than unstructured exploration.) Although some people might see this inactivity as one reason for childhood obesity, Louv had an entirely different concern: a disconnection from the natural world. It seemed impossible to believe that boys and girls would prefer to spend time indoors with technology rather than outside catching fireflies, watching meteor showers, following butterflies through fields of wildflowers, making snow angels, building forts, watching frogs, or fishing at the nearest pond. He discovered that, by and large, kids of the twenty-first century would rather play video games and watch television than spend actual time outside making discoveries in a field of grass or finding out what's hiding under a brookside rock. This phenomenon is a classic case of a "nature disconnect." The implications are startling.

Becoming well aware that people are not spending much time outdoors and the poor health implications of these findings, the gaming industry has taken notice. The 2016 video game Pokémon GO was designed

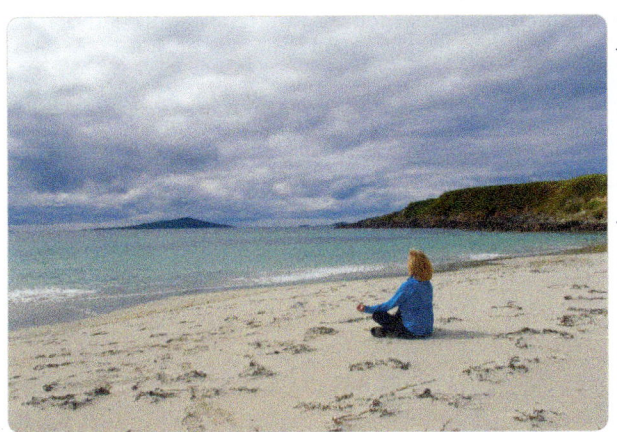

© Inspiration Unlimited. Used with permission.

FIGURE 28.1 Making a habit of spending quality alone time (solitude) in nature is a great way to calm the mind and bring a better sense of perspective to your life.

Stress with a Human Face

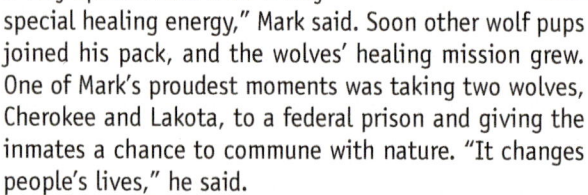

To get to the Rocky Mountain Wildlife Foundation (RMWF), a wolf rescue sanctuary, you head west on Route 24 from Colorado Springs. It's best to call for directions because some of the roads in these parts have yet to be charted on your favorite mapping site or GPS device. The reason to visit the sanctuary, of course, is to commune with wolves. If you're lucky, you might just get a wolf kiss.

Mark Johnson heads up the RMWF, a project he started in 2001. It began when he found himself the caretaker of a young wolf pup named Cheyenne. Mark's heart is as big as the Rocky Mountains themselves. His goal in raising Cheyenne was to teach people that wolves play an essential role in our ecosystem, and as such, they have much to teach us. Cheyenne became famous for her ability to befriend people, particularly people in need of physical, mental, or spiritual healing.

"Before she passed away, Cheyenne had met over 22,000 people and kissed over 1,900 people. She even had the unique ability to discern those people who had a chronic illness and spend extra time with them. She was a very special wolf with a very special healing energy," Mark said. Soon other wolf pups joined his pack, and the wolves' healing mission grew. One of Mark's proudest moments was taking two wolves, Cherokee and Lakota, to a federal prison and giving the inmates a chance to commune with nature. "It changes people's lives," he said.

As word spread about Cheyenne, Mark found himself taking care of more wolves and half-breeds (wolf and malamute or husky mixes). Some people might call Mark a wolf-whisperer, but he will tell you that he never whispers. He uses a combination of body language and voice commands—never any hand strikes. If you were to visit the wolf sanctuary today, Mark would first give you an educational lecture about wolves and the history of the RMWF. Afterward you would meet several wolves and wolf half-breeds, many of which long for your affection. If you're lucky, you might get a kiss or two, much like the one Lakota is giving Mark in the photo.

specifically to get people outdoors (despite the mixed message of being outdoors with screen devices).

In his best-selling book, *Last Child in the Woods* (2005), Louv coined the term **nature-deficit disorder**, a now-common behavior (affliction) where people simply don't get outside enough, hence losing touch with the natural world and all of its wonder and healing properties. He was quick to learn that it's not just kids who are afflicted; adults (parents) rarely get outside either, and kids model their behavior after that of their parents.

Yale scholar Steven Kellert, author of *Birthright* (2012), cites that the average person spends over 95 percent of his or her day inside. Kellert explains that this behavior is against our nature; specifically, it goes against the wisdom of our DNA. Being in nature (e.g., forests, beaches, gardens, and parks) is as important as the air we breathe. Without it, health will suffer. Kellert's colleague and renowned Harvard naturalist E.O. Wilson recoined the term **biophilia** to describe human beings' emotional affiliation to other living organisms. Kellert embraces this idea, stating that humans have an inherent connection and affinity to the natural world. Once this birthright is abandoned or forfeited, health issues—both personal and planetary—ensue.

There was a time not too many decades ago when people couldn't wait to get away from their work in offices, as well as mills and factories, and head out of town on a vacation to the nearest seaside beach or mountain forest. It's been this way for over a hundred years. Renowned naturalist John Muir put it this way back in the late nineteenth century: "Thousands of tired, nerve-shaken, over-civilized people are beginning to find out that going to the mountains is going home; that wildness is necessity; that mountain parks and reservations are useful not only as fountains of timber and irrigating rivers, but as fountains of life." Things have only become more

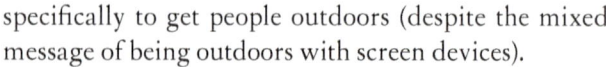

Nature-deficit disorder: A term coined by Richard Louv to describe a now-common behavior (affliction) where people (particularly children) simply don't get outside enough, hence losing touch with the natural world and all of its wonder.

Biophilia: Human beings' emotional affiliation to other living organisms (e.g., plants, trees, animals, birds, dolphins, and whales) and planet Earth as well.

complex, high tech, and stressful since he uttered these words. Moreover, people are now taking their smartphones and laptops (their virtual work desks) with them on vacations, denying themselves the true natural connection they should try to form.

Americans are not the only ones to be overstressed at work and nature deprived. The Japanese are famous for putting in long hours at the office. In fact, they coined a term to describe those who literally die from job stress: *karoshi*. Many Europeans are equally nature deprived. In fact, in 2008 an odd milestone was achieved in the history of humanity: For the first time ever, more people lived in urban cities than in rural areas. As more and more cultures adopt a Western lifestyle confined to an indoor routine, more cultures fall prey to this nature disconnect. As more people spend less time in nature, their indifference (some say apathy) regarding environmental issues dramatically increases. According to the 2008 *Proceedings of the National Academy of Sciences*, since the late 1980s, Americans have decreased their nature-based outdoor recreation by 35 percent (Cordell 2008). Based on their compilation and analysis of the data, the authors predicted serious impending health issues (Cordell 2008). Today, researchers from Japan, South Korea, China, and the United States are beginning to examine the effects of nature on various aspects of health, specifically stress levels. All over Japan you can now find "forest therapy" trails for what the Japanese call *shinrin-yoku*, or "forest bathing." The direct translation: "Let nature enter your spirit through the five senses." Although many Americans run or walk outside, more often than not, they are tethered to their smartphones all the while (**FIG. 28.2**). With their mind still attached to work or other responsibilities, they negate the "outdoor effect" considerably (Reynolds 2012).

◼ Physiological Effects of Ecotherapy

In their thought-provoking book, *Your Brain on Nature* (2012), authors Eva Selhub and Alan Logan compiled a strong body of research data from all corners of the earth and several disciplines to reveal just how important spending time in nature (or with representations of nature) is to our physical, mental, and emotional well-being. Highlights include the following:

- People shown images of nature had an increase in alpha waves in their brains and a corresponding increase in serotonin levels (the happy hormone).

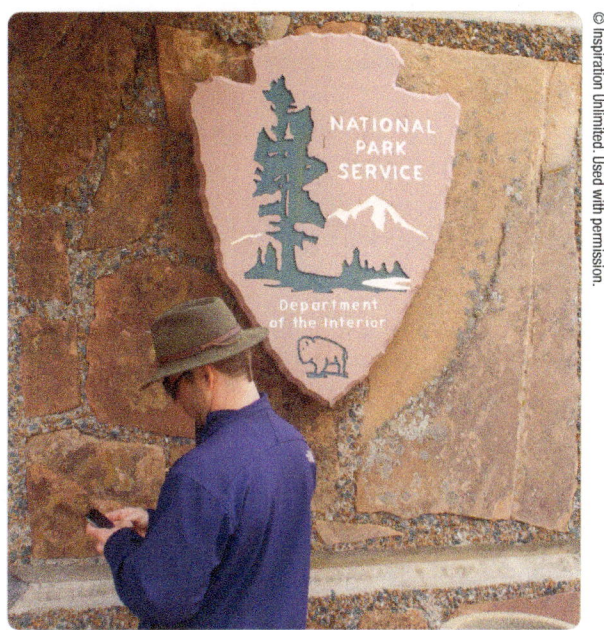

FIGURE 28.2   A vacationer checks his text messages and voicemail while in Rocky Mountain National Park.

- People shown photos of nature reported a decreased sense of anger, whereas photos of urban city life increased levels of frustration, as corroborated by functional magnetic resonance imaging [fMRI] scans of the brain's amygdala.

- Patients who had potted plants in their hospital rooms reported a greater sense of joy and happiness than those patients who had no plants. Similarly, people who have plants in their houses show decreased stress levels and improved stress moderation.

- People who viewed aesthetically pleasing images of nature had increased activity in the parahippocampal gyrus region of the brain, tissue that is rich in opioid receptors associated with the neuropeptide dopamine.

According to Selhub and Logan (2012), "If simply viewed in isolation, it might be easy for critics to dismiss some of the research. But when viewed together [subjective and objective data] the picture of nature's influence emerges. Our perception of stress, our mental state, our immunity, our happiness, and our resiliency are all chemically influenced by the nervous system and its response to the natural environment."

It may seem intuitive that a walk in nature might decrease stress levels, but today many researchers are finding out exactly what happens to your body as you leave technology behind and acclimate to the rhythms of the natural world. This research not only is fascinating, but also supports what philosophers and therapists have been saying for generations: Repeated exposure to the natural elements is good for you. Here are some other recent findings:

- A 2-hour walk in the forest was shown to improve sleep quality (Morita et al. 2011).

- Leisurely walks in a forested area (**FIG. 28.3**) decreased cortisol levels by 12.4 percent and significantly decreased resting heart rate and blood pressure (Miyazaki 2011; Park et al. 2010).

- Time spent in nature has been shown to increase the number of natural killer cells and anticancer proteins, sometimes by as much as 40 percent (Li et al. 2008).

- Exposure to phytoncides (aromatic scents) emitted by evergreen trees is associated with increased natural killer cells and decreased stress levels (Li et al. 2009).

- Exposing cancer cells grown in Petri dishes to phytoncides increased anticancer proteins and proteases, granzymes A and B, and perforin—substances known to destroy cancerous tumors (Li et al. 2009).

- Hospital patients who had a view of nature (e.g., trees) recovered more quickly from surgery than those who had a view of a brick wall (Ulrich 1984).

- Exposure to sunlight increases the production of white blood cells, which boost the immune system, and red blood cells, which increase oxygen-carrying capacity (Williams 2012).

- Repeated natural sunlight exposure (ultraviolet rays) converts cholesterol in your skin to vitamin D (hence sunlight's nickname, the "sunshine vitamin"). Lack of exposure to natural sunlight is known to increase cholesterol levels (Liberman 1991).

The health benefits of ecotherapy have not gone unnoticed by the medical profession. In light of a 2017 review of over 64 studies that hailed the benefits of nature therapy in the *Journal of Environmental Research and Public Health*, many physicians in the United States and Scotland are now prescribing nature prescriptions ("Outdoor Rx"), for their patients to reduce stress, depression, anxiety and blood pressure. Many physicians are now leading "Walk with a Doc" programs in communities and parks across the country.

Entrainment: A Symphony in Natural Rhythms

As the last person took their seat, the evening's keynote speaker, composer Steven Halpern, approached the stage and began to speak. It was the last keynote event at the Science and Consciousness Conference in Santa Fe, New Mexico. Halpern's presentation was on the topic of the healing power of music. For the next several minutes he explained that all aspects of nature have a healing rhythm, including the live potted plant on the stage next to the podium. Explaining some basic concepts of physics (such as that everything is energy and everything has a vibration), he began to speak about the vibrations one encounters in a forest, and how humans entrain on these vibrations (through sympathetic resonance) by direct contact. He then attached an electrode to a leaf of the potted plant. Through the magic of audio technology, with the electrode wires plugged into a transducer, a melody came from the speakers; it was an incredible harmonic melody that astounded the audience. "This is just one leaf of a plant," he said. "Can you imagine if I had an electrode attached to all the leaves? Can you imagine what your body senses at the energetic levels as you simply walk through a forest? This is the healing power of nature. Welcome to the healing power of entrainment in nature," he said.

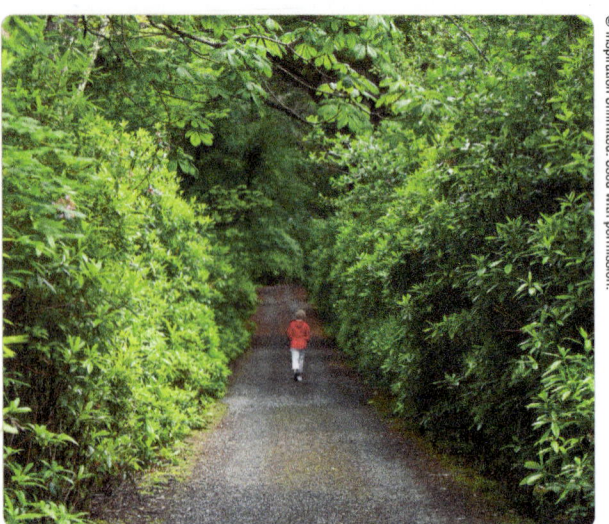

FIGURE 28.3 You don't have to be a tree hugger to gain the benefits of "forest bathing." A simple walk in the woods or park does wonders for one's health.

Waterfalls, whale songs, and scores of other natural wonders that make up the world we live in produce a vibration of 7.8 Hz. Also known as the Schumann resonance, this energy vibration is now considered to be the vibration of homeostasis. When separated from this vibration (or when we are in closer proximity to a higher vibration, such as the constant hum of our laptop computers), our bodies become out of sync with the natural energetic rhythms that help keep our health in check. This disruption affects everything from melatonin production for quality of sleep to the metabolic processes that regulate optimal health. Following the assumption that objects entrain to vibrations, the idea that spending time in nature to "bathe in the natural rhythms of the world" as a way to recalibrate the body's natural rhythms begins to make sense.

Circadian Rhythms and Physical Health

You may have heard of the term "biorhythms" before, but the correct scientific term is "circadian rhythms." From the Latin root *circa,* which means "about a day," **circadian rhythms** are the various body rhythms that take place in a 24-hour period. Simply stated, circadian rhythms define the body's internal clock. It is this clock that regulates everything from the release of melatonin (the sleep hormone) in the evening to the increase in activity of the gastrointestinal tract. These rhythms are based on Earth's 24-hour rotation on its axis and the corresponding cycles of light and dark; these rhythms have been ingrained in our DNA since the dawn of humanity. In today's world, they are every bit as important as when humans first evolved, yet they are often disturbed, because of our reliance on artificial light and our frequent exposure to glowing television and computer screens.

Research in the field of circadian rhythms suggests that our bodies do best when kept to a regular schedule with regard to sleep, meals, and exercise—for example, eating breakfast, lunch, and dinner at the same times each day; going to bed and waking up at the same times every day; and exercising at approximately the same time every day. People who keep their body on a regular schedule and who are in tune with these rhythms tend to live longer, healthier lives.

Conversely, when we get off schedule, our body's physiology has a hard time adjusting—disrupting circadian rhythms is a form of stress. Over time the result is a greater propensity toward disease and illness, as well as more rapid biological aging. Oncologists will tell you that cancer cells respond best to chemotherapy in the mid-morning hours as compared to early evening hours. Athletes will tell you that their best competitions are held at the same time as their practice workouts. The human body craves habitual routines for optimal health.

Psychological Effects of Ecotherapy

A clever line for an outdoor camping ad states: *Think outside. No box required.* The message is simple: Get outside! One need look no further to see the healing power of nature than in the scores of poems, books, and essays from people of all walks of life describing nature's best attributes (**BOXES 28.1** and **28.2**). Throughout history, philosophers, sages, and wisdom keepers the world over have looked to nature to help solve all kinds of problems. If nothing more, the vastness of nature, not to mention the stunning beauty, from her ocean beaches and cathedral forests to majestic mountain ranges, put into perspective the common, everyday problems of each individual. Being outdoors simply helps clear the mind and reduces personal issues to a manageable size. Perhaps John Muir said it best this way: "I only went out for a walk and finally concluded to stay out till sundown, for going out, I found, was really going in." Carl Jung also noticed that nature provided a canvas on which to explore the mind's landscape. He often wrote of the benefits of walks in nature and how immersion in nature benefits the yearning for wholeness; he offered dire warnings through his writings that when the connection to nature is severed, serious repercussions would result in harm to the psyche of the individual (Jung 2002).

In the book *Refuge* (1992), author and naturalist Terry Tempest Williams describes a parallel storyline between her mother's fight with cancer (which was a result of nuclear testing) and the Great Salt Lake floods that destroyed much wildlife in 1983. Williams is not alone

Circadian rhythms: Biological rhythms that occur or cycle within a 24-hour period (e.g., body temperature) that create the body's internal clock; also known as chronobiology. These can be affected by stress, causing a disruption that is even more stressful to the body.

> **BOX 28.1   The Voices of Healing Waters Are Many**
>
> The voices of healing waters are many,
>
> Her streams echo to the rising cliffs she once trespassed,
>
> Her waves sing a constant refrain to the beaches,
>
> Her moist clouds whisper incessantly to the trees and mountains,
>
> Soon cascading white ribbons refrain with misty rainbows,
>
> There is music in all of these songs,
>
> And this music dampens my dry heart like a spring rain.
>
> Yet the song I like best is the silent melody of gentle falling snow,
>
> Sometimes her voice is a thunderous roar that begs for my attention,
>
> But mostly water's song is a celebration of life and I celebrate with it.
>
> I long to hear the voices of water as I dangle my feet in a cool lake,
>
> Or wade in the shallow ocean surf, or drink from a cold mountain stream.
>
> The voices of healing waters are many and I sing with them.
>
> —Brian Luke Seaward

> **BOX 28.2   Nature Therapy Poems**
>
> You ask
>
> why I perch
>
> on a jade green mountain?
>
> I laugh
>
> but say nothing.
>
> My heart, free
>
> like a peach blossom,
>
> in the flowering stream,
>
> going by,
>
> in the depths,
>
> in another world,
>
> not among men.
>
> —Li Po (ancient Chinese poet)
>
> When the wind blows . . .
>
> This is my medicine
>
> When the sky rains,
>
> This is my medicine
>
> When the heavens are filled with snow,
>
> This is my medicine
>
> When the skies become clear after a storm,
>
> This is my medicine
>
> —Native American prayer

in her attempt to connect the parallels of nature to our own lives. Over 2,000 years ago the Chinese philosopher Lao Tzu created a philosophy of life based on living in the rhythms and cycles of nature, which he called Taoism and eloquently described in his classic book *The Tao Te Ching.*

Do your physical surroundings affect your thoughts and behavior? Students of psychology might be interested to learn of the *Journal of Environmental Psychology,* which reports on the influences of nature, space, design, and architecture on various aspects of cognition, memory, attention span, concentration, and behavior. Investigations into the relationship between nature and cognition include work by Rachel and Stephen Kaplan from the University of Michigan that led to their "attention restoration" theory. Apartment dwellers who were given a view of the natural elements (e.g., trees) were reported to show significant increases in concentration skills when compared to residents who did not have natural element views. Through their extensive body of research, the Kaplans advocate nurturing a strong bond with nature as a means of promoting mental health (Kaplan 1995, 2001).

Nature and the Art of Solitude

Experts in the field of sociology agree that modern life is not only fast paced, but also crowded and noisy. Taking time to separate yourself from the cacophony of civilization and seek quiet solitude is a time-honored prescription for inner peace. In spending time alone, one gets the chance to clear the mind of mental clutter and put problems and issues in perspective. One also gains clarity in honoring the simplicity of life rather than the human-made complexities to which we have become so accustomed. Solitude is a different concept from isolation. Although many people have become isolated behind a computer screen, **solitude**—the intentional act of separation from friends and family—is anything but isolation. More than cleansing the mind, solitude becomes, for some, a spiritual experience. Early nineteenth-century British poet Lord Byron described it this way in his poem "Solitude":

> To sit on rocks, to muse o'er flood and fell,
>
> To slowly trace the forest's shady scene,
>
> Where things that own not man's dominion dwell,
>
> And mortal foot hath ne'er or rarely been;
>
> To climb the trackless mountain all unseen,
>
> With the wild flock that never needs a fold;
>
> Alone o'er steeps and foaming falls to lean;
>
> This is not solitude, 'tis but to hold
>
> Converse with Nature's charms, and view her stores unrolled.

■ Spiritual Moments

To have a hummingbird gently perch on your finger as it drinks nectar from the cup of your palm, to swim alongside a baby humpback whale in the crystal blue waters of Tahiti (**FIG. 28.4**), or to spot an elk or gaze at the aurora borealis with curtains of green, yellow,

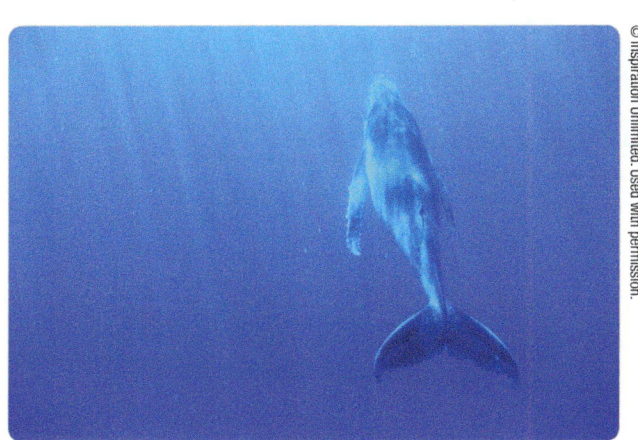

© Inspiration Unlimited. Used with permission.

FIGURE 28.4 Swimming alongside a 2-week old, 12-foot baby humpback whale in the Tahitian island lagoon of Moorea is considered by many to be nothing less than a spiritual experience.

and red lights flashing across the winter sky is more than a brief connection to nature; by all accounts it's a spiritual experience. Quite simply, these moments take your breath away. In a stress-filled world it is easy to become myopic, if not egocentric, with a score of work and life responsibilities that obscure our vision to the bigger world we live in. These spiritual moments in nature serve as a gentle reminder that we are part of a much bigger universe; making this humbling realization puts our lives back in perspective. The awareness of the diurnal cycles and seasonal changes offers a tangible reminder to move with the flow of nature, rather than in opposition to it. In survey after survey, people cite ocean beaches, lakes, and mountain streams as being the most relaxing places to be in nature—anywhere there is water. Just as the human body has rivers of energy called meridians, so, too, does the planet have rivers of energy (often located by bodies of water) called ley-lines. Although wisdom keepers will tell you that the entire planet is sacred, it is common to find many energetic spots on the planet deemed particularly spiritual that some call heaven on earth.

■ Earning "Nature Points"

No one is keeping score, but racking up nature points is a good idea as a means to bring balance back into your life. How often do you get outside? If you answer "every day," but you are plugged into an electronic device or talking on your phone the whole time, you don't score any nature points. (However, using your phone to take a few photos of nature will earn you a few points.) There are no nature points for having a dog or cat, but if you walk your dog outside, you do get points. If you see (and even more importantly, can identify) wildlife species, you definitely get nature points. In what phase is the moon tonight? If you have to look at a calendar for the answer, no nature points. If you make a point to watch the Perseid meteor showers or lunar eclipse, this scores you lots of nature points.

Securing nature points outdoors involves the use of all five senses at the same time; it requires you to be fully present in the moment of the experience. And although there is no official scorecard for nature points, scoring lots of points each day makes you a winner.

> **Solitude:** The intentional act of seeking alone time in a quiet space, away from family, friends, and daily distractions as a means of seeking inner peace.

■ Best Application of Ecotherapy

The message of ecotherapy is clear. We need to spend more time outside in nature. Going for a walk or a run in the woods, taking time to watch the sunset or sunrise, or turning off your smartphone or tablet and going outside at night to become familiar with the constellations, phases of the moon, and occasional meteor showers are just some of the many ways you can return to the surroundings of your natural world.

So is getting a bird feeder in your backyard (**FIG. 28.5**). In doing any one of these things, you begin to see your life in correct proportion to the bigger picture of life. Dedicating time each day outdoors, even if it involves nothing more than getting some exposure to the sun to recalibrate your circadian rhythms, is as important as brushing your teeth or paying your bills. Nature can be found anywhere, including city parks and local floral greenhouse nurseries. Find some nature near you, and get to know it!

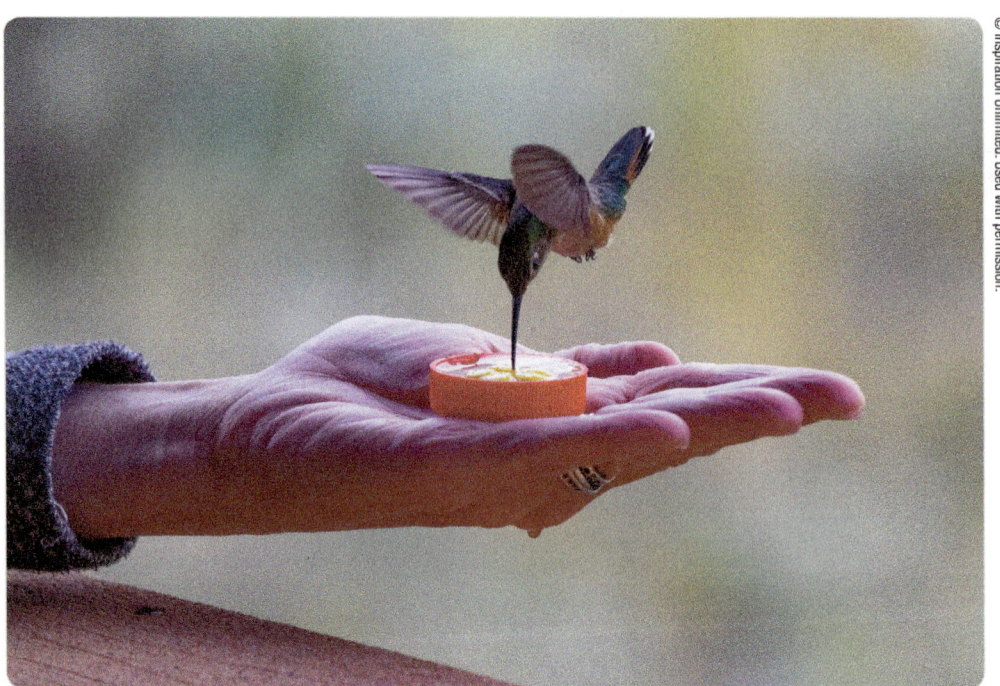

© Inspiration Unlimited. Used with permission.

FIGURE 28.5   We are part of nature, and nature is a part of us. When we realize and act on this inherent connection, and the need to maintain it, we reap the benefits of optimal health on many levels.

SUMMARY

- For millennia, philosophers have touted nature as a great healing agent for mind, body, and spirit.

- Ecotherapy, originally a discipline of psychology, promotes mind-body-spirit health effects through the repeated exposure to nature.

- Nature-deficit disorder is a term coined to explain the lack of exposure to nature due to people's love affair with technology.

- The physiological effects of spending time in nature include decreases in resting heart rate, blood pressure, and cortisol and increases in white blood cell count and biochemicals that have calming effects on the brain.

- Exposure to nature has a calming effect on the mind and human spirit. Being in the presence of a force greater than yourself puts things in perspective by reducing the scale of personal problems.

- Circadian rhythms are based on a 24-hour cycle of Earth's rotation on its axis; these rhythms affect countless physiological aspects of health, including sleep patterns and various metabolic processes.

- Nature affects us both objectively (e.g., raising dopamine and serotonin levels, and decreasing cortisol levels) and subjectively (giving us a feeling of peace, wonder, and awe).

- Routinely exposing yourself to nature enhances mental cognition, including attention span and possibly memory and concentration skills.

STUDY GUIDE QUESTIONS

1. What is ecotherapy?

2. What is nature-deficit disorder?

3. What is biophilia?

4. List three effects of nature on human physiology.

5. How does the concept of entrainment correspond to ecotherapy?

6. How do disruptions of circadian rhythms affect health and stress levels?

7. Explain how ecotherapy affects both mind and body.

8. Describe how solitude can be therapeutic.

9. Give three examples of how you earn nature points in your present weekly routine. Then describe changes to your routine that would allow you to score more points in the future.

REFERENCES AND RESOURCES

Buzzell, L., and C. Chalquist. 2009. *Ecotherapy: Healing with Nature in Mind*. San Francisco, CA: Sierra Club Books.

Chalquist, C. 2009. "Ecotherapy: A Look at Ecotherapy Research Evidence." http://cliftoncommunitypartnership .org/uploads/articles/2009/08/2009080315530099 /ecotheraphyeco.2009.0003.lowlink.pdf_v03.pdf.

Clifford, A. 2018. *Your Guide to Forest Bathing*. Newburyport, MA: Conari Press.

Cordell, H. K. 2008. "The Latest Trends in Nature-Based Outdoor Recreation." *Forest History Today,* Spring. http:// foresthistory.org/Publications/FHT/FHTSpring2008 /Cordell.pdf.

Ducharme, J. 2018. "A Prescription You Can't Fill at the Pharmacy." *Time*, November 19.

Fleischer, E. 2018. "Doctors in Scotland Can Now Prescribe Nature to Their Patients." Big Think, October 12. https:// bigthink.com/personal-growth/doctors-in-shetland- can-now-prescribe-a-walk-in-nature?rebelltitem=1# rebelltitem1.

Halpren, S. 2000. "A Report on the Second Annual International Conference on Science and Consciousness (ICSC)." Albuquerque, New Mexico, April 29–May 3. http:// realityshifters.com/pages/articles/2000icscreport.html.

Ivans, S. 2018. *Forest Therapy: Seasonal Ways to Embrace Nature for a Happier You*. Lebanon, IN: Da Capo Lifelong Book.

Jung, C. 2002. *The Earth Has a Soul: The Nature Writings of Jung*. Edited by M. Sabini. Berkeley, CA: North Atlantic Books.

Kaplan, R. 2001. "The Nature of the View from Home. Psychological Benefits." *Environment and Behavior* 33(4): 507–542.

Kaplan, S. 1995. "The Restorative Benefits of Nature." *Journal of Environmental Psychology* 15: 169–182.

Kellert, S. 2012. *Birthright: People and Nature in the Modern World*. New Haven, CT: Yale University Press.

Kellert, S. 2012. Living on Earth [Interview], December 14.

Li, Q., M. Kobayashi, Y. Wakayama, et al. 2009. "Effect of Phytoncide from Trees on Human Natural Killer Cell Function." *International Journal of Immunopathology Pharmacology* 4: 951–959.

Li, Q., K. Morimoto, M. Kobayashi, et al. 2008. "A Forest Bathing Trip Increases Human Natural Killer Cell Activity and Expression of Anti-cancer Proteins in Female Subjects." *Journal of Biological Regulators and Homeostatic Agents* 22(1): 45–55.

Liberman, J. 1991. *Light: Medicine of the Future*. Sante Fe, NM: Bear and Company.

Louv, R. 2005. *Last Child in the Woods*. Chapel Hill, NC: Algonquin Books.

Louv, R. 2011. *The Nature Principle: Reconnecting with Life in a Virtual World*. Chapel Hill, NC: Algonquin Books.

Mao, G. 2012. "Effects of Short-Term Forest Bathing on Human Health in a Broad-Leaved Evergreen Forest in Zhejiang Province, China." *Biomedical Environmental Science* 25(3): 317–324.

Miyazaki, Y. 2011. "Science of Natural Therapy." http://www.marlboroughforestry.org.nz/mfia/docs/naturaltherapy.pdf.

Morita, E., M. Imai, M. Okawa, T. Miyaura, and S. Mizyazaki. 2011. "A Before and After Comparison of the Effects of Forest Walking on Sleep of a Community-Based Sample of People with Sleep Complaints." *Biopsychosocial Medicine* 5(13).

Muir, J. 2015. *John Muir's Ultimate Collection: Travel Memoirs, Wilderness Essays, Environmental Studies and Letters*. e-artnow.

Park, B. J., Y. Tsunetsugu, T. Kasetani, T. Kagawa, and Y. Miyazaki. 2010. "The Physiological Effects of *Shinrin-yoku* (Taking in the Forest Atmosphere or Forest Bathing): Evidence from Field Experiments in 24 Forests Across Japan." *Environmental Health and Preventive Medicine* 15(1): 18–26.

Perrottet, T. 2013. "Birthplace of the American Vacation." *Smithsonian,* April, pp. 68–75.

Reynolds, G. 2012. "The 'Outside' RX: Six Natural Prescriptions for Improving Your Body and Mind." *Outside,* December. http://www.outsideonline.com/fitness/wellness/The-Outside-RX.html.

Roberts, E., and E. Amidon. 1991. *Earth Prayers*. New York: Harper Collins.

Roszak, T. (Ed.). 1995. *Ecopsychology, Restoring the Earth, Healing the Mind*. San Francisco, CA: Sierra Club Books.

Seaward, B. L. 2010. *Earth Songs: Mountains, Water and the Healing Power of Nature* (DVD). Boulder, CO: White Light Pictures.

Seaward, B. L. 2011. *A Beautiful World: The Earth Songs Journals*. Boulder, CO: White Light Publications.

Selhub, E., and A. Logan. 2012. *Your Brain on Nature*. New York: John Wiley and Sons.

Sifferlin, A. 2016. "The Healing Power of Nature." *Time,* July 25, p. 24.

Swanson, J. 2001. *Communing with Nature: A Guidebook for Enhancing Your Relationship with the Living Earth*. Corvalis, OR: Illahee Press.

Ulrich, R. 1984. "View Through a Window May Influence Recovery from Surgery." *Science* 224(4647): 420–421.

Williams, F. 2012. "The Nature Cure: Take Two Hours of Pine Forest and Call Me in the Morning." *Outside,* December, pp. 79–92.

Williams, F. 2017. *The Nature Fix: Why Nature Makes Us Happier, Healthier, and More Creative*. New York: W. W. Norton and Company.

Williams, T. 1992. *Refuge*. New York: Vintage Books.

Creating Your Own Stress Management Program

Human beings are like tea bags. You don't know your strength until you're put in hot water.

—Bruce Laingen,
Former Chargé D'affaires,
American Embassy in Iran

The coronavirus pandemic of 2020 and its aftermath put a lot of people in hot water. Nearly everyone faced lockdowns, self-quarantines, loss of personal income, and uncertain futures. Those on the front lines of health care had hotter water than most. What we learned from those on the front lines, moving from a mindset of survival to one of thriving, is the hallmark of a holistic stress management program.

Because everyone is so different (even under the same stressors), creating a stress management program is a very individual undertaking. There is no set formula or series of dogmatic guidelines, only suggestions. If there is a secret to successful stress management, it is to cultivate and utilize your inner resources. Just like Dorothy, who all along had the ability to leave Oz and return home, you have the power of your inner resources. Inner resources are those abstract qualities and characteristics that become a tangible bridge over the chasm of chaos. These include, among others, intuition, creativity, willpower, faith, humor, love, courage, self-reliance, and optimism.

After these are nurtured, how does one access inner resources? The answer begins with awareness and the desire to grow. From this desire comes a greater consciousness of yourself and the events and circumstances in your environment. Ultimately, these circumstances contribute to your growth and maturation. Awareness and desire serve as catalysts for positive change.

No one relaxation technique works for everyone. Nor is one coping strategy applicable in every stressful situation. Both focus on a wide range of functions. Exposure to an array of coping strategies and relaxation techniques allows you to pick and choose those that are most appropriate and will ensure the greatest returns. The initial purpose of this book was to do just that: to provide as great an exposure as possible. Now, knowledge can certainly be gained by reading a book such as this; our educational system is based on this premise. But it has been demonstrated time and time again that people are less likely to forget something when they have experienced it for themselves. Thus, putting the concepts in this book into practice is where the real learning will take place. *The Art of Peace and Relaxation Workbook*, which can be found online, is perhaps the best template to build your foundation of a personal stress management program.

Having taught stress management for nearly 40 years, and interviewing scores of people who have been through hell and back and done so quite gracefully, the following are my best suggestions for constructing the best personal stress management program in the effort to move from a motivation of fear-based thinking and behaviors to compassion-based thoughts and behaviors:

1. *Make a habit of spending some quality time each day to get to know yourself.* Take perhaps half an hour every day for self-exploration, whether in the form of journal writing, art therapy, music therapy, exercise, or something else. Be selfish. Believe that you deserve this time, and you will find it takes priority in your life. Time management is one of the major cornerstones of a successful stress management program; allocate time for this self-development. Keep in mind that there is a fixed amount of time in a day and that when a new activity is planned, an old one must be edited out of the daily agenda. Survey your daily routine to note where you can squeeze in a block of time for this purpose. If half an hour seems too long, start with 5 minutes

and build from there. And remember that the occasion when you feel you do not have time for self-exploration is when you need it most.

2. *Make a habit of reading your emotional barometer.* Recognize the times when you feel angry, frustrated, anxious, and guilty. When you catch yourself feeling a certain emotion, ask yourself: What triggered this response? Why did this emotion surface? What is the most appropriate action or behavior to resolve the feeling? Emotional well-being is the ability to feel and express the full range of emotions, but it also means being able to control these emotions. On average, people laugh 15 times a day. Make sure you fill this quota.

3. *Practice the art of unconditional love.* Self-esteem is so critical to effective stress management that it should be given top priority in the design of your stress management program. Focus on your positive attributes, not what you perceive to be your negative ones, and work to enhance these. Don't just think of yourself as a physical entity; appreciate your intellectual, emotional, and spiritual aspects, as well. Self-esteem is the seed of unconditional love. To say hello, to smile, to share a song, to give positive feedback—these are all expressions of love. And when these behaviors are practiced, they seem to double our own sense of self-esteem and self-love.

4. *Nurture your creativity skills.* Creativity is second in importance only to self-esteem as a means to manage stress. Creativity plays a direct role in problem solving and an indirect role in distracting attention from stressful episodes during moments of "play." Don't let childhood memories suffocate your creative abilities.

5. *Balance all components of your well-being and take time to nurture them.* Stress is often expressed in terms of things being out of balance. In physiological terms, this is called lack of homeostasis. But our mental, emotional, and spiritual components can also lack homeostasis. Search out and practice ways to help you achieve mental homeostasis by learning how to either stimulate or desensitize your intellect, depending on its current state. Be attentive to your emotional component, as well, by being aware of emotional states as they arise. Learn to express, not suppress, your emotions, but do it in a way that

is both therapeutic and diplomatic. Take good care of your body. Exercise it regularly. Feed it good nutrients, and get adequate amounts of sleep. Finally, give attention to your spirit by taking steps to enhance the maturation of your higher consciousness. Practice centering, emptying, grounding, and connecting on a regular basis. Search for and fulfill your purpose in life.

6. *Be like a child.* Children, like adults, experience acute stress, but they have not yet learned to be self-conscious about giggling or to suppress their tears. Before children are taught to conform to adult expectations, they are rich in curiosity, imagination, and creativity. These and other characteristics of young children can be relearned if we take the time to do so.

Designing and implementing a stress management program of your own may not seem easy at first, but it doesn't have to be difficult. It just takes a little desire, some discipline, and the realization that you are worth the effort. Most important, you don't have to be hit with an avalanche of stressors to begin the process of creating a sense of calm in your life. You can begin right now, gradually, one step at a time.

The following strategic plan takes into account insights and wisdom from the previous chapters in the book. As you take yourself through the progression of steps, feel free to embellish this plan to make it as personal for your situation as possible.

Step 1. Identify Your Stressors. List your top five stressors (from most stressful to least stressful) and explain each with a sentence. The purpose of this exercise is to identify the problem, which is the first step in resolving it.

1. _____

2. _____

3. _____

4. _____

5. _____

Step 2. Interventions. Now, look at your list of stressors. Ask yourself which problems trigger a sense of fear and mark these with an *F*. Next, ask yourself which of these issues promote feelings of anger (and remember—anger can surface in a great many ways, from impatience to rage and hostility). Place an *A* next to all of these. It's okay if you mark one or more items on your list with both an *A* and an *F*. Remember, after you have identified the underlying emotion associated with the problem, it becomes easier to address and resolve it.

Step 3. Integration. Stress affects all aspects of our being: mind, emotions, body, and spirit.

■ *Mind:* Do you feel overwhelmed or bored with your problems? If you feel overwhelmed, this is a sign that there is too much on your plate; some things need to be edited out or eliminated. If you feel bored, your threshold of stimulation probably is not being reached, and you might want to consider changing or adding something to achieve this balance. Mental well-being also involves attitudes and perceptions.

Describe one thing you can do to find mental balance. _____

_____

■ *Emotions:* The spectrum of stress-based emotions is rather wide, yet each emotion can be traced to some element of fear or anger. In the course of your day, ask yourself how you feel (not think, but feel). If you find that stress emotions occupy more than 50 percent of your time on a regular basis, this indicates an emotional imbalance.

Describe one thing you can do to find mental balance. _____

_____

■ *Body:* As you have learned throughout this book, stress can and will affect physical well-being. Do you have any health problems that you can associate with stress?

Describe one thing you can do to establish mental balance. _____

_____

■ *Spirit:* Take a look at your current list of stressors. How many of your stressors involve relationships, values (or value conflicts), and a meaningful purpose in life? Spiritual balance can be attained in a great many ways, from time spent alone in meditation to support groups or prayer.

Describe one thing you can do to find mental balance. _____

_____

Self-esteem is a part of spiritual well-being. Low self-esteem sets the stage for problems ranging from a bad hair day to the day from hell.

Describe one thing you can do to find mental balance. _____

_____

Step 4. Your Personal Stress Management Strategy. *Coping skills* are mental and emotional skills that help you change a threatening perception to a nonthreatening perception. Humor, reframing, time management, creativity, prayer, and social orchestration are just a few examples of coping skills.

Take a look at the list of stressors that you completed in step 1. Try to match at least three effective coping skills with each stressor.

Skills that you are now using:

1. _____
2. _____
3. _____
4. _____
5. _____
6. _____

Skills that you would like to incorporate:

1. _____
2. _____
3. _____
4. _____
5. _____
6. _____

Relaxation skills include any and all activities that return you to a sense of calm and tranquility.

Skills that you are now using:

1. _____
2. _____
3. _____
4. _____
5. _____
6. _____

Skills that you would like to incorporate:

1. _____
2. _____
3. _____
4. _____
5. _____
6. _____

Time management plays a huge role in putting stress-management strategies to wor
niques. Here is an important question to ask yourself: Where can I find a block of time (15 to 30 m...
lie down comfortably and relax?

REFERENCES

Carlson, R. 1998. *Don't Sweat the Small Stuff*. New York: Hyperion Books.

Kirsta, A. 1987. *The Book of Stress Survival: How to Relax and Live Positively*. New York: Simon and Schuster.

Seaward, B. L. 1999. *The Art of Calm: Relaxation through the Five Senses*. Deerfield Beach, FL: Health Communications.

Seaward, B. L. 2000. *Stressed Is Desserts Spelled Backward*. Duluth, MN: Whole Person Books.

Wheeler, C. M. 2007. *10 Simple Solutions to Stress*. Oakland, CA: New Harbinger Publications.

Index